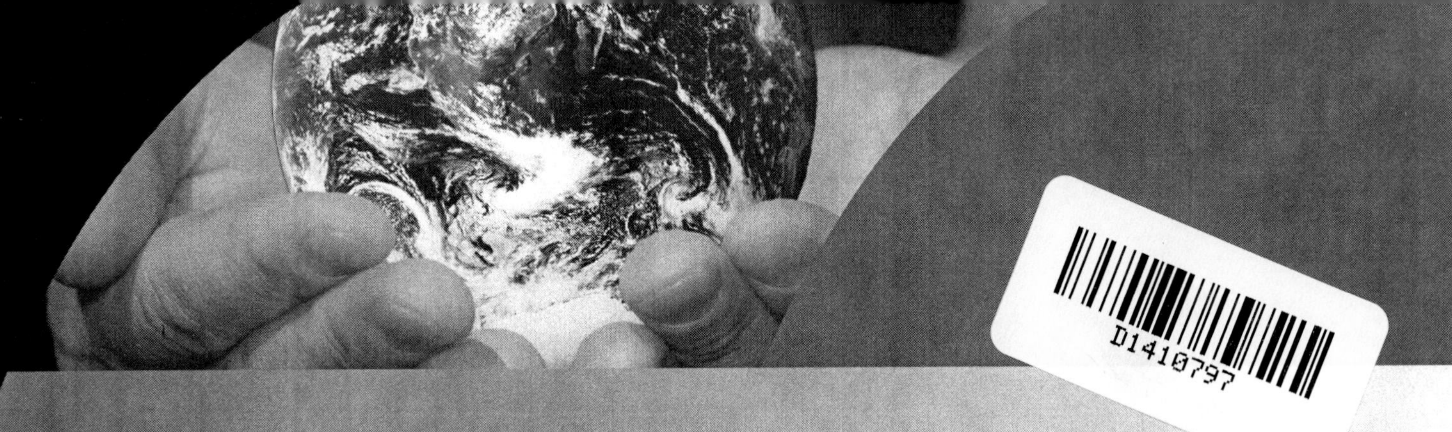

Public and Global Health Essentials

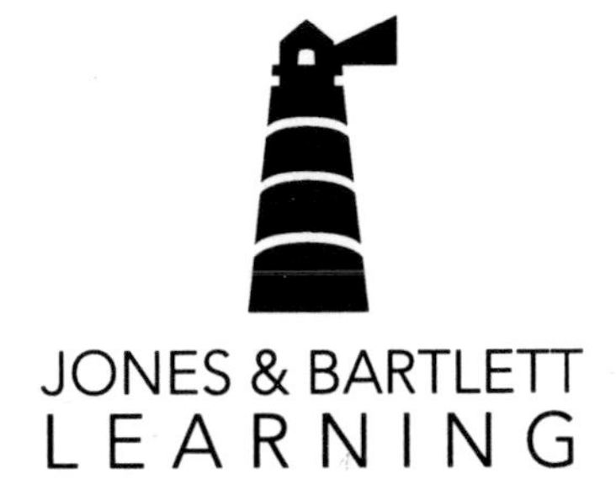

World Headquarters
Jones & Bartlett Learning
40 Tall Pine Drive
Sudbury, MA 01776
978-443-5000
info@jblearning.com
www.jblearning.com

Jones & Bartlett Learning
Canada
6339 Ormindale Way
Mississauga, Ontario L5V 1J2
Canada

Jones & Bartlett Learning
International
Barb House, Barb Mews
London W6 7PA
United Kingdom

Jones & Bartlett Learning books and products are available through most bookstores and online booksellers. To contact Jones & Bartlett Learning directly, call 800-832-0034, fax 978-443-8000, or visit our website www.jblearning.com.

Substantial discounts on bulk quantities of Jones & Bartlett Learning publications are available to corporations, professional associations, and other qualified organizations. For details and specific discount information, contact the special sales department at Jones & Bartlett Learning via the above contact information or send an email to specialsales@jblearning.com.

Production Credits
Publisher: Michael Brown
Acquisitions Editor: Katey Birtcher
Editorial Assistant: Teresa Reilly
Production Director: Amy Rose
Associate Production Editor: Tina Chen
Senior Marketing Manager: Sophie Fleck
Manufacturing and Inventory Control Supervisor: Amy Bacus
Composition: Publishers' Design and Production Services, Inc.
Cover Design: John Garland
Cover Images: Clockwise, from top: © Vitaly M/ShutterStock, Inc.; Courtesy of Chief Mass Communication Specialist Don Bray/U.S. Navy; © Jaimie Duplass/ShutterStock, Inc.; Courtesy of Tom Watanabe/U.S. Navy; Courtesy of Airman Jordan R. Beesley/U.S. Navy. Back cover: © Vitaly M/ShutterStock, Inc. Chapter openers: © Vitaly M/ShutterStock, Inc.
Printing and Binding: Malloy, Inc.
Cover Printing: Malloy, Inc.

ISBN 978-1-4496-2195-7

6048

Printed in the United States of America
14 13 12 11 10 10 9 8 7 6 5 4 3 2 1

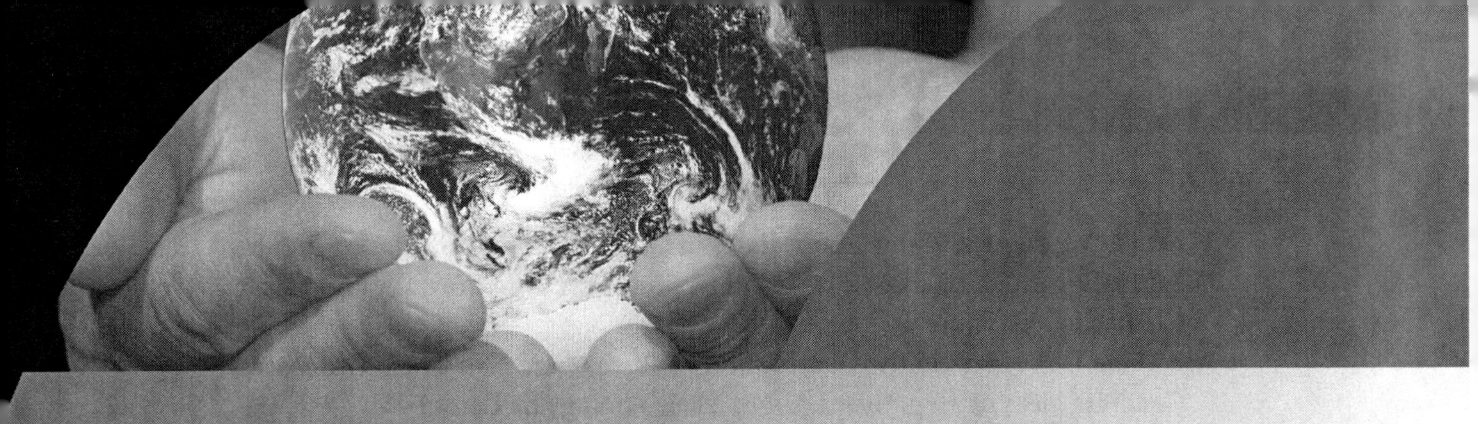

Table of Contents

Chapter 1	Public Health: The Population Health Approach	1
	Learning Objectives	1
	What Do We Mean by Public Health?	2
	How Has the Approach of Public Health Changed Over Time?	3
	What Is Meant by Population Health?	5
	Should We Focus on Everyone or On Vulnerable Groups?	7
	What Are the Approaches Available to Protect and Promote Health?	8
	What Factors Determine the Occurrence of Disease, Disability, and Death?	9
	Key Words	12
	Discussion Question	13
	References	13
Chapter 2	Health Determinants, Measurements, and Trends	15
	Learning Objectives	15
	Vignettes	15
	The Importance of Measuring Health Status	16
	The Determinants of Health	16
	Key Health Indicators	18
	Measuring the Burden of Disease	22
	The Global Burden of Disease	24
	Risk Factors	29
	The Demographic and Epidemiological Transitions	30
	Case Study	33
	Main Messages	35
	Discussion Questions	36
	References	37
Chapter 3	Evidence-based Public Health	39
	Learning Objectives	39
	How Can We Describe a Health Problem?	40

What Do We Need to Know About Rates in Order to Describe a Health Problem? 40
What Is the Burden of Disease in Terms of Morbidity and Mortality and Has It Changed Over Time? 41
Are There Differences in the Distribution of Disease and Can These Differences Generate Ideas or Hypotheses About Their Etiology or Cause? 42
Are the Differences or Changes Used to Suggest Group Associations Artifactual or Real? 43
What Is the Implication of a Group Association? 43
Etiology: How Do We Establish Contributory Cause? 44
What Can We Do If We Cannot Demonstrate All Three Requirements to Definitively Establish Contributory Cause? 45
What Does Contributory Cause Imply? 47
Recommendations: What Works to Reduce the Health Impact? 49
Implementation: How Do We Get the Job Done? 52
What Happens After Implementation? 54
Key Words 56
Discussion Questions 57
References 57

Chapter 4 Public Health Institutions and Systems 59
Learning Objectives 59
What Are the Goals and Roles of Governmental Public Health Agencies? 59
What Are the Ten Essential Public Health Services? 60
What Are the Roles of Local and State Public Health Agencies? 60
What Are the Roles of Federal Public Health Agencies? 65
What Are the Roles of Global Health Organizations and Agencies? 65
How Can Public Health Agencies Work Together? 68
What Other Government Agencies Are Involved in Health Issues? 69
What Roles Do Nongovernmental Organizations Play in Public Health? 70
How Can Public Health Agencies Partner with Health Care to Improve the Response to Health Problems? 70
How Can Public Health Take the Lead in Mobilizing Community Partnerships to Identify and Solve Health Problems? 71
Key Words 73
Discussion Questions 74
References 74

Chapter 5 Ethical and Human Rights Concerns in Global Health 75
Learning Objectives 75
Vignettes 75
The Importance of Ethical and Human Rights Issues in Global Health 75
The Foundations for Health and Human Rights 76
The "Rights Based Approach" 77
Selected Human Rights Issues 78
The Foundations for Research on Human Subjects 80
Key Human Research Cases 81
Ethical Issues in Making Investment Choices in Health 83

Key Challenges for the Future 84
Discussion Questions 86
References 87

Chapter 6 The Public Health Workforce 89
Learning Objectives 89
Public Health Work and Public Health Workers 90
Size and Distribution of the Public Health Workforce 90
Composition of the Public Health Workforce 93
Public Health Worker Ethics, Skills, and Competencies 94
Characteristics of Public Health Occupations 97
Public Health Practitioner Competencies 108
Public Health Workforce Development 112
Conclusion 114
Discussion Questions 116
References 116

Chapter 7 Non-communicable Diseases 117
Learning Objectives 117
Vignettes 117
The Importance of Non-communicable Disease 117
Key Definitions 118
The Burden of Non-communicable Diseases 118
The Costs and Consequences of Non-communicable Diseases, Tobacco Use, and Alcohol Abuse 123
Addressing the Burden of Non-communicable Disease 124
Case Studies 127
Future Challenges 131
Main Messages 132
Discussion Questions 133
References 134

Chapter 8 Communicable Diseases 137
Learning Objectives 137
Vignettes 137
The Importance of Communicable Diseases 137
Key Terms, Definitions, and Concepts 138
The Burden of Communicable Diseases 139
The Costs and Consequences of Communicable Diseases 146
Addressing the Burden of Disease 148
Case Studies 152
Avian Influenza 155
Future Challenges to the Control of Communicable Diseases 156
Main Messages 158
Discussion Questions 160
References 161

Chapter 9 The Environment and Health 163
Learning Objectives 163
Vignettes 163
The Importance of Environmental Health 163
Key Concepts 165
Key Environmental Health Burdens 166
The Burden of Environmentally-Related Diseases 167
The Costs and Consequences of Key Environmental Health Problems 168
Reducing the Burden of Disease 169
Future Challenges 173
Main Messages 173
Discussion Questions 175
References 176

Chapter 10 Natural Disasters and Complex Humanitarian Emergencies 177
Learning Objectives 177
Vignettes 177
The Importance of Natural Disasters and Complex Emergencies to Global Health 177
Key Terms 178
The Characteristics of Natural Disasters 180
The Characteristics of Complex Emergencies 181
The Health Burden of Natural Disasters 181
The Health Effects of Complex Humanitarian Emergencies 182
Addressing the Health Effects of Natural Disasters 184
Addressing the Health Effects of Complex Humanitarian Emergencies 185
Case Studies 187
Future Challenges in Meeting the Health Needs of Disasters 188
Main Messages 189
Discussion Questions 190
References 191

Chapter 11 Working Together to Improve Global Health 193
Learning Objectives 193
Vignettes 193
Introduction 194
Cooperating to Improve Global Health 194
Key Actors in Global Health 194
Non-governmental Organizations 200
Partnerships Related to WHO 201
Other Partnerships and Special Programs 201
Trends in Global Health Efforts 204
Setting the Global Health Agenda 205
Future Challenges 206
Case Study 207
Main Messages 208

Discussion Questions 210
References 211

Chapter 12 Culture and Health 213
Learning Objectives 213
Vignettes 213
The Importance of Culture to Health 213
The Concept of Culture 214
Health Beliefs and Practices 215
Health Behaviors and Behavior Change 218
Understanding and Engendering Behavior Change 221
Social Assessment 222
Main Messages 223
Discussion Questions 225
References 226

Glossary 227

Index 239

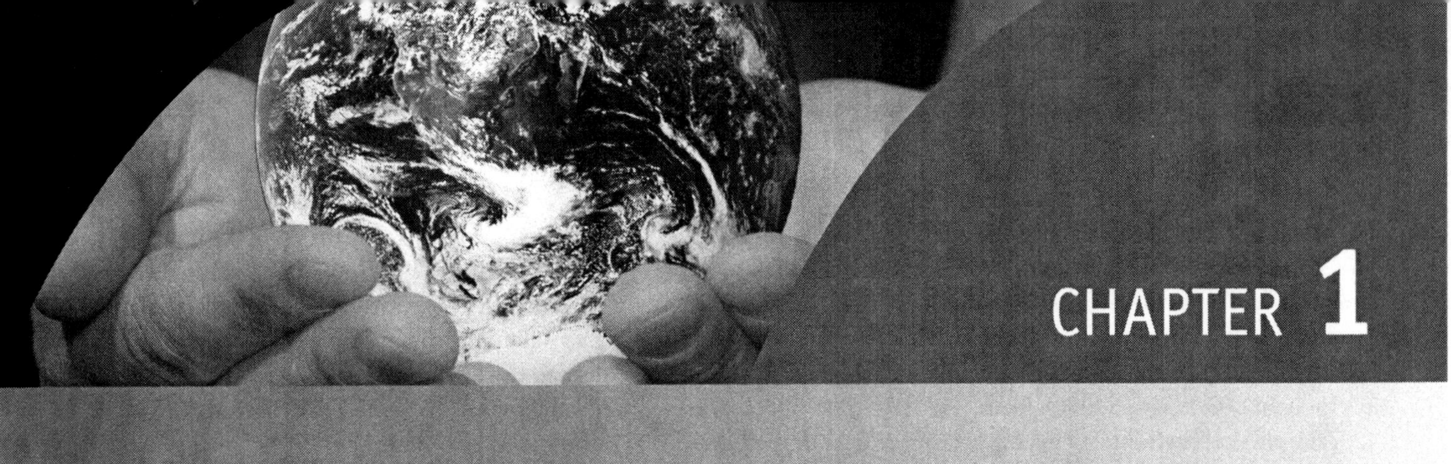

Public Health: The Population Health Approach

Learning Objectives:

By the end of this chapter the student will be able to:

- identify multiple ways that public health affects daily life.
- define eras of public health from ancient times to the early 21st century.
- define the meaning of population health.
- illustrate the uses of health care, traditional public health, and social interventions in population health.
- identify a range of determinants of disease.

I woke up this morning, got out of bed, and went to the bathroom where I used the toilet, washed my hands, brushed and flossed my teeth, drank a glass of water, and took my blood pressure medicine, cholesterol medication, and an aspirin. Then, I did my exercises and took a shower.

On the way to the kitchen, I didn't even notice the smoke detector I passed or the old ashtrays in the closet. I took a low fat yogurt out of the refrigerator and prepared hot cereal in the microwave oven for my breakfast.

Then, I walked out my door into the crisp clean air and got in my car. I put on my seat belt, saw the light go on for the air bag, and safely drove to work. I got to my office where I paid little attention to the new defibrillator at the entrance, the "no smoking" signs, or the absence of asbestos. I arrived safely in my well-ventilated office and got ready to teach Public Health 101.

It wasn't a very eventful morning, but then it's all in a morning's work when it comes to public health.

This rather mundane morning is made possible by a long list of achievements that reflect the often-ignored history of public health.[1] We take for granted the fact that water chlorination, hand washing, and indoor plumbing largely eliminated the transmission of common bacterial disease, which so often killed the young and not-so-young for centuries. Don't overlook the impact of prevention on our teeth and gums. Teeth brushing, flossing, and fluoridation of water have made a dramatic impact on dental health of children and adults.

The more recent advances in the prevention of heart disease have been a major public health achievement. Preventive successes include: the reduction of blood pressure and cholesterol, cigarette cessation efforts, use of low-dose aspirin, an understanding of the role of exercise, and the widespread availability of defibrillators. These can be credited with at least half the dramatic reductions in heart disease that have reduced the death rate from coronary artery disease by approximately 50 percent in the United States and most other developed countries in the last half century.

The refrigerator was one of the most important advances in food safety which illustrates the impact of social change and innovation not necessarily intended to improve health. Food and product safety are public health achievements that require continued attention. It was public pressure for food safety that in large part brought about the creation of the U.S. Food and Drug Administration. The work of this public health agency continues to affect all of our lives from the safety of the foods we eat to the drugs and cosmetics we use.

Radiation safety, like radiation itself, usually goes unnoticed from the regulation of microwave ovens to the reduction of radon in buildings. We rarely notice when disease does not occur.

Highway safety illustrates the wide scope of activities required to protect the public's health. From seat belts, child restraints, and air bags to safer cars, highways, designated driver programs and enforcement of drunk driving laws, public health efforts require collaboration with professionals not usually thought of as having a health focus.

The physical environment too has been made safer by the efforts of public health. Improvement in the quality of the air we breathe both outdoors and indoors has been an ongoing accomplishment of what we will call "population health." Our lives are safer today because of interventions ranging from installation of smoke detectors to removal of asbestos from buildings. However, the challenges continue. Globalization increases the potential for the spread of existing and emerging diseases and raises concerns about the safety of the products we use. Climate change and ongoing environmental deterioration continue to produce new territory for "old" diseases, such as malaria. Overuse of technologies, such as antibiotics, have encouraged the emergence of resistant bacteria.

The 20th century saw an increase in life expectancy of almost 30 years in most developed countries, much of it due to the successes of public health initiatives.[2] We cannot assume that these trends will continue indefinitely. The epidemic of obesity already threatens to slow down or reverse the progress we have been making. The challenges of 21st century public health include protection of health and continued improvement in its quality, not just its quantity.

To understand the role of public health in these achievements and ongoing challenges, let us start at the beginning and ask: what do we mean by public health?

WHAT DO WE MEAN BY PUBLIC HEALTH?

Ask your parents what public health means and they might say "health care for the poor." Well, they are right that public health has always been about providing services for those with special vulnerabilities either directly or through the healthcare system. But that is only one of the ways that public health serves the most needy and vulnerable in our population. Public health efforts often focus on the most vulnerable populations from reducing exposure to lead paint in deteriorating buildings to food supplementation to prevent birth defects and goiters. Addressing the needs of vulnerable populations has always been a cornerstone of public health. As we will see, however, the definition of vulnerable populations continues to change as do the challenges of addressing their needs.

Ask your grandparents what public health means and they might say "washing your hands." Well, they are right too—public health has always been about determining risks to health and providing successful interventions that are applicable to everyone. But hand washing is only the tip of the iceberg. The types of interventions that apply to everyone and benefit everyone span an enormous range: from food and drug safety to controlling air pollution; from measures to prevent the spread of tuberculosis to vaccinating against childhood diseases; from prevention and response to disasters to detection of contaminants in our water.

The concerns of society as a whole are always in the forefront of public health. These concerns keep changing and the methods for addressing them keep expanding. New technologies and global, local, and national interventions are becoming a necessary part of public health. To understand what public health has been and what it is becoming, let us look at some definitions of public health. The following are two definitions of public health—one from the early 20th century and one from more recent years.

> *Public health is ". . . the science and art of preventing disease, prolonging life and promoting health . . . through organized community effort. . . ."*[3]

> *The substance of public health is the "organized community efforts aimed at the prevention of disease and the promotion of health."*[4]

These definitions show how little the concept of public health changed in the 20th century, however the concept of public health in the 21st century is beginning to undergo important changes in a number of ways including:

- The goal of prolonging life is being complemented by an emphasis on the quality of life.
- Protection of health when it already exists is becoming a focus along with promoting health when it is at risk.
- Use of new technologies, such as the Internet, are redefining "community," as well as offering us new ways to communicate.
- The enormous expansion in the options for intervention, as well as the increasing awareness of potential harms and costs of intervention programs, require a new science of "evidence-based" public health.
- Public health and clinical care, as well as public and private partnerships, are coming together in new ways to produce collaborative efforts rarely seen in the 20th century.

Thus, a new 21st century definition of public health is needed. One such definition might read as follows:

> *The totality of all evidence-based public and private efforts that preserve and promote health and prevent disease, disability, and death.*

This broad definition recognizes public health as the umbrella for a range of approaches which need to be viewed as a part of a big picture or population perspective. Specifically, this definition enlarges the traditional scope of public health to include:

- An examination of the full range of environmental, social, and economic determinants of health—not just those traditionally addressed by the public health and clinical health care
- An examination of the full range of interventions to address health issues, including the structure and function of healthcare delivery systems, plus the role of public policies that affect health even when health is not their intended effect

If you are asked by your children what is public health, you might respond: "*It is about the big picture issues that affect our own health and the health of our community every day of our lives. It is about protecting health in the face of disasters; preventing disease from addictions such as cigarettes; controlling infections such as the human immunodeficiency virus (HIV); and developing systems to ensure the safety of the food we eat and the water we drink.*"

A variety of terms have been used to describe this big picture perspective that takes into account the full range of factors that affect health and considers their interactions.[5] A variation of this approach has been called the social-ecological model, systems thinking, or the **population health approach**. We will use the latter term. Before exploring what we mean by the population health approach, let us examine how the approaches to public health have changed over time.[a]

HOW HAS THE APPROACH OF PUBLIC HEALTH CHANGED OVER TIME?

Organized community efforts to promote health and prevent disease go back to ancient times.[6,7] The earliest human civilizations integrated concepts of prevention into their culture, their religion, and their laws. Prohibitions against specific foods—including pork, beef, and seafood—plus customs for food preparation, including officially-designated methods of killing cattle and methods of cooking, were part of the earliest practices of ancient societies. Prohibitions against alcohol or its limited use for religious ceremony have long been part of societies' efforts to control behavior, as well as prevent disease. Prohibition of cannibalism, the most universal of food taboos, has strong grounding in the protection of health.[b]

Sexual practices have been viewed as having health consequences from the earliest civilizations. Male circumcision, premarital abstinence, and marital fidelity have all been shown to have impacts on health.

Quarantine or isolation of individuals with disease or exposed to disease has likewise been practiced for thousands of years. The intuitive notion that isolating individuals with disease could protect individuals and societies led to some of the earliest organized efforts to prevent the spread of disease. At times they were successful, but without a solid scientific basis. Efforts to separate individuals and communities from epidemics sometimes led to misguided efforts, such as the unsuccessful attempts to control the black plague by barring outsiders from walled towns and not recognizing that it was the rats and fleas that transmitted the disease.

During the 18th and first half of the 19th century individuals occasionally produced important insights into the prevention of disease. In the 1740s, British naval commander James Lind demonstrated that lemons and other citrus fruit could prevent and treat scurvy, a then-common disease of sailors whose daily nourishment was devoid of citrus fruit, the best source of vitamin C.

In the last years of the 18th century, English physician Edward Jenner recognized that cowpox, a common mild ailment of those who milked cows, protected those who developed it against life-threatening smallpox. He developed what came to be called a vaccine—derived from the Latin "*vacs*," meaning cows. He placed fluid from cowpox sores under the skin of recipients, including his son, and exposed them to smallpox. Despite the success of these smallpox prevention efforts, widespread use of vaccinations was slow to develop partially because at that time there was not an adequate scientific basis to explain the reason for its success.

All of these approaches to disease prevention were known before organized public health existed. Public health awareness began to emerge in Europe and America in the mid-19th century. The American public health movement had its origins in Europe where concepts of disease as the consequence of social conditions took root in the 1830s and 1840s. This movement, which put forth the idea that disease emerges from social conditions of inequality, produced the concept of

[a] Turnock[2] has described several meanings of public health. These include the system and social enterprise, the profession, the methods, the government services, and the health of the public. The population health approach used in this book may be thought of as subsuming all of these different perspectives on public health.

[b] In recent years, this prohibition has been indirectly violated by feeding beef products containing bones and brain matter to other cattle. The development of "mad cow" disease and its transmission to humans has been traced to this practice, which can be viewed as analogous to human cannibalism.

social justice. Many attribute public health's focus on vulnerable populations to this tradition.

While early organized public health efforts paid special attention to vulnerable members of society, they also focused on the hazards that affected everyone: contamination of the environment. This focus on sanitation and public health was often called the hygiene movement, which began even before the development of the germ theory of disease. Despite the absence of an adequate scientific foundation, the hygiene movement made major strides in controlling infectious diseases, such as tuberculosis, cholera, and waterborne diseases largely through alteration of the physical environment.

The fundamental concepts of epidemiology also developed during this era. In the 1850s, John Snow, often called the father of epidemiology, helped establish the importance of careful data collection and documentation of rates of disease before and after an intervention to evaluate effectiveness. He is known for his efforts to close down the Broad Street pump, which supplied water contaminated by cholera to a district of London. His actions quickly terminated that epidemic of cholera. John Snow's approach has become a symbol of the earliest epidemiological thinking.

Semmelweis, an Austrian physician, used much the same approach in the mid-19th century to control puerperal fever—or fever of childbirth—then a major cause of maternal mortality. Noting that physicians frequently went from autopsy room to delivery room without washing their hands, he instituted a hand washing procedure and was able to document a dramatic reduction in the frequency of puerperal fever. Unfortunately, he was unable to convince many of his contemporaries to accept this intervention without a clear mechanism of action. Until the acceptance of the germ theory of disease, puerperal fever continued to be the major cause of maternal deaths in Europe and North America.

The mid-19th century in England also saw the development of birth and death records, or vital statistics, which formed the basis of population-wide assessment of health status. From the beginning, there was controversy over how to define the cause of death. Two key figures in the early history of organized public health took opposing positions that reflect this continuing controversy. Edwin Chadwick argued that specific pathological conditions or diseases should be the basis for the cause of death. William Farr argued that underlying factors, including what we would today call risk factors and social conditions, should be seen as the actual causes of death.

Thus, the methods of public health were already being established before the development of the germ theory of disease by Louis Pasteur and his European colleagues in the mid-1800s. The revolutions in biology that they ignited ushered in a new era in public health. American physicians and public health leaders often went to Europe to study new techniques and approaches and brought them back to America to use at home.

After the Civil War, American public health began to produce its own advances and organizations. In 1872, the American Public Health Association (APHA) was formed. According to its own historical account, "the APHA's founders recognized that two of the association's most important functions were advocacy for adoption by the government of the most current scientific advances relevant to public health, and public education on how to improve community health."[8]

The biological revolution of the late 19th and early 20th centuries that resulted from the germ theory of disease laid the groundwork for the modern era of public health. An understanding of the contributions of bacteria and other organisms to disease produced novel diagnostic testing capabilities. For example, scientists could now identify tuberculosis cases through skin testing, bacterial culture, and the newly discovered chest X-ray. Concepts of vaccination advanced with the development of new vaccines against toxins produced by tetanus- and diphtheria-causing bacteria. Without antibiotics or other effective cures, much of public health in this era relied on prevention, isolation of those with disease, and case-finding methods to prevent further exposure.

In the early years of the 20th century, epidemiology methods continued to contribute to the understanding of disease. The investigations of pellagra by Goldberger and the United States Public Health Service overthrew the assumption of the day that pellagra was an infectious disease and established that it was a nutritional deficiency that could be prevented or easily cured with vitamin B-6 (niacin) or a balanced diet. Understanding of the role of nutrition was central to public health's emerging focus on prenatal care and childhood growth and development. Incorporating key scientific advances, these efforts matured in the 1920s and 1930s and introduced a growing alphabet of vitamins and nutrients to the American vocabulary.

A new public health era of effective intervention against active disease began in force after World War II. The discovery of penicillin and its often miraculous early successes convinced scientists, public health practitioners, and the general public that a new era in medicine and public health had arrived.

During this era, public health's focus was on filling the holes in the healthcare system. In this period, the role of public health was often seen as assisting clinicians to effectively deliver clinical services to those without the benefits of private medical care and helping to integrate preventive efforts into the practice of medicine. Thus, the great public health success of organized campaigns for the eradication of polio was mistakenly seen solely as a victory for medicine. Likewise, the successful passage of Medicaid and Medicare, outgrowths of public health's commitment to social justice, was simply viewed as efforts to expand the private practice of medicine.

This period, however, did lay the foundations for the emergence of a new era in public health. Epidemiological methods designed for the study of noncommunicable diseases demonstrated the major role that cigarette smoking plays in lung cancer and a variety of other diseases. The emergence of the randomized clinical trial and the regulation of drugs, vaccines, and other interventions by the Food and Drug Administration developed the foundations for what we now call evidence-based public health and evidence-based medicine.

The 1980s and much of the 1990s were characterized by a focus on individual responsibility for health and interventions at the individual level. Often referred to as health promotion and disease prevention, these interventions targeted individuals to effect behavioral change and combat the risk factors for diseases. As an example, to help prevent coronary artery disease, efforts were made to help individuals address high blood pressure and cholesterol, cigarette smoking, and obesity. Behavioral change strategies were also used to help prevent the spread of the newly emerging HIV/AIDS epidemic. Efforts aimed at individual prevention and early detection as part of medical practice began to bear some fruit with the widespread introduction of mammography for detection of breast cancer and the worldwide use of Pap smears for the detection of cervical cancer. Newborn screening for genetic disease became a widespread and often legally-mandated program, combining individual and community components.

Major public health advances during this era resulted from the environmental movement, which brought public awareness to the health dangers of lead in gasoline and paint. The environmental movement also focused on reducing cancer by controlling radiation exposure from a range of sources including sunlight and radon, both naturally-occurring radiation sources. In a triumph of global cooperation, governments worked together to address the newly-discovered hole in the ozone layer. In the United States, reductions in air pollution levels and smoking rates during this era had an impact on the frequency of chronic lung disease, asthma, and most likely coronary artery disease.

The heavy reliance on individual interventions that characterized much of the last half of the 20th century changed rapidly in the beginning of the 21st century. A new era in public health that is often called "population health" has begun to transform professional and public thought about health. From the potential for bioterrorism to the high costs of health care to the control of pandemic influenza and AIDS, the need for community-wide or population-wide, public health efforts have become increasingly evident. This new era is characterized by a global perspective and the need to address international health issues. It includes a focus on the potential impacts of climate change, emerging and reemerging infectious diseases, and the consequences of trade in potentially contaminated or dangerous products, ranging from food to toys.

Table 1-1 outlines these eras of public health, identifies their key defining elements, and highlights important events that symbolize each era.[9]

Thus, today we have entered an era in which a focus on the individual is increasingly coupled with a focus on what needs to be done at the community and population level. This era of public health can be viewed as "the era of population health."

WHAT IS MEANT BY POPULATION HEALTH?

The concept of population health has emerged in recent years as a broader concept of public health that includes all the ways that society as a whole or communities within society are affected by health issues and how they respond to these issues. Population health provides an intellectual umbrella for thinking about the wide spectrum of factors that can and do affect the health of individuals and the population as a whole. Figure 1-1 provides an overview of what falls under the umbrella of population health.

Population health also provides strategies for considering the broad range of potential **interventions** to address these issues. By intervention we mean the full range of strategies designed to protect health, and prevent disease, disability, and death. Interventions include: preventive efforts, such as nutrition and vaccination; curative efforts, such as antibiotics and cancer surgery; and efforts to prevent complications and restore function—from chemotherapy to physical therapy. Thus, population health is about *healthy people and healthy populations.*

The concept of population health can be seen as a comprehensive way of thinking about the modern scope of public health. It utilizes an evidence-based approach to analyze the determinants of health and disease and the options for intervention to preserve and improve health. Population health requires us to define what we mean by **health issues** and what we mean by **population(s)**. It also requires us to define what we mean by **society's shared health concerns**, as well as **society's vulnerable groups**.

To understand population health, we therefore need to define what we mean by each of these four components:

- Health issues
- Population(s)
- Society's shared health concerns
- Society's vulnerable groups

TABLE 1-1 Eras of Public Health

Eras of public health	Focus of attention/ Paradigm	Action framework	Notable events and movements in public health and epidemiology
Health protection (Antiquity–1830s)	Authority-based control of individual and community behaviors	Religious and cultural practices and prohibited behaviors	Quarantine for epidemics; sexual prohibitions to reduce disease transmission; dietary restrictions to reduce food-borne disease
Hygiene movement (1840–1870s)	Sanitary conditions as basis for improved health	Environmental action on a community-wide basis distinct from health care	Snow on Cholera; Semmelweis and puerperal fever; collection of vital statistics as empirical foundation for public health and epidemiology
Contagion control (1880–1940s)	Germ theory: demonstration of infectious origins of disease	Communicable disease control through environmental control, vaccination, sanatoriums, and outbreak investigation in general population	Linkage of epidemiology, bacteriology, and immunology to form TB sanatoriums; outbreak investigation, e.g., Goldberger and pellagra
Filling holes in the medical care system (1950s–mid-1980s)	Integration of control of communicable diseases; modification of risk factors; and care of high-risk population as part of medical care	Public system for care of and control of specific infectious diseases and vulnerable populations distinct from general health care system; Integrated health maintenance organizations with integration of preventive services into general health care system	Antibiotics; randomized clinical trials; concept of risk factors; Surgeon General reports on cigarette smoking; Framingham study on cardiovascular risks; health maintenance organizations and community health centers with integration of preventive services into general healthcare system
Health promotion/ Disease prevention (Mid-1980–2000)	Focus on individual behavior and disease detection in vulnerable and general populations	Clinical and population-oriented prevention with focus on individual control of decision making and multiple interventions	AIDS epidemic and need for multiple interventions to reduce risk; reductions in coronary heart disease through multiple interventions
Population health (21st century)	Coordination of public health and health care delivery based upon shared evidence-based systems thinking	Evidence-based recommendations and information management; focus on harms and costs as well as benefits of interventions; globalization	Evidence-based medicine and public health; information technology; medical errors; antibiotic resistance; global collaboration, e.g., SARS, tobacco control, climate change

Source: Awofeso N. What's new about the "New Public Health"? *American Journal of Public Health.* 2004;94(5):705–709.

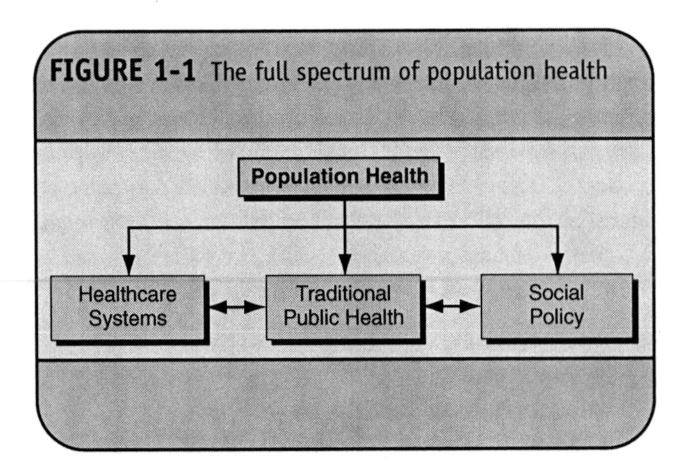

FIGURE 1-1 The full spectrum of population health

What Are the Implications of Each of the Four Components of Population Health?

All four of the key components of public health have changed in recent years. Let us take a look at the historical, current, and emerging scopes of each component and consider their implications.

For most of the history of public health, the term "health" focused solely on physical health. Mental health has now been recognized as an important part of the definition; conditions such as depression and substance abuse make enormous contributions to disability in populations throughout the world. The boundaries of what we mean by health continue to expand and the limits of health are not clear. Many novel medical interventions, including modification of genes and treatments to increase height, improve cosmetic appearance, and improve sexual performance, confront us with the question: are these health issues?

The definition of a population, likewise, is undergoing fundamental change. For most of recorded history, a population was defined geographically. Geographic communities, such as cities, states, and countries, defined the structure and functions of public health. The current definition of population has expanded to include the idea of a global community, recognizing the increasingly interconnected issues of global health. The definition of population is also focusing more on nongeographic communities. Universities now include the distance-learning community; health care is delivered to members of a health plan; and the Internet is creating new social communities. All of these new definitions of a population are affecting the thinking and approaches needed to address public health issues.

What about the meaning of society-wide concerns—have they changed as well? Historically, public health and communicable disease were nearly synonymous, as symbolized by the field of epidemiology which actually derives its name from the study of communicable disease epidemics. In recent decades, the focus of society-wide concerns has greatly expanded to include toxic exposures from the physical environment, transportation safety, and the costs of health care. However, communicable disease never went away as a focus of public health and the 21st century is seeing a resurgence in concern over emerging infectious diseases, including HIV/AIDS, pandemic flu, and newly drug-resistant diseases, such as staph infections and tuberculosis. Additional concerns, ranging from the impact of climate change to the harms and benefits of new technologies, are altering the meaning of society-wide concerns.

Finally, the meaning of vulnerable populations continues to transform. For most of the 20th century, public health focused on maternal and child health and high risk occupations as the operational definition of vulnerable populations. While these groups remain important to public health, additional groups now receive more attention, including the disabled, the frail elderly, and those without health insurance. Attention is also beginning to focus on the immune-suppressed among those living with HIV/AIDS, who are at higher risk of infection and illness, and those whose genetic code documents their special vulnerability to disease.

Public health has always been about our shared health concerns as a society and our concerns about vulnerable populations. These concerns have changed over time, and new concerns continue to emerge. Table 1-2 outlines historical, current, and emerging components of the population health approach to public health. As is illustrated by communicable diseases, past concerns cannot be relegated to history.

SHOULD WE FOCUS ON EVERYONE OR ON VULNERABLE GROUPS?

Public health is often confronted with the potential conflict of focusing on everyone and addressing society-wide concerns

TABLE 1-2 Components of Population Health

	Health	Population	Examples of society-wide concerns	Examples of vulnerable groups
Historical	Physical	Geographically limited	Communicable disease	High risk maternal and child, high risk occupations
Current	Physical and mental	Local, state, national, global, governmentally-defined	Toxic substances, product and transportation safety, communicable diseases, costs of health care	Disabled, frail elderly, uninsured
Emerging	Cosmetic, genetic, social functioning	Defined by local, national, and global communications	Disasters, climate change, technology hazards, emerging infectious diseases	Immune-suppressed, genetic vulnerability

versus focusing on the needs of vulnerable populations.[10] This conflict is reflected in the two different approaches to addressing public health problems. We will call them the **high-risk approach** and the **improving-the-average approach**.

The high-risk approach focuses on those with the highest probability of developing the disease and aims to bring their risk close to the levels experienced by the rest of the population. Figure 1-2A illustrates the high risk approach.

The success of the high-risk approach, as shown in Figure 1-2B, assumes that those with a high probability of developing disease are heavily concentrated among those with exposure to what we call **risk factors**. Risk factors include a wide range of exposures from cigarette smoke and other toxic substances to high risk sexual behaviors.

The improving-the-average approach focuses on the entire population and aims to reduce the risk for everyone. Figure 1-3 illustrates this approach.

The improving-the-average approach assumes that everyone is at some degree of risk and the risk increases with the extent of exposure. In this situation, most of the disease occurs among the large number of people who have only modestly increased exposure. The successful reduction in average cholesterol levels through changes in the American diet and the anticipated reduction in diabetes via a focus on weight reduction among children illustrate this approach.

FIGURE 1-2A High risk

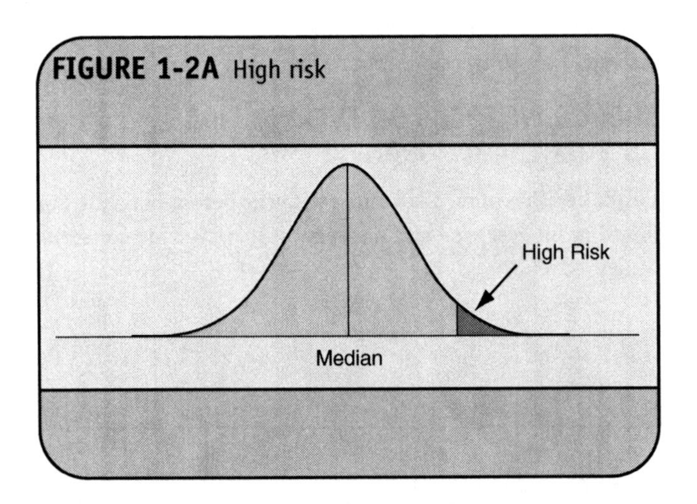

FIGURE 1-2B Reducing high risk

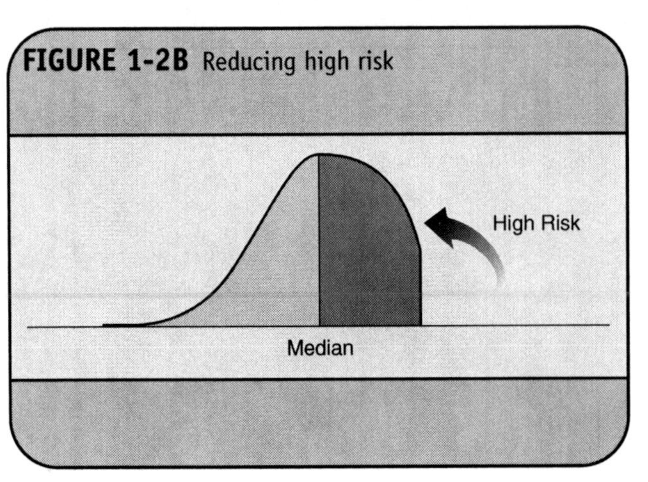

FIGURE 1-3 Improving the average

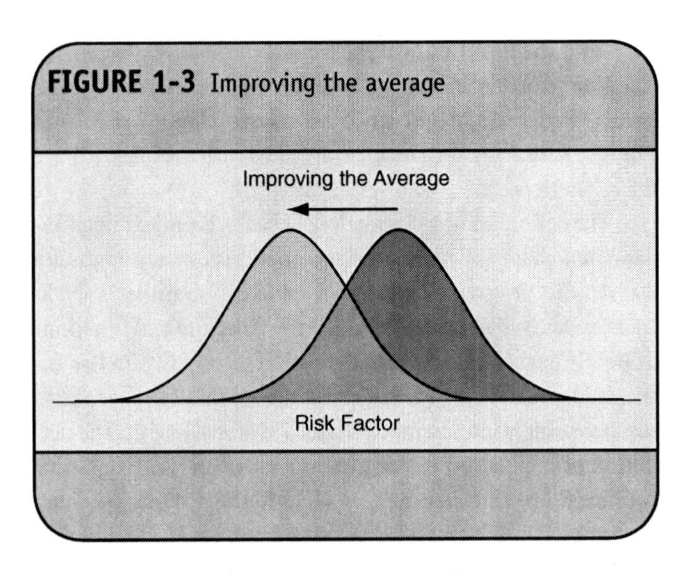

One approach may work better than the other in specific circumstances, but in general both approaches are needed if we are going to successfully address today's and tomorrow's health issues. These two approaches parallel public health's longstanding focus on both the health of vulnerable populations and society-wide health concerns.[c]

Now that we understand what is meant by population health, let us take a look at the range of approaches that may be used to promote and protect health.

WHAT ARE THE APPROACHES AVAILABLE TO PROTECT AND PROMOTE HEALTH?

The wide range of strategies that have been, are being, and will be used to address health issues can be divided into three general categories: health care, traditional public health, and social interventions.

Health care includes the delivery of services to individuals on a one-on-one basis. It includes services for those who are sick or disabled with illness or diseases, as well as for those who are asymptomatic. Services delivered as part of clinical prevention have been categorized as vaccinations, behav-

[c] An additional approach includes reducing disparities by narrowing the curve. For instance, this might be accomplished by transferring financial and/or health services from the low risk to the high risk category through taxation or other methods. Depending on the distribution of the factors affecting health, this approach may or may not reduce the overall frequency of disease more than the other approaches. The distribution of risk in Figures 1-1 and 1-2 assumes a bell-shaped or normal distribution. The actual distribution of factors affecting health may not follow this distribution.

ioral counseling, screening for disease, and preventive medications.[11]

Traditional public health efforts have a population-based preventive perspective utilizing interventions targeting communities or populations, as well as defined high risk or vulnerable groups. Communicable disease control, reduction of environmental hazards, food and drug safety, and nutritional and behavioral risk factors have been key areas of focus of traditional public health approaches.

Both health care and traditional public health approaches share a goal to directly affect the health of those they reach. In contrast, social interventions are primarily aimed at achieving other nonhealth goals, such as increasing convenience, pleasure, economic growth, and social justice. Social interventions range from improving housing, improving education and services for the poor, to increased global trade. These interventions may have dramatic and sometimes unanticipated positive or negative health consequences. Social interventions, like increased availability of food, may improve health, while the availability of high-fat or high-calorie foods may pose a risk to health.

Table 1-3 describes the characteristics of health care, traditional public health, and social approaches to population health and provides examples of each approach.

None of these approaches is new. However, they have traditionally been separated or put into silos in our thinking process with the connections between them often ignored. As we will see in subsequent chapters, connecting the pieces is an important part of the 21st century challenge of defining public health.

Now that we have explained what we mean by public health and seen the scope and methods that we call population health, let us continue our big-picture approach by taking a look at what we mean by the determinants of health and disease.

WHAT FACTORS DETERMINE THE OCCURRENCE OF DISEASE, DISABILITY, AND DEATH?

To complete our look at the big picture issues in public health, we need to gain an understanding of the forces that determine disease and the outcome of disease including what in public health has been called morbidity (disability) and mortality (death).[d]

As we will see in Chapter 3, we need to establish what are called contributory causes based on evidence. **Contributory causes** can be thought of as causes of disease. For instance, the HIV virus and cigarette smoking are two well-established contributory causes of disease, disability, and death. They produce disease, as well as disability and death. However, knowing these contributory causes of disease is often not enough. We need to ask: what determines whether people will smoke or come in contact with the HIV virus? What determines their course once exposed to cigarettes or HIV? In public health we use the term **determinants** to identify these underlying factors that ultimately bring about disease.

Determinants look beyond the known contributory causes of disease to factors that are at work often years before

[d] We will use the term "disease" as shorthand for the broad range of outcomes that includes injuries and exposures that result in death and disability.

TABLE 1-3 Approaches to Population Health

	Characteristics	Examples
Health care	Systems for delivering one-on-one individual health services including those aimed at prevention, cure, palliation, and rehabilitation	Clinical preventive services including: vaccinations, behavioral counseling, screening for disease, and preventive medications
Traditional public health	Group- and community-based interventions directed at health promotion and disease prevention	Communicable disease control, control of environmental hazards, food and drug safety, reduction in risk factors for disease
Social	Interventions with another nonhealth-related purpose, which have secondary impacts on health	Interventions that improve the built environment, increase education, alter nutrition, or address socioeconomic disparities through changes in tax laws; globalization and mobility of goods and populations

a disease develops.[12,13] These underlying factors may be thought of as "upstream" forces. Like great storms, we know the water will flow downstream, often producing flooding and destruction along the way. We just don't know exactly when and where the destruction will occur.

There is no official list or agreed-upon definition of what is included in determinants of disease.[e] Nonetheless, there is wide agreement that the following factors are among those that can be described as determinants in that they increase or at times decrease the chances of developing conditions that threaten the quantity and/or quality of life.

Behavior
Infections
Genetics

Geography
Environment
Medical care
Socio-economic-cultural

BIG GEMS provides a convenient device for remembering these determinants of disease. Let's see what we mean by each of the determinants.

Behavior—Behavior implies actions that increase exposure to the factors that produce disease or protect individuals from disease. Actions such as cigarette smoking, exercise, diet, alcohol consumption, unprotected intercourse, and seat belt use are all examples of the ways that behaviors help determine the development of disease.

Infection—Infections are often the direct cause of disease. In addition, we are increasingly recognizing that early or long-standing exposures to infections may contribute to the development of disease or even protection against disease. Diseases as diverse as gastric and duodenal ulcers, gallstones, and hepatoma or cancer originating in the liver, are increasingly suspected to have infection as an important determinant of the disease. Early exposure to infections may actually reduce diseases ranging from polio to asthma.

Genetics—The revolution in genetics has focused our attention on roles that genetic factors play in the development and outcome of disease. Even when contributory causes, such as cigarettes, have been clearly established as producing lung cancer, genetic factors also play a role in the development and progression of the disease. While genetic factors play a role in many diseases, they are only occasionally the most important determinant of disease.

Geography—Geographic location influences the frequency and even the presence of disease. Infectious diseases such as malaria, Chagas disease, schistosomiasis, and Lyme disease occur only in defined geographic areas. Geography may also imply local geological conditions, such as those that produce high levels of radon—a naturally-occurring radiation that contributes to the development of lung cancer.

Environment—Environmental factors determine disease and the course of disease in a number of ways. The unaltered or "natural" physical world around us may produce disability and death from sudden natural disasters, such as earthquakes and volcanic eruptions, to iodine deficiencies due to low iodine content in the food-producing soil. The altered physical environment produced by human intervention includes exposures to toxic substances in occupational or nonoccupational settings. The physical environment built for use by humans—the **built environment**—produces determinants ranging from indoor air pollution, to "infant-proofed" homes, to hazards on the highway.

Medical care—Access to and the quality of medical care can be a determinant of disease. When a high percentage of individuals are protected by vaccination, nonvaccinated individuals in the population may be protected as well. Cigarette smoking cessation efforts may help smokers to quit, and treatment of infectious disease may reduce the spread to others. Medical care, however, often has its major impact on the course of disease by attempting to prevent or minimize the disability and death once disease develops.

Social-economic-cultural—In the United States, socioeconomic factors have been defined as education, income, and occupational status. These measures have all been shown to be determinants of diseases as varied as breast cancer, tuberculosis, and occupational injuries. Cultural and religious factors are increasingly being recognized as determinants of diseases because beliefs sometimes influence decisions about treatments, in turn affecting the outcome of the disease. While most diseases are more frequent in lower socioeconomic groups, others such as breast cancer are often more common in higher socioeconomic groups.

We will return to determinants again and again as we explore the work of population health. Historically, understanding determinants has often allowed us to prevent diseases and their consequences even when we did not fully understand the

[e] Health Canada[12] has identified 12 determinants of health that are: 1) income and social status; 2) employment; 3) education; 4) social environments; 5) physical environments; 6) healthy child development; 7) personal health practices and coping skills; 8) health services; 9) social support networks; 10) biology and genetic endowment; 11) gender; and 12) culture. Many of these are subsumed under socio-economic-cultural determinants in the BIG GEMS framework. The World Health Organization's Commission on Social Determinants of Health has also produced a list of determinants that is consistent with the BIG GEMS framework.[13]

mechanism by which the determinants produced their impact. For instance:

- Scurvy was controlled by citrus fruits well before vitamin C was identified.
- Malaria was partially controlled by clearing swamps before the relationship to mosquito transmission was appreciated.
- Hepatitis B and HIV infections were partially controlled even before the organisms were identified through reduction in use of contaminated needles and blood transfusions.
- Tuberculosis death rates were greatly reduced through less crowded housing, the use of TB sanitariums, and better nutrition.

Using asthma as an example, Box 1-1 illustrates the many ways that determinants can affect the development and course of a disease.

Thus, population health focuses on the big picture issues and the determinants of disease. Increasingly, public health also emphasizes a focus on the research evidence as a basis for understanding the cause or etiology of disease and the intervention that can improve the outcome.

BOX 1-1 Asthma and the Determinants of Disease.

Jennifer, a teenager living in an urban rundown apartment in a city with high levels of air pollution, develops severe asthma. Her mother also has severe asthma, yet both of them smoke cigarettes. Her clinician prescribed medications to prevent asthma attacks, but she takes them only when she experiences severe symptoms. Jennifer is hospitalized twice with pneumonia due to common bacterial infections. She then develops an antibiotic-resistant infection. During this hospitalization, she requires intensive care on a respirator. After several weeks of intensive care and every known treatment to save her life, she dies suddenly.

Asthma is an inflammatory disease of the lung coupled with an increased reactivity of the airways, which together produce a narrowing of the airways of the lungs. When the airways become swollen and inflamed, they become narrower, allowing less air through to the lung tissue and causing symptoms such as wheezing, coughing, chest tightness, breathing difficulty, and predisposition to infection. Once considered a minor ailment, asthma is now the most common chronic disorder of childhood. It affects over six million children under the age of 18 in the United States alone.

Jennifer's tragic history illustrates how a wide range of determinants of disease may affect the occurrence, severity, and development of complications of a disease. Let's walk through the BIG GEMS framework and see how each determinant impacts in Jennifer's story.

Behavior—Behavioral factors play an important role in the development of asthma attacks and in their complications. Cigarette smoking makes asthma attacks more frequent and more severe. It also predisposes individuals to developing infections such as pneumonia. Treatment for severe asthma requires regular treatments along with more intensive treatment when an attack occurs. It is difficult for many people, especially teenagers, to take medication regularly, yet failure to adhere to treatment greatly complicates the disease.

Infection—Infection is a frequent precipitant of asthma and asthma increases the frequency and severity of infections. Infectious diseases, especially pneumonia, can be life-threatening in asthmatics requiring prompt and high quality medical care. The increasing development of antibiotic-resistant infections pose special risks to those with asthma.

Genetics—Genetic factors predispose people to childhood asthma. However, many children and adults without a family history develop asthma.

Geography—Asthma is more common in geographic areas with high levels of naturally occurring allergens due to flowering plants. However, today even populations in desert climates in the United States are often affected by asthma, as irrigation results in the planting of allergen-producing trees and other plants.

Environment—The physical environment, including that built for use by humans, has increasingly been recognized as a major factor affecting the development of asthma and asthma attacks. Indoor air pollution is the most common form of air pollution in many developing countries. Along with cigarette smoke, air pollution inflames the lungs acutely and chronically. Cockroaches often found in rundown buildings have been found to be highly allergenic and predisposing to asthma. Other factors in the built environment, including mold and exposure to pet dander, can also trigger wheezing in susceptible individuals.

(continues)

BOX 1-1 continued.

Medical care—The course of asthma can be greatly affected by medical care. Management of the acute and chronic effects of asthma can be positively affected by efforts to understand an individual's exposures, reducing the chronic inflammation with medications, managing the acute symptoms, and avoiding life-threatening complications.

Socio-economic-cultural—Disease and disease progression are often influenced by an individual's socioeconomic status. Air pollution is often greater in lower socioeconomic neighborhoods of urban areas. Mold and cockroach infestations may be greater in poor neighborhoods. Access to and quality of medical care may be affected by social, economic, and cultural factors.

Thus, asthma is a condition which demonstrates the contributions made by the full range of determinants included in the BIG GEMS framework. No one determinant alone explains the bulk of the disease. The large number of determinants and their interactions provide opportunities for a range of health care, traditional public health, and social interventions.

Key Words

- Population health approach
- Social justice
- Interventions
- Health issues
- Population(s)
- Society's shared health concerns
- Society's vulnerable groups
- High-risk approach
- Improving-the-average approach
- Risk factor
- Contributory causes
- Determinants
- Built environment
- Behavior
- Infections
- Genetics
- Geography
- Environment
- Medical care
- Socio-economic-cultural

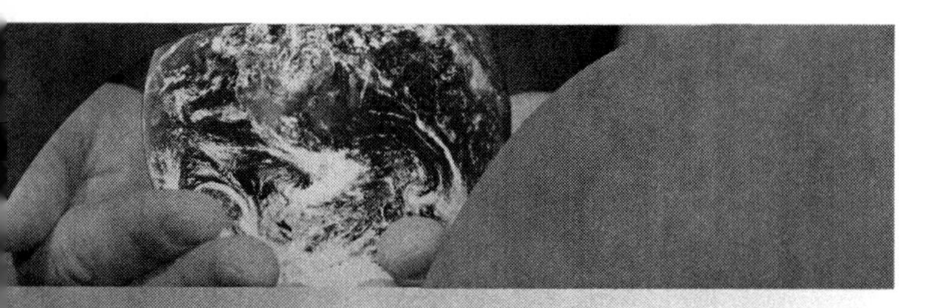

Discussion Question

1. Think about a typical day in your life and identify ways that public health affects it.

REFERENCES

1. Pfizer Global Pharmaceuticals. *Milestones in Public Health: Accomplishments in Public Health over the Last 100 Years.* New York: Pfizer Global Pharmaceuticals; 2006.
2. Turnock BJ. *Public Health: What It Is and How It Works,* 4th ed. Sudbury, MA: Jones and Bartlett Publishers; 2009.
3. Winslow CEA. The untilled field of public health. *Mod. Med.* 1920; 920;2:183–191.
4. Institute of Medicine. *The Future of Public Health.* Washington, DC: National Academy Press; 1988:41.
5. Young TK. *Population Health: Concepts and Methods.* New York: Oxford University Press; 1998.
6. Rosen G. *A History of Public Health.* Baltimore: Johns Hopkins University Press; 1993.
7. Porter D. *Health, Civilization, and the State: A History of Public Health from Ancient to Modern Times.* Oxford: Rutledge; 1999.
8. American Public Health Association. APHA History and Timeline. Available at: http://www.apha.org/about/news/presskit/aphahistory.htm?NRMODE=Published&NRNODEGUID=%7b8AF0A3FE-8B29-4952-87EF-2757B9B2668F%7d&NRORIGINALURL=%2fabout%2fnews%2fpresskit%2faphahistory.htm&NRCACHEHINT=NoModifyGuest&PF=true. Accessed March 12, 2009.
9. Awofeso N. What's new about the "New Public Health"? *American Journal of Public Health.* 2004;94(5):705–709.
10. Rose G, Khaw KT, Marmot M. *Rose's Strategy of Preventive Medicine.* New York: Oxford University Press; 2008.
11. Agency for Healthcare Research and Quality. Preventive Services. Available at: http://www.ahrq.gov/. Accessed March 12, 2009.
12. Public Health Agency of Canada. Population Health Approach—What Determines Health? Available at: http://www.phac-aspc.gc.ca/ph-sp/determinants/index-eng.php. Accessed March 12, 2009.
13. Commission on Social Determinants of Health. *Closing the gap in a generation: health equity through action on the social determinants of health. Final Report of the Commission on Social Determinants of Health.* Geneva: World Health Organization; 2008.

CHAPTER 2

Health Determinants, Measurements, and Trends

LEARNING OBJECTIVES

By the end of this chapter the reader will be able to:

- Describe the determinants of health
- Define the most important health indicators
- Discuss the differences between incidence and prevalence; morbidity, disability, and mortality; and non-communicable and communicable diseases
- Discuss the concepts of Health Adjusted Life Expectancy (HALE), Disability Adjusted Life Years (DALYs), and the burden of disease
- Describe the leading causes of death in low-, middle-, and high-income countries
- Describe the demographic and epidemiological transitions

VIGNETTES

Shawki is a 60-year-old Jordanian man who lives in Jordan's capital of Amman. Unfortunately, Shawki's health has deteriorated in the last year. His blood pressure and cholesterol are too high. He has developed diabetes. He is sometimes short of breath. What are the causes of his ill and declining health? Do these problems stem from any genetic issues? Could they come from a lack of understanding about a healthy lifestyle and diet? Could it be that Shawki lacks the income he needs to eat properly and to ensure that he gets health checkups when he needs them?

Life expectancy in Botswana prior to the spread of HIV/AIDS was about 65 years.[1] Today, it is about 40 years.[1] Life expectancy in Russia in 1985 was about 64 years for males and 74 years for females. In 2001, however, it had fallen to about 59 years for males and 72 years for females.[2] What does life expectancy measure? What are the factors contributing to its decline in both of these countries? What has happened to trends in life expectancy in other countries? Which countries have the longest and shortest life expectancies and why?

In Cambodia today, families have, on average, four children and those children, on average, will live about 57 years.[3] Many children will die in their first month of life, and the leading causes of infant and child death will be diarrhea and pneumonia. Thirty years ago, the demographic and epidemiological profile of Thailand looked a lot like Cambodia looks today. Today, however, Thai families have on average about two children and those children on average will live 71 years.[3] Children in Thailand rarely die, and when they do, 50 percent of them die from injury.[4] What causes these shifts in fertility and mortality? Do they occur consistently as countries develop economically? How long will it take before Cambodia has the same fertility and disease burden that Thailand has today?

In Peru, the people who are poor tend to live in the mountains, be indigenous people, be less educated, and have worse health status than other people. In Eastern Europe, the same issues occur among their ethnic groups that are of lower socioeconomic status, such as the Roma people. In the United States, there are also enormous health disparities, as seen in the relative health status of African Americans and Native Americans. If one wants to understand and address differences in health status among different groups, then how do we have to measure health status? Do we measure it by age? By gender? By socioeconomic status? By level of education? By ethnicity? By location?

THE IMPORTANCE OF MEASURING HEALTH STATUS

If we want to understand the most important global health issues and what can be done to address them, then we must understand what factors have the most influence on health status, how health status is measured, and what key trends in health status have occurred historically. We must, in fact, be able to answer the questions that are posed in the narratives above.

This chapter, therefore, covers four distinct, but closely related topics. The first section concerns what are called "the determinants of health." That section examines the most important factors that relate to people's health status. The second section reviews some of the most important indicators of health status and how they are used. The third section discusses the burden of disease worldwide and how it varies across countries. The last section looks at how fertility and mortality change as countries become more developed and what this means for the types of health problems countries face.

THE DETERMINANTS OF HEALTH

Why are some people healthy and some people not healthy? When asked this question, many of us will respond that good health depends on access to health services. Yet, as you will learn, whether or not people are healthy depends on a large number of factors, many of which are interconnected, and most of which go considerably beyond access to health services.

There has been considerable writing about the "determinants of health" and one way of depicting these **determinants** is shown in Figure 2-1. The next section largely follows the approach to the determinants of health that is discussed in "What Determines Health" by the Public Health Agency of Canada.[5]

The first group of factors that helps to determine health relates to the personal and inborn features of individuals. These include genetic makeup, sex, and age. Our genetic makeup has much to do with what diseases we get and how healthy we live. One can inherit, for example, a genetic marker for a particular disease, such as Huntington's disease, which is a neurological disorder. One can also inherit the genetic component of a disease that has multiple causes, such as breast cancer. Sex also has an important relationship with health. Men and women are physically different, for example, and may get different diseases. Women face the risk of childbearing. They also get cervical and uterine cancers that men do not get. Women also have higher rates of certain health conditions, such as thyroid and breast cancers. For similar reasons, age is also an important determinant of health. Young children in developing countries often die of diarrheal disease, while older people are much more likely to die of heart disease, to cite one of many examples of the relationship between health and age.

Social and cultural issues also play important roles in determining health. Social status is an important health determinant. There is good evidence that people of higher social status have more control over their lives than people of lower status, and people of higher social status also tend to have higher incomes and education, both of which are strongly correlated with better health.[6] In addition, the gender roles that are ascribed to women in many societies also have an important impact on health. In such environments, women may be less well treated than men and this, in turn, may mean that women have less income, less education, and fewer opportunities to engage in safe employment. All of these militate against their good health.

The extent to which people get social support from family, friends, and community has also been shown to have an important link with health.[6] The stronger the social networks and the stronger the support that people get from those networks, the healthier people will be. Of course, culture is also an extremely important determinant of health.[6] Culture helps to determine how one feels about health and illness, how one uses health services, and the health practices in which one engages.

The environment, both indoor and outdoor, is also a powerful determinant of health. Related to this is the safety of the environment in which people work. Although many people know about the importance of outdoor air pollution to health, few people are aware of the importance of indoor air pollution to health. In many developing countries, women cook indoors with very poor ventilation, thereby creating an indoor environment that is full of smoke and that encourages respiratory illness and asthma. The lack of safe drinking water and sanitation is a major contributor to ill health in poor countries. In addition, many people in those same countries work in environments that are very unhealthy. Because they lack skills, social status, and opportunities, they may work without sufficient protection with hazardous chemicals, in polluted air, or in circumstances that expose them to occupational accidents.

Education is a powerful determinant of health for several reasons. First, it brings with it knowledge of good health practices. Second, it provides opportunities for gaining skills, getting better employment, raising one's income, and enhancing one's social status, all of which are also related to health. Studies have shown, for example, that the single best predictor of the birth weight of a baby is the level of educational attainment of the mother.[7] Most of us already know that throughout the world, there is an extremely strong and positive correlation between the level of education and all key health indicators. People who are better educated eat better, smoke less, are less obese, have fewer children, and take better care of their children's health than do people with less education. It is not a surprise, therefore, that they and their children live longer and healthier lives than do less well educated people and their children.

Of course, people's own health practices and behaviors are also critical determinants of their health. Being able to identify when you or a family member is ill and needs health care can be critical to good health. As noted previously, however, one's health also depends on how one eats, or if one smokes, drinks too much alcohol, or drives safely. We also know that being active physically and getting exercise regularly is better for one's health than is being sedentary.

Another important determinant of future health is the way in which infants and young children are cared for and nourished and the manner in which their health is attended. Being born premature or of low birthweight can have important negative consequences on health. There is a strong correlation between the nutritional status of infants and young children and the extent to which they meet their biological potentials, enroll in school, or stay in school. In addition, poor nutritional status in infancy and young childhood may be linked with a number of chronic diseases, including diabetes and heart disease. [8]

Of course, one's health does depend on access to appropriate healthcare services. Even if one is born healthy, raised healthy, and engages in good health behaviors, there will still be times when one has to call on a health system for help. The more likely you are to access services of appropriate quality, the more likely you are to stay healthy. To address the risk of dying from a complication of pregnancy, for example, one must have access to health services that can carry out an emergency cesarean section if necessary. Even if the mother has had the suggested level of prenatal care and has prepared well in all other respects for the pregnancy, in the end, certain complications can only be addressed in a healthcare setting.

Finally, one should note that the approach that governments take to different policies and programs in the health sector and in other sectors has an important bearing on people's health. People living in a country that promotes high educational attainment, for example, will be healthier than people in a country that does not promote widespread education of appropriate quality, because better educated people engage in healthier behaviors. A country that has universal

FIGURE 2-1 Key Determinants of Health

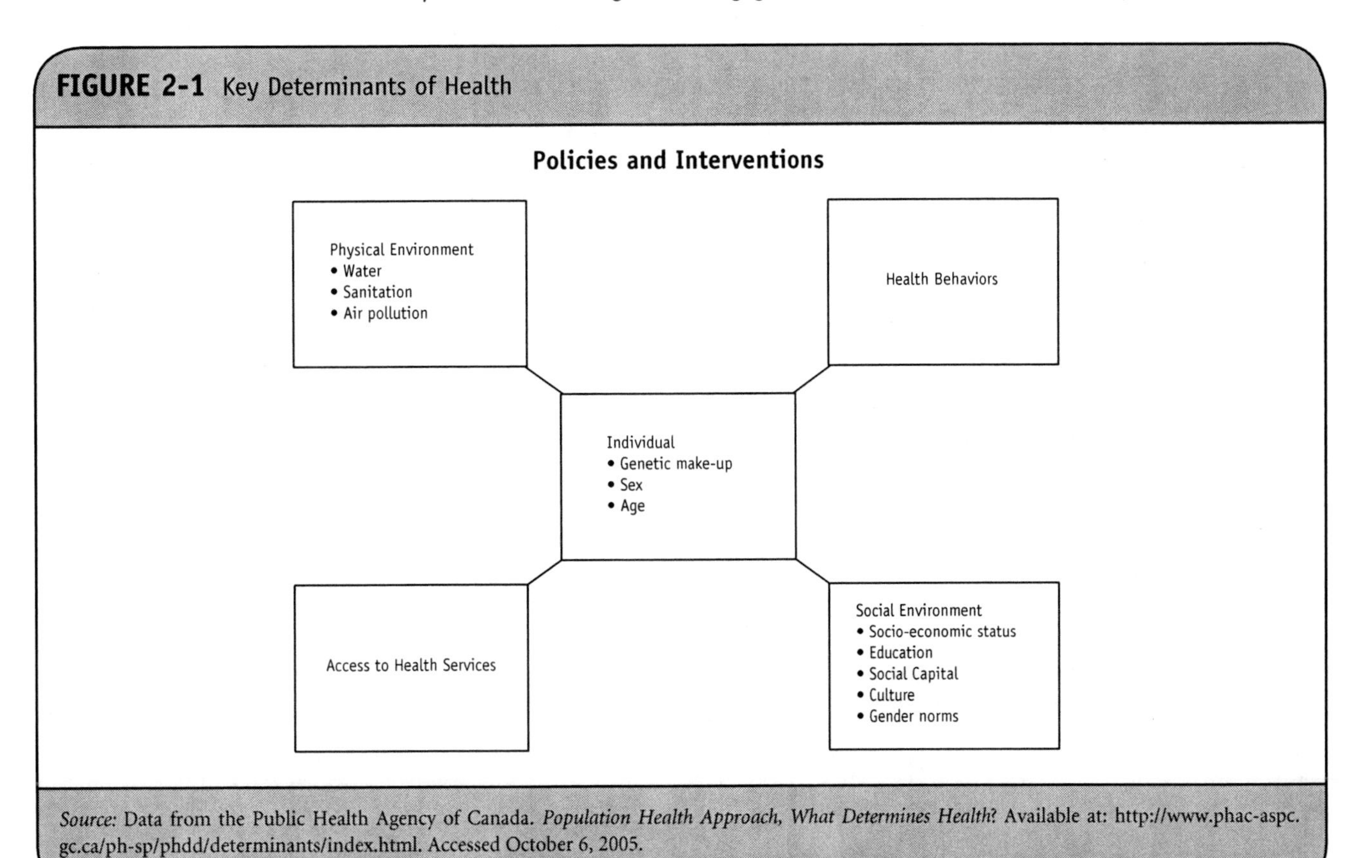

Source: Data from the Public Health Agency of Canada. *Population Health Approach, What Determines Health?* Available at: http://www.phac-aspc.gc.ca/ph-sp/phdd/determinants/index.html. Accessed October 6, 2005.

health insurance is likely to have healthier people than a country that does not insure all of its people, because the uninsured may lack needed health services. The same would be true, for example, for a country that promoted safe water supply for all of its people, compared to one that does not.

KEY HEALTH INDICATORS

It is critical that we use data and evidence to understand and address key global health issues. Some types of health data concern the health status of people and communities, such as measures of life expectancy and infant and child mortality, as discussed further hereafter. Some concern health services, such as the number of nurses and doctors per capita in a certain country or the indicators of coverage for certain health services, such as immunization. Other data concern the financing of health, such as the amount of public expenditure on health or the share of national income represented by health expenditure. This book also provides only a limited discussion of health financing, which is also primarily in the chapter on health systems.

There are a number of very important uses of data on health status, which we shall explore further and discuss throughout the book.[9] We need data, for example, to know what are the health conditions from which people suffer. We also need to know the extent to which these conditions cause people to be sick, to be disabled, or to die. We need to gather data to carry out disease surveillance. This helps us to understand if particular health problems such as influenza, polio, or malaria are occurring, where they are infecting people, who is getting these diseases, and what might be done to address them. Other forms of data also help us to understand the burden of different health conditions, the relative importance of them to different societies, and the importance that should be attached to dealing with them.

If we are to use data in the previously mentioned ways, then it is important that we use a consistent set of indicators to measure health status. In this way, we can make comparisons across people in the same country or across different countries. There are, in fact, a number of indicators that are used most commonly by those who work in global health and in development work, as well, as noted later. These are listed and defined in Table 2-1 and are discussed briefly below.

Among the most commonly used indicators of health status is life expectancy at birth. **Life expectancy at birth** is "the average number of additional years a newborn baby can be expected to live if current mortality trends were to continue for the rest of that person's life."[10] In other words, it measures how long a person born today can expect to live, if there were no change in their lifetime in the present rate of death for people of different ages. The higher the life expectancy at birth, the better the health status of a country. In the United States, life expectancy at birth is about 77 years; in a middle-income country, such as Jordan, life expectancy is 72 years; in a very poor country, such as Mali, the life expectancy is 48 years. Figure 2-2 shows life expectancy at birth by region.[3]

Another important and widely used indicator is the infant mortality rate. The **infant mortality rate** is "the number of deaths of infants under age 1 per 1000 live births in a given year."[10] This rate is usually expressed in deaths per 1000 live births. In other words, it measures how many children younger than 1 year of age will die for every 1000 who were born alive that year. Each country seeks as low a rate of infant mortality as possible, but we will see that the rate varies largely with the income status of a country. Some of the poorer countries, such as Niger, have infant mortality rates as high as 150 infant deaths for every 1000 live births, whereas in Sweden only about 3 infants die for every 1000 live births.[12] (See Figure 2-3).

Although the infant mortality rate is a powerful indicator of health status of a country, most children younger than 1 year of age who die actually die in the first month of life. Thus, the **neonatal mortality rate** is also an important health status indicator. This rate measures "the number of deaths to infants younger than 28 days of age in a given year, per 1000 live births in that year."[10] Like the infant mortality rate, this rate will generally vary directly with the

TABLE 2-1 Key Health Status Indicators

Infant Mortality Rate—The number of deaths of infants under age 1 per 1000 life births in a given year

Life Expectancy at Birth—The average number of years a newborn baby could expect to live if current mortality trends were to continue for the rest of the newborn's life

Maternal Mortality Ratio—The number of women who die as a result of pregnancy and childbirth complications per 100,000 live births in a given year

Neonatal Mortality Rate—The number of deaths to infants under 28 days of age in a given year per 1000 live births in that year

Under Five Mortality Rate (Child Mortality Rate) —The probability that a newborn baby will die before reaching age five, expressed as a number per 1000 live births.

Source: Haupt A, Kane TT. Population Handbook. Washington, DC: Population Reference Bureau; 2004; World Bank. Beyond Economic Growth: Glossary. http://www.worldbank.org/depweb/english/beyond/global/glossary.html. Accessed April 15, 2007.

FIGURE 2-2 Life Expectancy at Birth, by Region, 2004

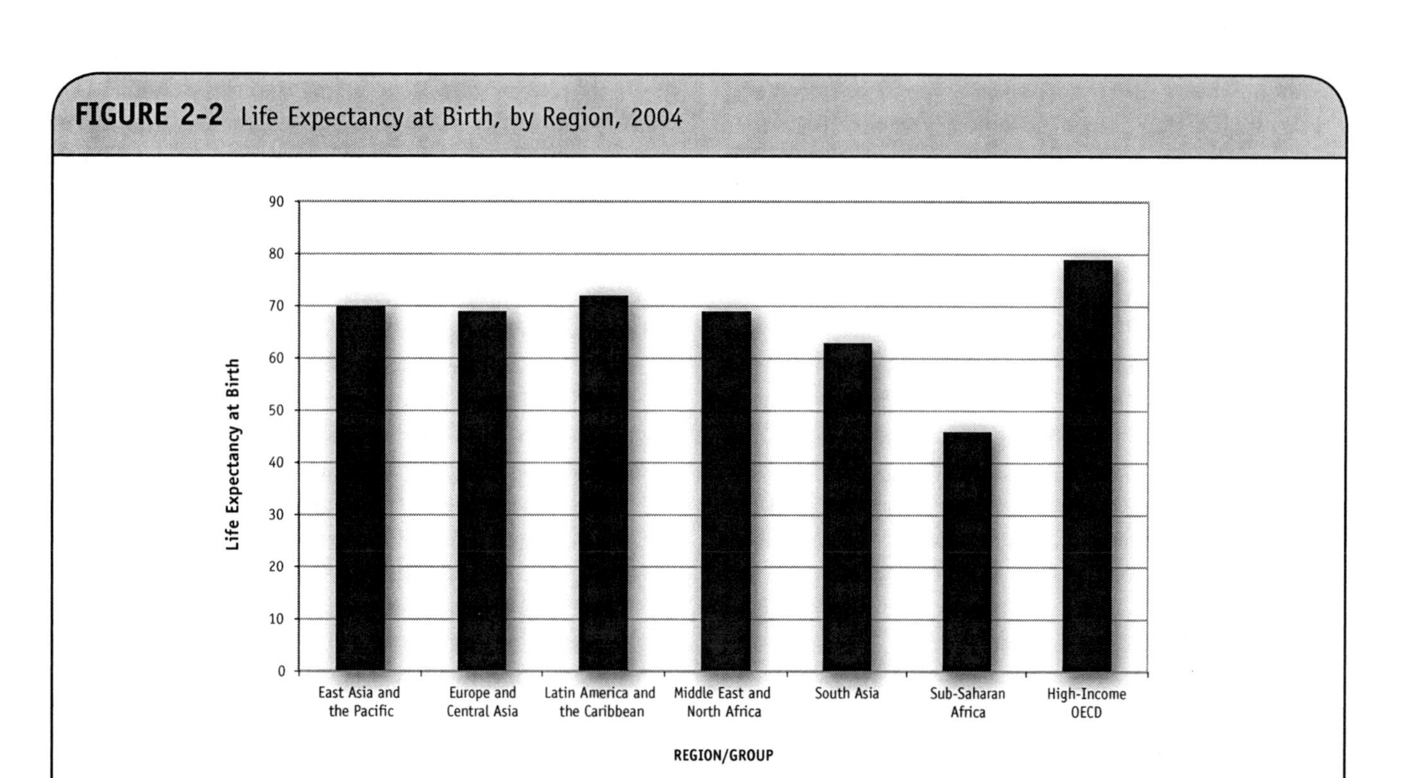

Source: Data from the World Bank. World Development Indicators, Data Query. Available at: http://devdata.worldbank.org. Accessed July 10, 2006.

FIGURE 2-3 Infant Mortality Rate, by Region, 2004

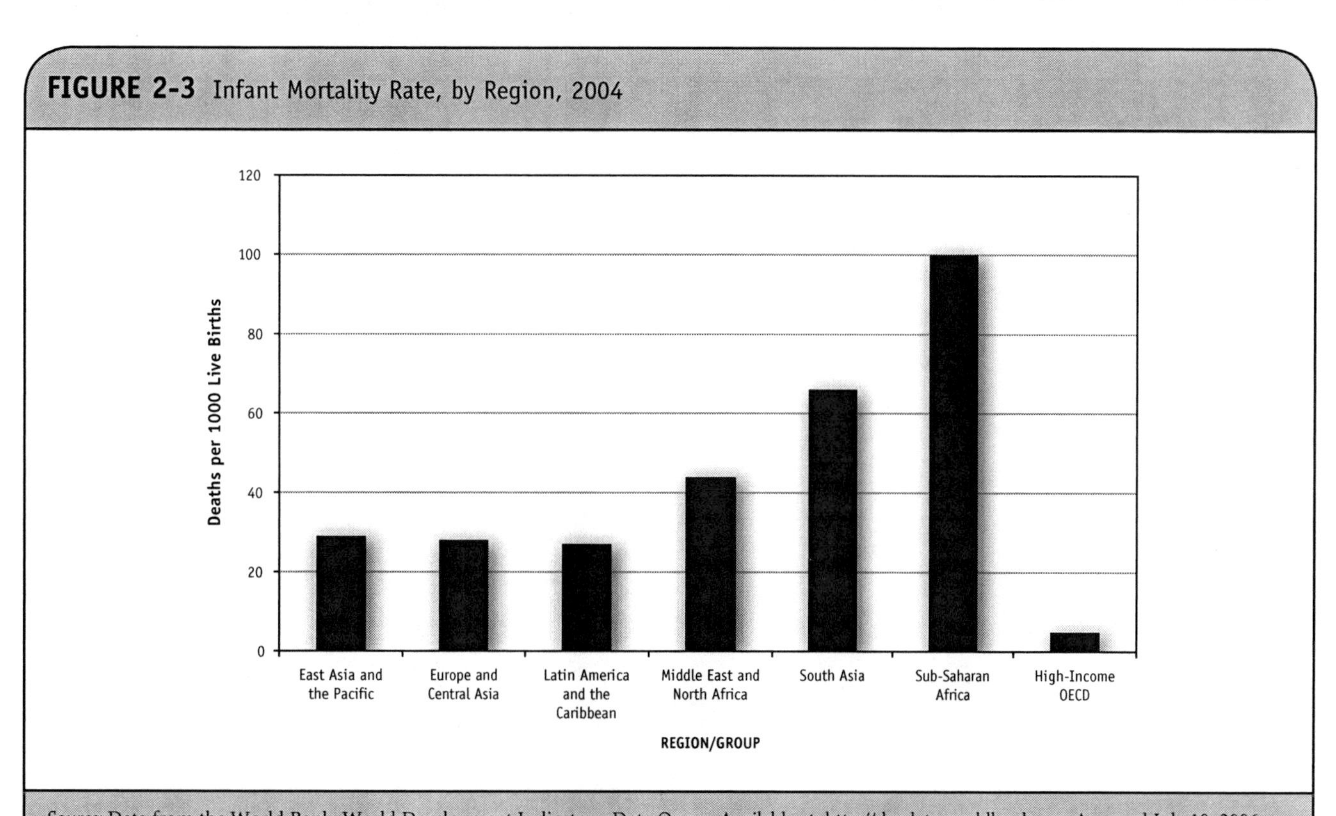

Source: Data from the World Bank. World Development Indicators, Data Query. Available at: http://devdata.worldbank.org. Accessed July 10, 2006.

level of income of different countries. Poorer countries will have a much higher neonatal mortality rate then the richer countries. The neonatal mortality rate is about 40 per 1000 live births in Sub-Saharan Africa but below 5 per 1000 live births in developed countries.[14] The neonatal mortality rate by region is portrayed in Figure 2-4.

The **under-five child mortality rate** is also called the "child mortality rate." This is "the probability that a newborn will die before reaching age five, expressed as a number per 1000 live births."[10] Like the infant mortality rate, this rate is also expressed per 1000 live births. Of course, this rate is very similar to the infant mortality rate, and here, too, the lower the rate the better. This rate also varies largely with the wealth of a country. In the developed countries the rate is about 20 per 1000 live births. However, in the poorest countries, the rate can be as high as 170 per 1000 live births, as in the Africa Region of the World Health Organization (WHO).[16] The under-five child mortality rate is depicted in Figure 2-5. As infant mortality declines, the under-five child mortality rate becomes a more important health indicator. The relative standing of different regions in under-five child mortality, as shown in Figure 2-5, looks very similar to that for infant mortality.

The **maternal mortality ratio** is a measure of the risk of death that is associated with childbirth. Because these deaths are more rare than infant and child deaths, the maternal mortality ratio is measured as 'the number of women who die as a result of pregnancy and childbirth complications per 100,000 live births in a given year.'[10] The rarity of maternal deaths and the fact that they largely occur in low-income settings also contributes to maternal mortality being quite difficult to measure. Very few women die in childbirth in rich countries and the maternal mortality rate in Sweden, for example, is 5 per 100,000 live births. On the other hand, in very poor countries, in which women have low status and there are few facilities for dealing with obstetric emergencies, the rates can be over 500 per 100,000 live births, as they are in Gabon, India, and Laos.[18] As you can see in Figure 2-6, the maternal mortality ratio is also very strongly correlated with a country's income.

There are a few other concepts and definitions that are important to understand as we think about measuring health status, and they are summarized in Table 2-3. The first is **morbidity**. Essentially, this means sickness or any departure, subjective or objective, from a psychological or physiological state of well-being. Second is **mortality**, which refers to death. A "death rate" is the number of deaths per 1000 population in a given year.[10] The third is **disability**. Although some conditions cause people to get sick or die,

FIGURE 2-4 Neonatal Mortality Rate, by WHO Region, 2000

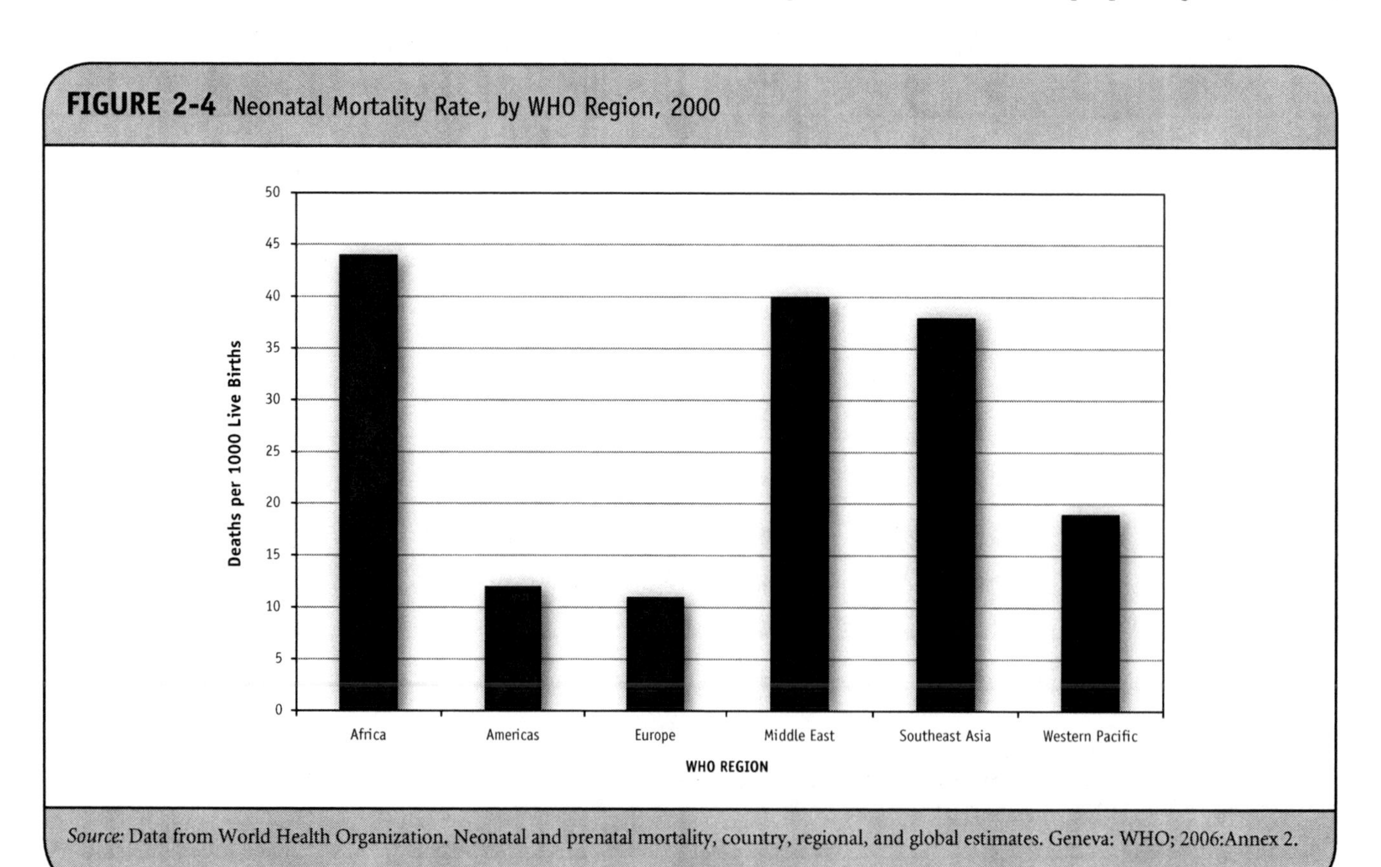

Source: Data from World Health Organization. Neonatal and prenatal mortality, country, regional, and global estimates. Geneva: WHO; 2006:Annex 2.

FIGURE 2-5 Under-five Child Mortality, by Region, 2006

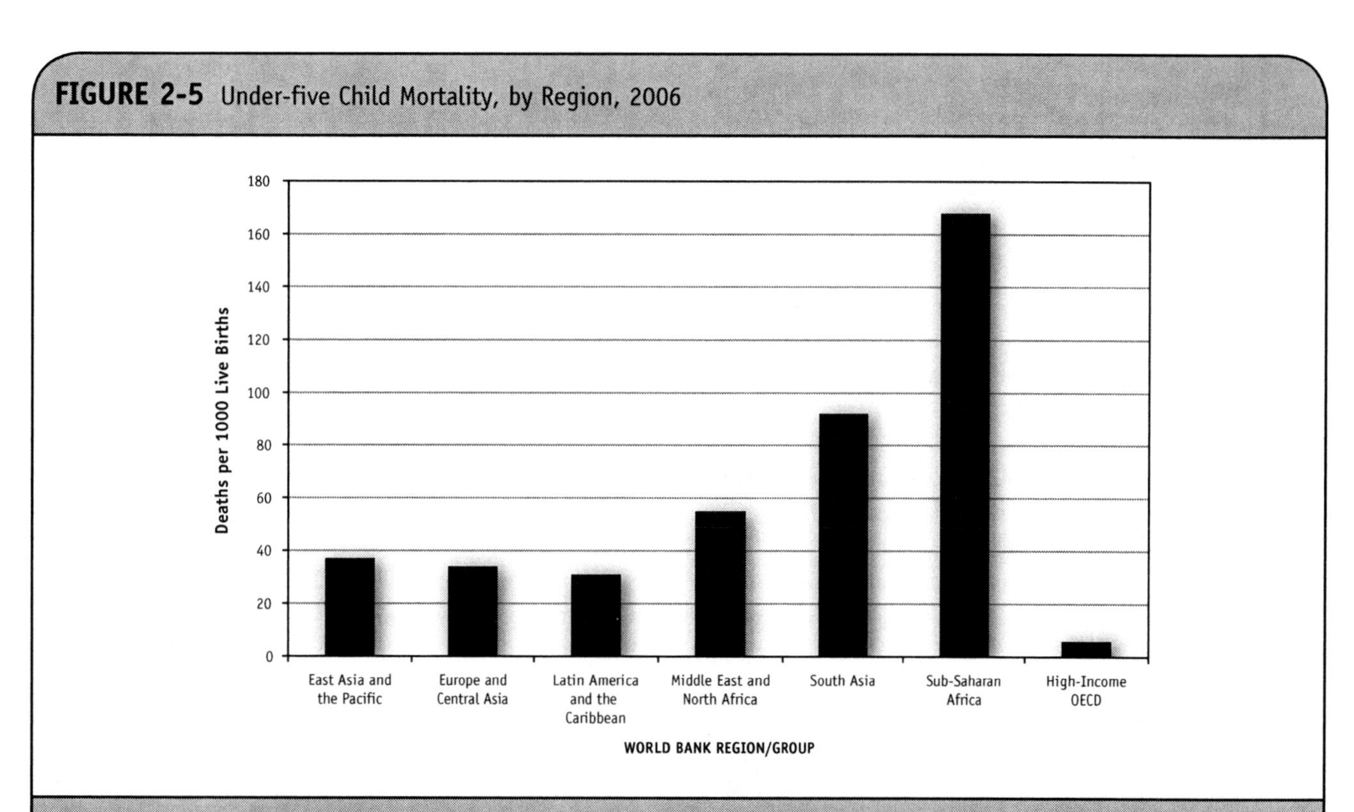

Source: Data from the World Bank. World Development Indicators, Data Query. Available at: http://devdata.worldbank.org. Accessed July 10, 2006.

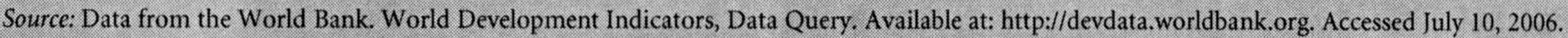

FIGURE 2-6 Maternal Mortality, by Region, 2000

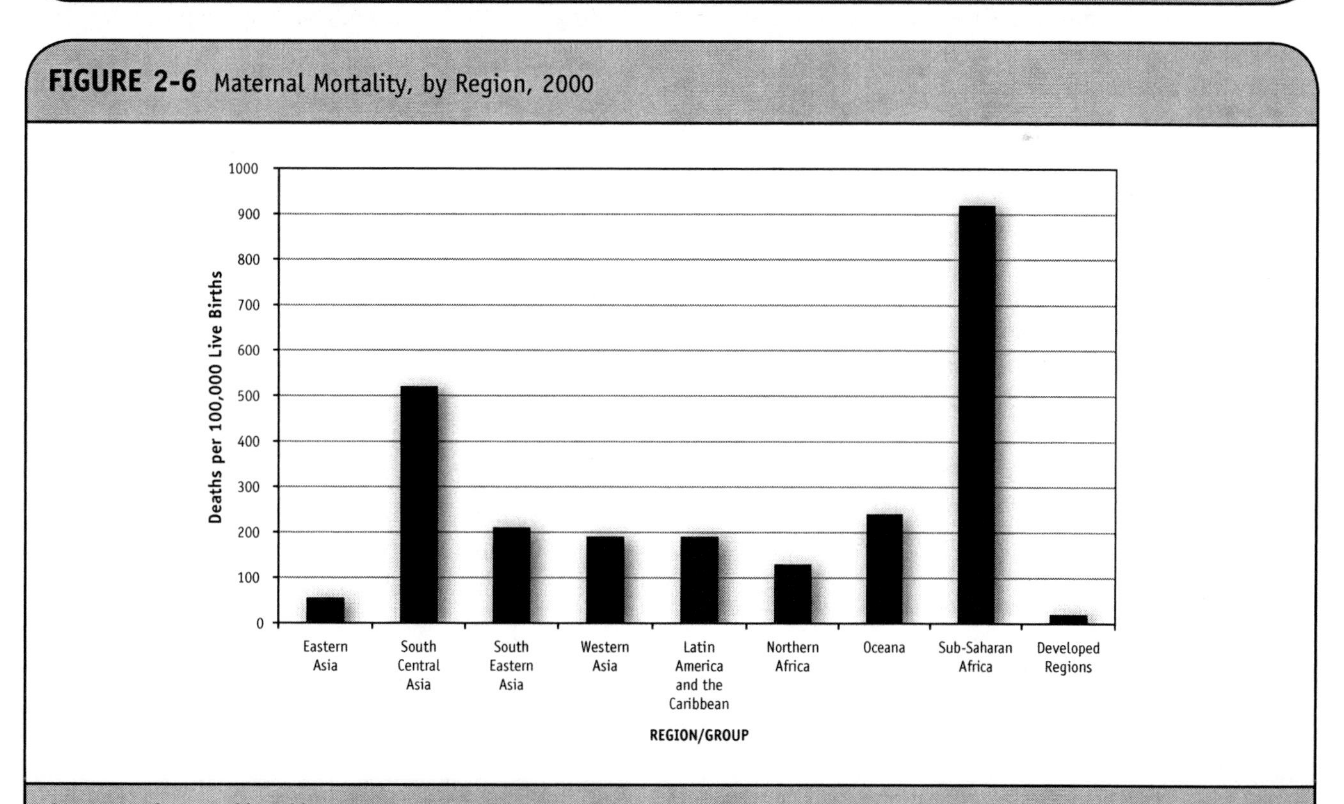

Source: Data from World Health Organization. Maternal Mortality in 2000, Estimates Developed by WHO, UNICEF & UNFPA. Available at: www.who.int/reproductive-health/publications/maternal_mortality. Accessed July 10, 2006.

they might also cause people to suffer the "temporary or long-term reduction in a person's capacity to function."[21]

There will also be considerable discussion in this book and most readings on global health of the **prevalence** of health conditions. This refers to the number of people suffering from a certain health condition over a specific time period. It measures the chances of having a disease. For global health work, one usually refers to "point prevalence" of a condition, which is "the proportion of the population that is diseased at a single point in time."[22] The point prevalence of HIV/AIDS among adults in South Africa, for example, is estimated to be between 17% and 21%. This means that today between 17% and 21% of all adults between the ages of 15 and 49 in South Africa are HIV positive.[23]

The **incidence rate** is also a very commonly used term. This refers to the rate at which new cases of a disease occur in a population. **Incidence** measures the chances of getting a disease. Incidence rate is "the number of persons contracting a disease per 1000 population at risk, for a given period of time."[10] It is usually specified as the number of people getting the disease over a year, per 100,000 people at risk. In India, for example, the incidence rate for TB is 168 per 100,000.[25] This means that for every 100,000 people in India, 168 in the last year got TB.

Many people confuse incidence rate and prevalence rate. It may be convenient to think of prevalence as the pool of people with a disease at a particular time and incidence as the flow of new cases of people with that disease each year into that pool. You should note, of course, that the size of the pool will vary as new cases flow into the pool and old cases flow out, as they die or are cured.

Finally, one needs to be familiar with how diseases get classified. When you read about health, there will be discussions of communicable diseases, non-communicable diseases, and injuries. **Communicable diseases** are also called infectious diseases. These are illnesses that are caused by a particular infectious agent and that spread directly or indirectly from people to people, animals to people, or people to animals.[26] Examples of communicable diseases include influenza, measles, and HIV. **Non-communicable diseases** are illnesses that are not spread by any infectious agent, such as hypertension, coronary heart disease, and diabetes. Another category of health conditions is **injuries**. These usually include, among other things, road traffic injuries, falls, self-inflicted injuries, and violence.[27]

MEASURING THE BURDEN OF DISEASE

The definition of health is "a state of complete physical, mental and social well-being and not merely the absence of disease or infirmity." Those who work on global health have attempted for a number of years to construct a single indicator that could be used to compare how far different countries are from the state of good health, as defined previously. Ideally, such an index would take account of morbidity, mortality, and disability; allow one to calculate the index by age, by gender, and by region; and, allow one to make comparisons of health status across regions within a country and across countries.[28] This kind of index would measure what is generally referred to as "the burden of disease."

One such indicator is **Health-Adjusted Life Expectancy**, or HALE. It is a "health expectancy measure." The HALE "summarizes the expected number of years to be lived in what might be termed the equivalent of good health."[29] This can also be seen as "the equivalent number of years in full health that a newborn can expect to live, based on current rates of ill health and mortality."[30] To calculate the HALE, "the years of ill health are weighted according to severity and subtracted from the overall life expectancy."[6]

WHO calculated HALEs for most countries, using a standard methodology. Table 2-2 shows life expectancy at birth in 2000 for a number of low-, middle-, and high-income countries and how its compares with HALEs for those countries in the same year. As you can see from Table 2-2, the greater the number of years that people in any population are likely to spend in ill health or with disability, the greater the difference will be between life expectancy at birth and health-adjusted life expectancy.

The composite indicator of health status that is most commonly used in global health work is called the **Disability Adjusted Life Year**, or DALY. This indicator was first used in conjunction with the 1993 World Development Report of the World Bank, and is a "health gap measure." It is now used in burden of disease studies. In the simplest terms, a DALY is:

> . . . a unit for measuring the amount of health lost because of a particular disease or injury. It is calculated as the present value of future years of disability free life that are lost as the result of the premature deaths or causes of disability occurring in a particular year.[31]

The DALY is a measure of premature deaths and losses due to illnesses and disabilities in a population. A DALY measures how many healthy years of life are lost between the population being measured and the "healthiest" possible population, which is used as a standard. It does this by adding together the losses of healthy years of life that occur from illness, disability, and death. The value of disability is

TABLE 2-2 Life Expectancy at Birth and Health Adjusted Life Expectancy, Selected Countries, 2004

Country	Life Expectancy/Health Adjusted Life Expectancy Males	Life Expectancy/Health Adjusted Life Expectancy Females
Afghanistan	42/35.3	42/35.8
Argentina	71/62.5	78/68.1
Bangladesh	62/55.3	63/53.3
Bolivia	63/53.6	66/55.2
Brazil	67/57.2	74/62.4
Cambodia	51/45.6	58/49.5
Cameroon	50/41.1	51/41.8
Canada	78/70.1	83/74.0
Chile	74/64.9	81/69.7
China	70/63.1	74/65.2
Costa Rica	75/65.2	80/69.3
Cuba	75/67.1	80/69.5
Denmark	75/68.6	80/71.1
Ethiopia	49/40.7	51/41.7
Ghana	56/49.2	58/50.3
Haiti	53/43.5	56/44.1
India	61/53.3	63/53.6
Indonesia	65/57.4	68/58.9
Jordan	69/59.7	73/62.3
Malaysia	69/61.6	74/64.8
Nepal	61/52.5	61/51.1
Niger	42/35.8	41/35.2
Nigeria	45/41.3	46/41.8
Pakistan	62/54.2	63/52.3
Peru	69/59.6	73/62.4
Philippines	65/57.1	72/61.5
Singapore	77/68.8	82/71.3
Sri Lanka	68/59.2	75/64.0
Turkey	69/61.2	73/62.8
United States of America	75/67.2	80/71.3
Vietnam	69/59.8	74/62.9

Source: Data from WHO. Core Health Indicators. Available at: http://www3.who.int/whosis/core/core_select_process.cfm. Accessed September 24, 2006.

based on values that have been established for the severity of different disabling conditions. The calculation of a DALY "discounts" losses so that losses from ill health, disability, and death in the future are worth less than losses that occur today, just as a dollar you get in the future will be worth less than one you would get today.[9, 32–34] This is why the DALY is referred to as a "present value."

For calculating DALYs, health conditions are generally broken down into three categories:[35]

Group 1—communicable, maternal, and perinatal conditions, (meaning in the first week after birth), and nutritional disorders

Group 2—non-communicable diseases

Group 3—injuries, including, among other things, road traffic accidents, falls, self-inflicted injuries, and violence

To get a better sense of the meaning of DALYs, it will be valuable to construct a few simple examples of what goes into their calculation and how they would be used. Consider, for example, that a male can expect under the standard used to live to be 80 years old. Now let us suppose that this person dies of a heart attack at 40 years of age. That person would have lost 40 years of life. The value of this loss, discounted to the present, would be part of the calculation of DALYs.

Let us also imagine that a woman, who is 40 years of age, has diabetes that has disabled her in a number of ways. In principle, she should live to the standard used of 82.5 years of age. In practice, however, the person's disability is so severe that her quality of life is equal to only about half of what it would be if she were in a "disease free" state. Even if she were to live to be 80 years of age, therefore, she would have lost about half of the quality of her last 42.5 years due to disability. The value of this loss, discounted to the present, would also be part of the calculation of DALYs.

The DALYs for the society in which the two people are living would be a composite of the data calculated from the losses due to the premature death of the first person and the disability of the second.

In reality, of course, many health conditions produce both disability and premature death. Let us suppose that a man gets TB at 45 years of age. In the absence of treatment, let us say that he dies at 47 years of age. He suffered two years of disability and lost 33 years of life due to his illness, compared to the standard used for longevity. A person who suffers a severe road traffic injury at age 50 may live, let us say, 10 years with severe disability due to his injuries and then at age 60 die due to those injuries. He would have lost quality of life years during the period of his disability and 20 years of life from premature death, compared to the standard against which DALYs are calculated.

A society that has more premature death, illness, and disability has more DALYs than a society that is healthier and has less illness, disability, and premature death. One of the goals of health policy is to avert these DALYS in the most cost-efficient manner possible. If, for example, a society is losing many hundreds of thousands of DALYs due to malaria that is not diagnosed and treated in a timely and proper manner, what steps can be taken to avert those DALYs at the lowest cost?

An important point to remember when considering DALYs, compared to measuring deaths, is that DALYs take account of periods in which people are living in ill health or with disability. By doing this, DALYs and other composite indicators try to give a better estimate than measuring deaths alone of the true "health" of a population. This is easy to understand. Most mental health problems, for example, are not associated with deaths. However, they cause an enormous amount of disability. Several parasitic infections, such as schistosomiasis, also cause very few deaths, but enormous amounts of illness and disability. If we measured the health of a population with an important burden of schistosomiasis and mental illness only by measuring deaths, we would miss a major component of morbidity and disability and would seriously overestimate the health of that population. The next section on the global burden of disease will make the concept of DALYs clearer to you, especially as you see how DALYs compare to deaths for a number of health conditions. Other sections of the book will also make extensive use of the concept of DALYs.

Indeed, calculating DALYs requires information on disease prevalence and incidence that is not always available. In addition, the health expectancy measures are more widely used in developed countries, given the health information available to them. A number of critiques of DALYs have been written.[36] Nonetheless, this book will repeatedly refer to DALYs because this measure is so extensively used in global health work. In addition, a considerable amount of important analysis has been carried out that is based on the use of DALYs for measuring overall health status and assessing the most cost-effective approaches to dealing with various health problems.

THE GLOBAL BURDEN OF DISEASE

Overview

As you start a review of global health, it is important to get a clear picture of the leading causes of illness, disability, and death in the world. As noted earlier, it is also very important to understand how they vary by age, sex, ethnicity, and socioeconomic status, both within and across countries. It is also essential to understand how these causes have varied over time and how they might change in the future. These topics are examined briefly below and in much greater detail throughout the book.

Table 2-3 shows the 10 leading causes of death and the 10 leading causes of DALYs lost for low- and middle-income countries and for high-income countries. Both deaths and DALYs are ranked in order of importance.

The table indicates that the leading causes of death in low- and middle-income countries are non-communicable diseases, which account for about 54% of all deaths. This is followed by communicable diseases at about 36% of all deaths and then injuries at about 10% of all deaths.[37]

In order of rank, heart attacks and strokes are the two leading causes of death in low- and middle-income countries. However, all but one of the next leading causes of death in these countries is communicable. The third leading cause of death is lower respiratory conditions, related to pneumonia, often in children. The fourth leading cause is HIV/AIDS. The next are perinatal conditions, linked with the death of newborns. TB, diarrheal disease, and malaria are also major killers.

TABLE 2-3 The 10 Leading Causes of Death and DALYs, 2001

Low- and middle-income countries		High-income countries	
Cause	Percentage of total deaths	Cause	Percentage of total deaths
1. Ischemic heart disease	11.8	1. Ischemic heart disease	17.3
2. Cerebrovascular disease	9.5	2. Cerebrovascular disease	9.9
3. Lower respiratory infections	7.0	3. Trachea, bronchus, and lung cancers	5.8
4. HIV/AIDS	5.3	4. Lower respiratory infections	4.4
5. Perinatal conditions	5.1	5. Chronic obstructive pulmonary disease	3.8
6. Chronic obstructive pulmonary disease	4.9	6. Colon and rectal cancers	3.3
7. Diarrheal diseases	3.7	7. Alzheimer's and other dementias	2.6
8. Tuberculosis	3.3	8. Diabetes mellitus	2.6
9. Malaria	2.5	9. Breast cancer	2.0
10. Road traffic accidents	2.2	10. Stomach cancer	1.9
Cause	Percentage of total DALYs	Cause	Percentage of total DALYs
1. Perinatal conditions	6.4	1. Ischemic heart disease	8.3
2. Lower respiratory infections	6.0	2. Cerebrovascular disease	6.3
3. Ischemic heart disease	5.2	3. Unipolar depressive disorders	5.6
4. HIV/AIDS	5.1	4. Alzheimer's and other dementias	5.0
5. Cerebrovascular disease	4.5	5. Trachea, bronchus, and lung cancers	3.6
6. Diarrheal Diseases	4.2	6. Hearing loss, adult onset	3.6
7. Unipolar depressive disorders	3.1	7. Chronic obstructive pulmonary disease	3.5
8. Malaria	2.9	8. Diabetes mellitus	2.8
9. Tuberculosis	2.6	9. Alcohol use disorders	2.8
10. Chronic obstructive pulmonary disease	2.4	10. Osteoarthritis	2.5

Source: Adapted with permission from The World Bank, Lopez AD, Mathers CD, Murray CJL. The burden of disease and mortality by condition: data, methods, and results for 2001. In: Lopez AD, Mathers CD, Ezzati M, Jamison DT, Murray CJL, eds. *Global Burden of Disease and Risk Factors.* New York: Oxford University Press; 2006.

Road traffic accidents are the 10th leading cause of death in low- and middle-income countries.[35]

Non-communicable diseases are also the leading causes of deaths in high-income countries. However, in other respects, the picture of deaths that emerges in high-income countries is quite different from that in low- and middle-income countries. In high-income countries almost 87% of the deaths are from non-communicable causes, 7.5% are from injuries, and only 5.7% are from communicable causes. In high-income countries, the first three leading causes of death are heart disease, stroke, and lung cancers. The fourth, and the only communicable cause among the leading causes of death, is lower respiratory infections, which is associated in high-income countries mostly with death from pneumonia of older people. Colon and rectal cancers are the fifth leading cause of death and diabetes is the sixth.[35]

If we look at DALYs, rather than deaths, for low- and middle-income countries, communicable diseases and injuries become slightly more important and non-communicable diseases somewhat less important in percentage terms than they were for deaths. In terms of individual conditions, diarrheal disease, malaria, and perinatal conditions become more important percentages than they were for deaths. However, the most significant difference is for unipolar depressive disorders (depression), which were not in the 10 leading causes of death, but which are in the 10 leading causes of DALYs. This stems from the fact that this mental illness is not associated with many deaths but is associated with an exceptional amount of disability in almost all countries. In fact, when we look at DALYs compared to deaths for high-income countries, the relative shares of DALYs by cause group is generally not very different than it is for deaths. However, for high-income countries, as well as low- and middle-income countries, unipolar depressive disorders become very important, as do Alzheimer's disease and other dementias.

Causes of Death by Region

As you would expect, the burden of disease varies by region, as shown in Table 2-4. In general, the higher the level of income within the region, the more likely it is that the leading causes of the burden of disease will be non-communicable. The lower the level of income, the more likely it is that the leading causes of the burden of disease will be communicable. What is most important to note is the remarkable extent to which the burden of disease in the Africa region remains dominated by communicable diseases. The relative impor-

TABLE 2-4 The Ten Leading Causes of the Burden of Disease in Low- and Middle-Income Countries by Region, 2001

East Asia and Pacific	Percentage of total DALYs	Europe and Central Asia	Percentage of total DALYs
1. Cerebrovascular disease	7.5	1. Ischemic heart disease	15.9
2. Perinatal conditions	5.4	2. Cerebrovascular disease	10.8
3. Chronic obstructive pulmonary disease	5.0	3. Unipolar depressive disorders	3.7
4. Ischemic heart disease	4.1	4. Self-inflicted injuries	2.3
5. Unipolar depressive disorders	4.1	5. Hearing loss, adult onset	2.2
6. Tuberculosis	3.1	6. Chronic obstructive pulmonary disease	2.0
7. Lower respiratory infections	3.1	7. Trachea, bronchus, and lung cancers	2.0
8. Road traffic accidents	3.0	8. Osteoarthritis	2.0
9. Cataracts	2.8	9. Road traffic accidents	1.9
10. Diarrheal diseases	2.5	10. Poisonings	1.9
Latin America and the Caribbean	**Percentage of total DALYs**	**Middle East and North Africa**	**Percentage of total DALYs**
1. Perinatal conditions	6.0	1. Ischemic heart disease	6.6
2. Unipolar depressive disorders	5.0	2. Perinatal conditions	6.3
3. Violence	4.9	3. Road traffic accidents	4.6
4. Ischemic heart disease	4.2	4. Lower respiratory infections	4.5
5. Cerebrovascular disease	3.8	5. Diarrheal diseases	3.9
6. Endocrine disorders	3.0	6. Unipolar depressive disorders	3.1
7. Lower respiratory infections	2.9	7. Congenital anomalies	3.1
8. Alcohol use disorders	2.8	8. Cerebrovascular disease	3.0
9. Diabetes mellitus	2.7	9. Vision disorders, age-related	2.7
10. Road traffic accidents	2.6	10. Cataracts	2.3
South Asia	**Percentage of total DALYs**	**Sub-Saharan Africa**	**Percentage of total DALYs**
1. Perinatal conditions	9.2	1. HIV/AIDS	16.5
2. Lower respiratory infections	8.4	2. Malaria	10.3
3. Ischemic heart disease	6.3	3. Lower respiratory infections	8.8
4. Diarrheal diseases	5.4	4. Diarrheal diseases	6.4
5. Unipolar depressive disorders	3.6	5. Perinatal conditions	5.8
6. Tuberculosis	3.4	6. Measles	3.9
7. Cerebrovascular disease	3.2	7. Tuberculosis	2.3
8. Cataracts	2.3	8. Road Traffic Accidents	1.8
9. Chronic obstructive pulmonary disease	2.3	9. Pertussis	1.8
10. Hearing loss, adult onset	2.0	10. Protein-energy malnutrition	1.5

Source: Adapted with permission from The World Bank, Lopez AD, Mathers CD, Murray CJL. The Burden of Disease and Mortality by Condition: Data, Methods, and Results for 2001. In: Lopez AD, Mathers CD, Ezzati M, Jamison DT, Murray CJL, eds. *Global Burden of Disease and Risk Factors.* New York: Oxford University Press 2006:91.

tance of communicable diseases in the South Asia Region also sets that region apart. Throughout the book, in fact, the relatively high burden of communicable diseases in South Asia and Sub-Saharan Africa will be highlighted.[38]

Causes of Death by Age

Tables 2-5 and 2-6 show the leading causes of death by age group for both low- and middle-income countries and high-income countries.

It is clear from Table 2-5 that children in low- and middle-income countries die overwhelmingly of communicable diseases that are no longer problems in the more developed countries. You can also see that HIV/AIDS and TB are among the leading causes of death in low- and middle-income countries among adults, while no communicable disease is among the 10 leading causes of death in the high-income countries.

TABLE 2-5 [1]The Ten Leading Causes of Death in Children Ages 0–14, by Broad Income Group, 2001

Low- and middle-income countries		High-income countries	
Cause	Percentage of total deaths	Cause	Percentage of total deaths
Perinatal conditions	20.7	Perinatal conditions	33.9
Lower respiratory infections	17.0	Congenital anomalies	20.0
Diarrheal diseases	13.4	Road traffic accidents	5.9
Malaria	9.2	Lower respiratory infections	2.5
Measles	6.2	Endocrine disorders	2.4
HIV/AIDS	3.7	Drownings	2.4
Congenital anomalies	3.7	Leukemia	1.9
Whooping cough	2.5	Violence	1.8
Tetanus	1.9	Fires	1.2
Road traffic accidents	1.5	Meningitis	1.2

Source: Adapted with permission from The World Bank, Lopez A, Begg S, Bos E. Demographic and Epidemiological Characteristics of Major Regions, 1990–2001. In: Lopez A, Mathers C, Ezzati M, Jamison D, Murray C, eds. *Global Burden of Disease and Risk Factors.* New York: Oxford University Press; 2006:70.

TABLE 2-6 The Ten Leading Causes of Death in Adults 15–59, by Broad Income Group, 2001

Low- and middle-income countries		High-income countries	
Cause	Percentage of total deaths	Cause	Percentage of total deaths
HIV/AIDS	14.1	Ischemic heart disease	10.8
Ischemic heart disease	8.1	Self-inflicted injuries	7.2
Tuberculosis	7.1	Road traffic accidents	6.9
Road traffic accidents	5.0	Trachea, bronchus, and lung cancers	6.8
Cerebrovascular disease	4.9	Cerebrovascular disease	4.4
Self-inflicted injuries	4.0	Cirrhosis of the liver	4.4
Violence	3.1	Breast cancer	4.0
Lower respiratory infections	2.3	Colon and rectal cancers	3.1
Cirrhosis of the liver	2.2	Diabetes mellitus	2.1
Chronic obstructive pulmonary disease	2.2	Stomach cancer	2.0

Source: Adapted with permission from The World Bank, Lopez A, Begg S, Bos E. Demographic and Epidemiological Characteristics of Major Regions, 1990–2001. In: Lopez A, Mathers C, Ezzati M, Jamison D, Murray C, eds. *Global Burden of Disease and Risk Factors.* New York: Oxford University Press; 2006:70.

Causes of Death by Gender

It is also important to examine deaths by gender. Table 2-7 shows deaths by gender for low- and middle-income countries.

For this group of countries, the causes of death among men and women are largely alike. However, it is important to note that, even in these countries, heart disease and stroke are the leading causes of death among both genders, that men die much more than women of road traffic accidents, and that diabetes has become the 10th leading cause of death among women.

Trends

Between 1960 and 2002, life expectancy at birth for the world as a whole increased from 50 to 67. In addition, as shown in Table 2-8 below, life expectancy at birth declined in Sub-Saharan Africa and stayed the same in Europe and Central Asia. The rise in life expectancy in most regions has been associated with overall economic development and some important improvements in the health of children, partly as a result of better coverage of health interventions for

TABLE 2-7 The Ten Leading Causes of Death Ordered by Sex, in Low- and Middle-Income Countries, 2001

Males		Females	
Cause	Percentage of total deaths	Cause	Percentage of total deaths
Ischemic heart disease	11.8	Ischemic heart disease	10.8
Cerebrovascular disease	8.5	Cerebrovascular disease	7.2
Lower respiratory Infections	6.7	Lower respiratory Infections	6.9
Perinatal conditions	5.4	HIV/AIDS	6.8
HIV/AIDS	5.4	Chronic obstructive pulmonary disease	4.4
Chronic obstructive pulmonary disease	4.7	Perinatal conditions	4.4
Tuberculosis	4.1	Diarrheal diseases	4.0
Diarrheal diseases	3.6	Malaria	3.1
Road traffic accidents	3.1	Tuberculosis	2.1
Malaria	2.3	Diabetes mellitus	2.0

Source: Adapted with permission from The World Bank, Lopez A, Begg S, Bos E. Demographic and Epidemiological Characteristics of Major Regions, 1990–2001. In: Lopez A, Mathers C, Ezzati M, Jamison D, Murray C, eds. *Global Burden of Disease and Risk Factors.* New York: Oxford University Press; 2006:70.

TABLE 2-8 Life Expectancy, 1960–2002, by World Bank Region

World Bank Region	Life expectancy (years) 1960	1990	2002
East Asia and the Pacific	39	67	70
Europe and Central Asia		69	69
Latin America and the Caribbean	56	68	71
Middle East and North Africa	47	64	69
South Asia	44	58	63
Sub-Saharan Africa	40	50	46
High-income countries	69	76	78

Source: Data with permission from The World Bank, Jamison DT. Investing in Health. In: Jamison Dt, Breman JG, Measham AR, et al., eds. *Disease Control Priorities in Developing Countries.* New York: Oxford University Press 2006:3–36.

No data for Europe and Central Asia for 1960

children under five years. The decline in life expectancy at birth in Sub-Saharan Africa from 1990 to 2002 is attributable to the spread of HIV/AIDS. The lack of improvement in life expectancy at birth in Europe and Central Asia is largely attributed to the social issues that arose in the former Soviet Union, including alcoholism, which has led to an increase in adult mortality, especially among men. These points are discussed in greater detail later.[38]

As we look forward, we can forecast that communicable diseases will continue to be very important to the burden of disease in South Asia and Sub-Saharan Africa. However, barring the advent of a new or emerging infectious disease, the exceptional worsening of the HIV/AIDS pandemic, or a continuing long-run failure of Sub-Saharan Africa to grow economically, the non-communicable diseases will become increasingly important everywhere.

The Burden of Deaths and Disease within Countries

As you consider causes of death and the burden of disease globally and by region, age, and sex, it is also important to consider how deaths and DALYs would vary within countries, by gender, ethnicity, and socioeconomic status. In most low- and middle-income countries, the answer to this is relatively simple:

- Rural people will be less healthy than urban people
- Disadvantaged ethnic minorities will be less healthy than majority populations
- Women will suffer a number of conditions that relate to their relatively weak social positions
- Poor people will be less healthy than better-off people
- Uneducated people will be less healthy than better educated people

In addition, people of lower socioeconomic status will have higher rates of communicable diseases, illness, and death related to maternal causes and malnutrition than will people of higher status. Lower socioeconomic status people will also suffer from a larger burden of disease related to smoking, alcohol, and diet than would be the case for better-off people. These points are fundamental to understanding global health and will also be highlighted throughout the book.

RISK FACTORS

As we discuss the determinants of health and how health status is measured, there will be many references to risk factors for various health conditions. A **risk factor** is "an aspect of personal behavior or life-style, an environmental exposure, or an inborn or inherited characteristic, that, on the basis of epidemiologic evidence, is known to be associated with health-related condition(s) considered important to prevent."[39] Risks that relate to health can also be thought of as "a probability of an adverse outcome, or a factor that raises this probability."[40] We are all familiar with the notion of risk factors from our own lives and from encounters with health services. When we answer questions about our health history, for example, we are essentially helping to identify the most important risk factors that we face ourselves. Do our parents suffer from any health conditions that might affect our own health? Are we eating in a way that is conducive to good health? Do we get enough exercise and enough sleep? Do we smoke or drink alcohol excessively? Are there any special stresses in our life? Do we wear seat belts when we drive?

If we extend the idea of risk factors to poor people in low- and middle-income countries, then we might add some other questions that relate more to the ways that they live. Does the family have safe water to drink? Do their house and community have appropriate sanitation? Does the family cook indoors in a way that makes the house smoky? Do the father and mother work in places that are safe environmentally? We might also have to ask if there is war or conflict in the country, because they are also important risk factors for illness, death, and disability.

If we are to understand how the health status of people can be enhanced, particularly poor people in low- and middle-income countries, than it is very important that we understand the risk factors to which their health problems relate. Table 2-9 shows the relative importance of different risk factors to deaths and DALYs in low- and middle-income countries, compared to high-income countries. These are shown in the table in order of their importance by category of risk.

When we consider low- and middle-income countries, the most striking factor is the extent to which malnutrition is a risk factor. Another important point is the extent to which other nutrition related risk factors are important for deaths and DALYs, such as high blood pressure and high cholesterol. Deaths and DALYs attributable to the risks of smoking and unsafe sex make up the other most significant risk factors in low- and middle-income countries.[41]

In high-income countries, there is little undernutrition but a considerable amount of overweight and obesity. It is not surprising, therefore, that three of the most important risk factors for both deaths and DALYs in high-income countries are high blood pressure, high cholesterol, and overweight and obesity. Nor is it surprising that, despite

TABLE 2-9 The Leading Risk Factors for the Burden of Disease, 2001, Low- and Middle-Income and High-Income Countries, Ranked in Order of Percent

Low- and Middle-Income Countries		High-Income Countries	
Deaths	**DALYs**	**Deaths**	**DALYs**
High blood pressure (12.9)	Childhood underweight (8.7)	Smoking (12.7)	Smoking (12.7)
Childhood underweight (7.5)	Unsafe sex (5.8)	High blood pressure (17.6)	High blood pressure (9.3)
Smoking (6.9)	High blood pressure (5.6)	High cholesterol (10.7)	Overweight and obesity (7.2)
High cholesterol (6.3)	Smoking (3.9)	Overweight and obesity (7.8)	High cholesterol (6.3)
Unsafe sex (5.8)	Unsafe water, sanitation, and hygiene (3.7)	Physical inactivity (4.8)	Alcohol use (4.4)
Low fruit and vegetable intake (4.8)	Alcohol use (3.6)	Low fruit and vegetable intake (4.2)	Physical inactivity (3.2)
Alcohol use (3.9)	High cholesterol (3.1)	Urban air pollution (1.0)	Low fruit and vegetable intake (2.7)
Indoor smoke from household use of solid fuels (3.7)	Indoor smoke from household use of solid fuels (3.0)	Illicit drug use (0.5)	Unsafe sex (0.6)
Overweight and obesity (3.6)	Low fruit and vegetable intake (2.4)	Unsafe sex (0.4)	Iron-deficiency anemia (0.5)
Unsafe water, sanitation, and hygiene (3.2)	Overweight and obesity (2.3)	Alcohol use (0.3)	Child sexual abuse (0.5)

Source: Data with permission from The World Bank, Lopez AD, Mathers CD, Ezzati M, Jamison DT, Murray CJ, eds. *Global Burden of Disease and Risk Factors*, 1990–2001. New York: Oxford University Press; 2006:10.

important progress in reducing the prevalence of smoking in some countries, tobacco remains the leading risk factor for both deaths and DALYs in high-income countries.[41]

THE DEMOGRAPHIC AND EPIDEMIOLOGICAL TRANSITIONS

The previous discussion has already suggested several very important trends that occur in total fertility, which is the number of children born alive to a woman over her lifetime,[42] in mortality, and in patterns of disease. The first trend is a change over time from patterns of high fertility and high mortality to a pattern of low fertility and low mortality. This is called the **demographic transition**. The second, and closely related, trend that occurs is called the **epidemiological transition**, and refers to the changing pattern of disease, from a burden of disease profile that is dominated primarily by communicable diseases to one that is dominated primarily by non-communicable diseases. Both of these important transitions are discussed further below.

Demographic Transition[43]

When we look back historically at the countries that are now high-income, we can see that they had long periods historically when fertility was high, mortality was high, and population growth was, therefore, relatively slow, or which might even have declined in the face of epidemics. Beginning around the turn of the nineteenth century, however, mortality in those countries began to decline as hygiene and nutrition improved and the burden of infectious diseases became less. In most cases, this decline in mortality went before much decline in fertility. As mortality declined, the population increased and the share of the population that was of younger ages also increased. Later, fertility began to decline and, as births and deaths became more equal, population growth slowed. As births and deaths stayed more equal, the share of the population that was of older ages increased.

The demographic transition is shown graphically in Figure 2-7.

The first population pyramid reflects a country with high fertility and high mortality. The second population pyramid is indicative of a country in which mortality has begun to decline but fertility remains high. This would be similar to the demographics one would find, for example, in a number of countries in Sub-Saharan Africa that are undergoing demographic transition. The third pyramid looks more like a cylinder than a pyramid. This reflects a population in which fertility has been reduced and in which there is a larger share of older people in the population than in the first and second pyramids. This would be similar to the demographics that one would find in a number of low fertility, aging populations in Western Europe.

The Epidemiologic Transition[44]

The epidemiologic transition is closely related to the demographic transition, as suggested throughout the previous discussion. Historically there has been a shift in the patterns of disease that follows the trends noted below:

- First, high and fluctuating mortality, related to very poor health conditions, epidemics, and famine
- Then, progressive declines in mortality, as epidemics become less frequent
- Finally, further declines in mortality, increases in life expectancy, and the predominance of non-communicable diseases

Figure 2-8 shows examples of two sets of countries. The first has a burden of disease profile that is pretransition. The second is of a developed country that has completed its epidemiological transition.

You can see in Figure 2-8 how the pattern of disease differs between the two types of countries. You can also see the changes that will occur over time, as the low-income country develops and the burden of disease moves from one that is predominantly communicable diseases to one that is predominantly non-communicable diseases.

The pace of the epidemiological transition in different societies depends on a number of factors related to the "determinants of health" that were discussed earlier. In its early stages, the transition appears to depend primarily on improvements in hygiene, nutrition, education, and socioeconomic status. Some improvements also stem from advances in public health and in medicine, such as the development of new vaccines and antibiotics.[45] Most of the countries that are now high-income went through epidemiologic transitions that were relatively slow, with the exception of Japan. Most

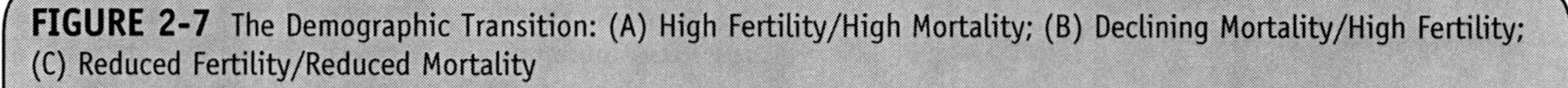
FIGURE 2-7 The Demographic Transition: (A) High Fertility/High Mortality; (B) Declining Mortality/High Fertility; (C) Reduced Fertility/Reduced Mortality

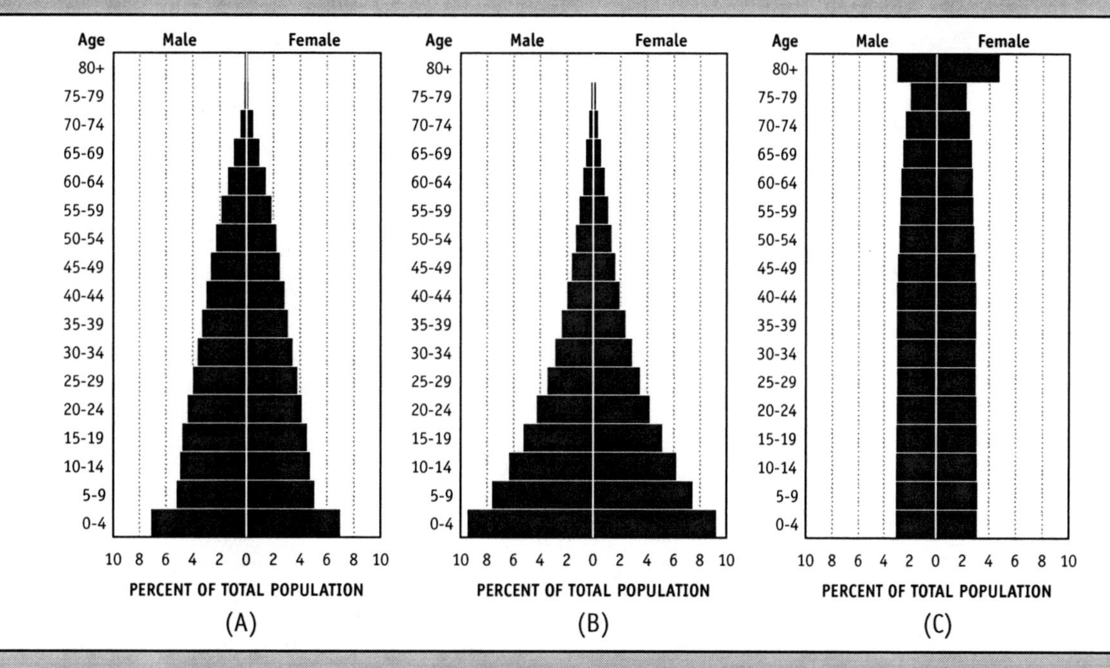

Source: Reprinted from U.S. Census Bureau. International population reports WP/02. *Global Population Profile: 2002.* Washington, DC: U.S. Government Printing Office; 2004:35.

FIGURE 2-8 The Burden of Disease by Group of Cause, Percent of Deaths, 2001

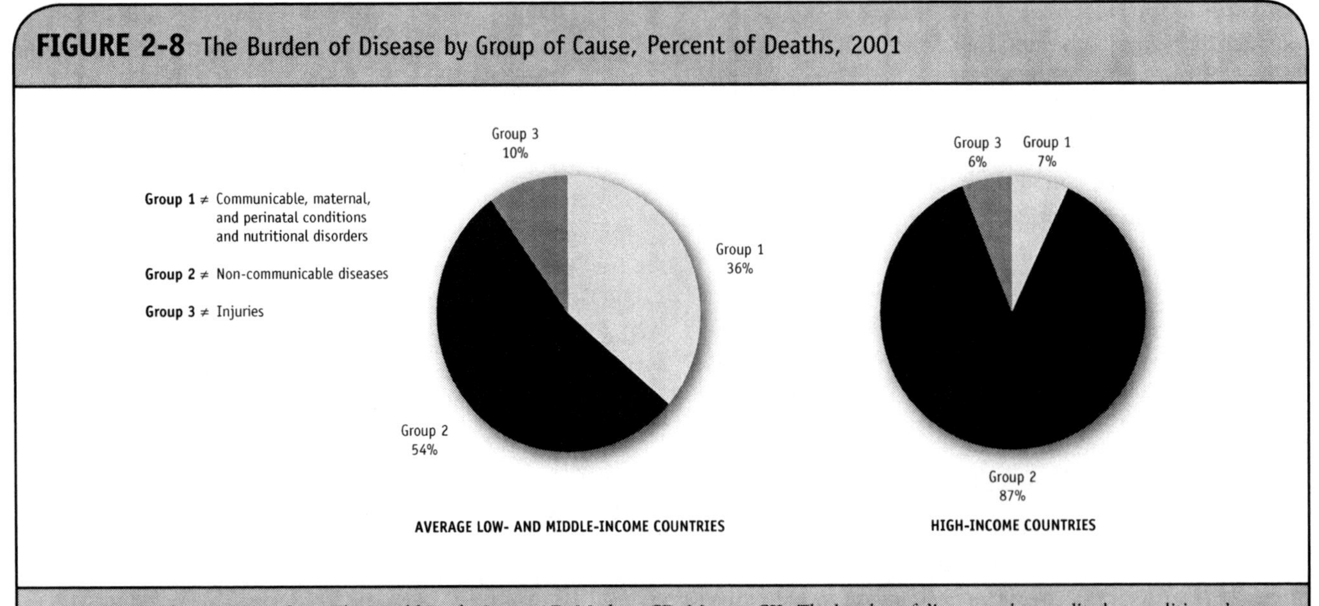

Source: Data with permission from The World Bank, Lopez AD, Mathers CD, Murray CJL. The burden of disease and mortality by condition: data, methods, and results for 2001. In: Lopez AD, Mathers CD, Ezzati M, Jamison DT, Murray CJL, eds. *Global Burden of Disease and Risk Factors.* New York: Oxford University Press; 2006.

developing countries have already begun their transition. However, it is still far from complete in most of them.

Implications of the Demographic and Epidemiological Transitions

There are several especially important points about these transitions that one must keep in mind.

- The large share of the population that is younger in relatively poor societies with high fertility has an enormous implication for the funds that countries must spend on education, health, and some other key investments.
- As countries age, they face pressure to fund the health of their older population, who tend to suffer from non-communicable diseases. They also face pressure on the funding of pension schemes for their older workers, because there is a large share of workers who have retired but a relatively smaller share of young people who pay taxes into the pension fund. This is now the case, for example, in much of Western Europe.
- Most low-income countries are in an ongoing epidemiologic transition and many of them, therefore, face significant burdens of communicable and non-communicable diseases, and injuries at the same time. This strains the capacity of the health system of many of these countries. It is also expensive for countries that are resource poor to address a substantial burden of all three of these types of diseases simultaneously.

In fact, the demographic and epidemiological transitions have many important implications for public policy, some of which were noted earlier. From the point of view of this text, however, one especially important question that policy makers in low-income countries face concerning these transitions is: "How can public policy help to speed the demographic and epidemiological transitions in our country at lowest possible cost, in a manner consistent with the social values of the country?"

Figure 2-9 shows national income of a sample of countries, plotted against life expectancy at birth for females in those countries.

From this figure, one can see that, generally, the health of a country does increase as national income rises. However, one can also see that there are some countries, such as China, Costa Rica, Cuba, and Sri Lanka, that have achieved higher average life expectancies at birth than one would have predicted for countries at their level of income.

To a large extent, countries like those above achieved these important health gains as a result of:

- Focusing on investing in nutrition, health, and education, particularly of their poor people
- Improving people's knowledge of good hygiene
- Making selected investments in health services that at

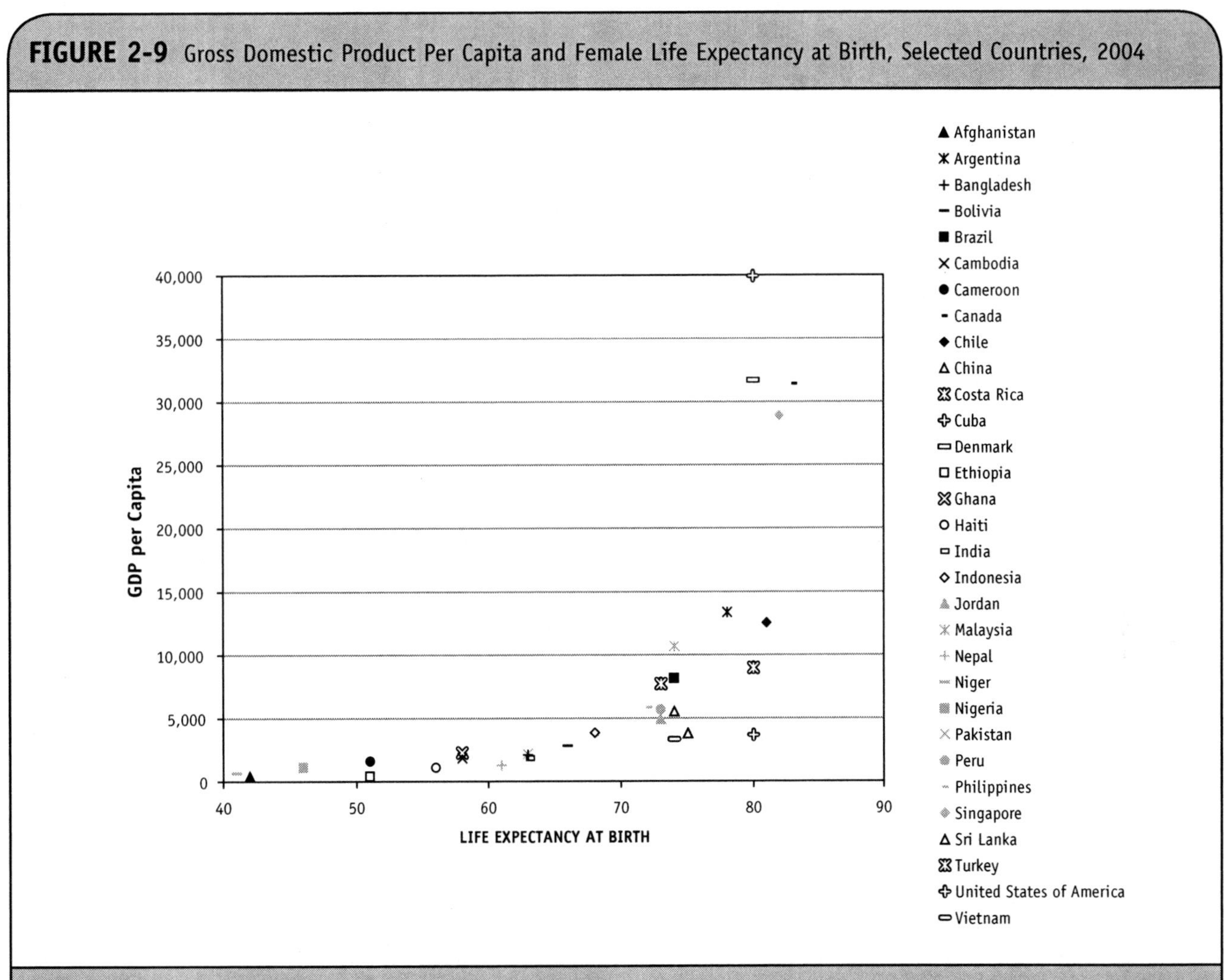

FIGURE 2-9 Gross Domestic Product Per Capita and Female Life Expectancy at Birth, Selected Countries, 2004

Source: Data from WHO. Core Health Indicators. Available at: http://www3.who.int/whosis/core/core_select_process.cfm. Accessed September 24, 2006.

low cost could have a high impact on health status, such as vaccination programs for children and TB control

These themes will also be discussed throughout this book.

Indeed, in the long run, economic progress *will* help to bring down fertility, reduce mortality from communicable diseases, and help to produce a healthier population. However, at the present rates of progress in improving health in most low-income countries, these changes will take a very long time to occur. One great public policy challenge for these countries and their governments, therefore, is how they can "short-circuit" this process and reach reduced levels of fertility, lower mortality, and better health for their people, even as they remain relatively poor.

CASE STUDY

The State of Kerala

Having begun to review health status and how countries can speed improvements in health, it will be valuable to end this chapter by examining a well-known case of a place that improved health status considerably, even at relatively low levels of income. One of the best known of such success stories concerns Kerala State in India.

Introduction

Kerala is a coastal state in Southwestern India with a population of more than 31 million people.[46] Despite having only slow rates of economic growth and a state per capita income lower than that of many other states in India, the health indicators for Kerala are the best in India and rival those in developed countries. What approach did Kerala take historically to produce such high levels of health, even in the face of relatively low income? What factors contributed to improvements in health status? What lessons does the Kerala experience suggest for other countries and for other states within India?

The Kerala Approach

One of the primary reasons why people in Kerala have such high levels of health has been the emphasis that the state put on education and the exceptionally widespread access to education in Kerala. The state introduced free primary and secondary education in the early part of 20th century.[47] In addition, Kerala has always put important emphasis on the education of females.

Kerala also made an early commitment to widespread health services for its people. The state created, for example, an extensive network of primary healthcare centers. This provided its citizens, throughout the state, with access to free basic health care and free family planning services. This was coupled with programs to promote exclusive breastfeeding and the improved nutrition of infants, children, and pregnant women. The central government supported the family planning program, the maternal and child health program, and the universal immunization program in all of India, but they were implemented far more effectively and efficiently in Kerala than in other states of India.[48]

The place of women in Kerala society also contributed to the uptake of education by females and improvements throughout Kerala in nutrition and health status. The role of women in many communities in Kerala differs from the roles ascribed to women in many other parts of India. In much of the rest of India, especially in parts of North India, women are regarded by families as liabilities rather than as assets. In most of India, this is partly represented in cultural terms by the fact that the family of a bride must pay a dowry to the family of the groom. In Kerala, however, women have been treated differently for over a century. They have been seen culturally much more as assets to families and they could inherit and own land, giving them a financial independence and power which was unrivalled among women elsewhere in India.[49]

It is also important to note that Kerala has historically been run by a government that has traditionally placed a premium on community mobilization on important social issues, such as education, greater empowerment of women, health, nutrition, and land reform. Many of these efforts were carried out in ways that raised social awareness about health and nutrition. In 1989, Kerala launched a total literacy campaign, for example, and by the start of the World Literacy Year in 1990, Ernakulam district in Kerala was declared India's first totally literate district.[50]

Given widespread education in Kerala and the place of women in society, it is not surprising that Kerala went through the demographic transition quite early and well before other places in India. Women with more education are more likely to work and marry later and thus have wider choice in economic and social pursuits. They also have a better knowledge of and easier access to family planning methods and lower fertility than do women with less education.[51]

The Impact

What were the impacts on health status of the emphasis that Kerala placed on education, health, nutrition, and the empowerment of women? Although it is not possible to scientifically indicate which policy contributed what share of better health, we can say that for many years the people of Kerala have enjoyed the best educational attainment of any group within India. In the last census, the literacy rates of people aged 7 years and above for India were about 65% on average, with about 76% for males and 54% for females. Kerala, however, had the highest literacy rate in the country, with about 91% overall and about 94% for males and 88% for females.[52] Kerala also boasts one of the highest newspaper readerships in the world, another feature that promotes the value of women, education, nutrition, and health. It also helps to raise political awareness and the demands of people for participation in and solutions to their concerns, such as education, health, and water.

Linked with this high level of education, especially of women and the promotion of nutrition and health, infant mortality in Kerala in 2001 was 14 per 1000, compared with 91 per 1000 for low-income countries generally and 68 per 1000 on average for India.[52] In India, about 2.1 million child deaths occur every year, which is the highest number within a single country worldwide.[53] The national under-five mortality rate is around 87 per 1000 live births with a wide variation between states. In Kerala, however, the mortality of children under five years is the best in India with an impressive rate of only 19 such deaths per 1000 births in 1998–1999.[54] In addition, maternal deaths in Kerala are much less common, at 87 per 100,000, than the Indian average of 407 per 100,000.[55] This partly reflects the extent to which deliveries take place in hospitals in Kerala. Indeed, Kerala's health care system garnered international acclaim when UNICEF and WHO designated it as the world's first "baby-friendly state." This was in recognition of the fact that more than 95% of Keralite births are hospital-delivered.[56]

Given these high health indicators, it is not surprising that nutritional status in Kerala is also much better than the Indian average, with 27% of the children younger than five years in Kerala being underweight, compared to the Indian average of 47%. Finally, one should note that life expectancy for men and women in Kerala is about the same at 73 years. This is closer to many developed countries like the United States, which had a life expectancy in 2004 of 78 years, than it is to life expectancy in most low- and middle-income countries.[57]

Lessons Learned

Kerala has long been cited, along with China, Costa Rica, Cuba, and Sri Lanka, as a model of a country or state within a country that has achieved high levels of education and health for its people, before achieving high levels of income. It appears that Kerala has achieved these impacts by politically supporting widespread access to education, nutrition, and health; mobilizing communities around the importance of these areas and of women's empowerment; and investing in low cost but high yielding areas of education, nutrition, and health. In a manner much like Sri Lanka, Kerala has also managed to achieve high levels of health status at relatively low cost.

Have the high levels of health and education in Kerala, however, been associated with high levels of growth of income in the state? The answer to that question is no. The annual per capita Gross Domestic Product (GDP) for the state in year 2001 was $469. This was close to the Indian average of $460. [58] It appears that the economic policies held by the state government over time in Kerala have not yielded high rates of economic growth or produced an environment in which domestic and foreign investors were prepared to work. Rather, the overall income of the state remains quite dependent on the money that workers from Kerala living abroad, especially in the Middle East, send back to their families in Kerala.[59]

What then are the messages to take away from Kerala in terms of the link between health and development? First, it is possible, even in the absence of high levels of income, to achieve high levels of health through political commitment, sound investments, and social mobilization. Second, however, in the absence of sound economic policies, the presence of a literate and healthy population alone will not be sufficient to promote rapid economic growth.

MAIN MESSAGES

To understand the most important global health issues, we must be able to understand the determinants of health, how health status is measured, and the meaning of the demographic and epidemiological transitions. There are a number of factors that influence health status. These include genetic makeup, sex, and age. Social and cultural issues and health behaviors are also closely linked to health status. The determinants of health also include education, nutritional status, and socio-economic status. The environment is also a powerful determinant of health, as is access to health services, and the policy approaches that countries take to their health sectors and to investments that could influence the health of their people.

It is also important to understand the most important risk factors that lead to ill health. In the low-income countries on which this book focuses considerable attention, some of the most important risk factors include nutritional status, the lack of safe water or appropriate sanitation, and tobacco smoking. Poor diets that relate to obesity, high blood pressure, high cholesterol, and cardiovascular disease are becoming increasingly important problems as well, even in low-income countries.

There are a number of uses of health data including measuring health status, carrying out disease surveillance, making decisions about investments in health, and assessing the performance of health programs. Those working in health use a common set of indicators to measure health status, including life expectancy, infant and neonatal mortality, under-five child mortality, and the maternal mortality ratio. They also use composite indices, such as DALYs, to measure the burden of disease.

Poorer countries have a relatively larger burden of disease from communicable diseases than from non-communicable diseases, compared to richer countries. As these poorer countries develop, fertility and mortality will decline, the population will age, and the burden of disease will shift toward the non-communicable diseases. These phenomena occur as countries go through what are referred to as the demographic transition and the epidemiological transition.

Life expectancy has improved in all regions of the world since 1990, except in Europe, Central Asia, and Sub-Saharan Africa. The leading cause of death worldwide has now become cardiovascular disease. However, communicable diseases remain relatively much more important in South Asia and Sub-Saharan Africa than in the rest of the world.

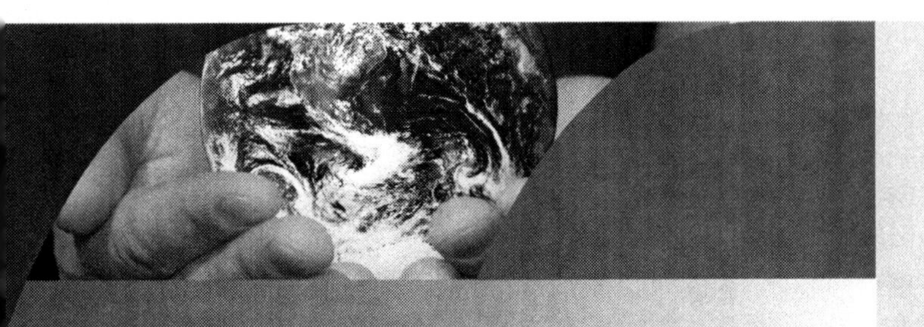

Discussion Questions

1. What are the main factors that determine your health?
2. What are the main factors that would determine the health of a poor person in a poor country?
3. If you could only pick one indicator to describe the health status of a poor country, which indicator would you use and why?
4. Why is it valuable to have composite indicators like DALYs to measure the burden of disease?
5. What is a HALE and how does it differ from just measuring life expectancy at birth?
6. As countries develop economically, what are the most important changes that occur in their burden of disease?
7. Why do these changes occur?
8. In your own country, what population groups have the best health indicators and why?
9. In your country, what population groups have the worst health status and why?
10. How would the population pyramid of Italy differ from that of Nigeria and why?

REFERENCES

1. A global emergency: a combined response *The world health report 2004 - changing history*. Geneva: World Health Organization; 2004:6.

2. Russia. Available at: http://www.prb.org/TemplateTop.cfm?Section=PRB_Country_Profiles&template=/customsource/country-profile/countryprofiledisplay.cfm&Country=470. Accessed June 29, 2006.

3. Key Development Data and Statistics. Internet Resource; Computer File Available at: http://web.worldbank.org/WBSITE/EXTERNAL/DATASTATISTICS/0,,contentMDK:20535285~menuPK:1192694~pagePK:64133150~piPK:64133175~theSitePK:239419,00.html. Accessed June 17, 2006.

4. Kozik CA, Suntayakorn S, Vaughn DW, Suntayakorn C, Snitbhan R, Innis BL. Causes of death and unintentional injury among schoolchildren in Thailand. *Southeast Asian J Trop Med Public Health*. Mar 1999;30(1):129-135.

5. Public Health Agency of Canada. Population Health Approach, What Determines Health? Available at: http://www.phac-aspc.gc.ca/ph-sp/phdd/determinants/index.html. Accessed October 6, 2005.

6. World Health Organization. WHO Issues New Healthy Life Expectancy Rankings: Japan Number One in New "Healthy Life" System. Available at: http://www.who.int/inf-pr-2000/en/pr2000-life.html. Accessed January 3, 2006.

7. Hobcraft J. Women's education, child welfare and child survival : a review of the evidence. *Health Transition Review*. 1993;3(2):159-173.

8. World Bank. *Repositioning Nutrition as Central to Development—A Strategy for Large-Scale Action*. Washington, DC: The World Bank; 2006.

9. Basch P. *Textbook of International Health*. 2nd ed. New York: Oxford University Press; 2001:73-113.

10. Haupt, A, Kane, TT, Population Handbook, Washington, DC: Population Reference Bureau. 2004.

11. Haupt, A, Kane, TT, Population Handbook, Washington, DC: Population Reference Bureau. 2004.

12. WDI Data Query. Available at: http://devdata.worldbank.org/data-query/. Accessed July 1, 2006.

13. Haupt, A, Kane, TT, Population Handbook, Washington, DC: Population Reference Bureau. 2004.

14. Zupan J. Perinatal mortality in developing countries. *N Engl J Med*. May 19 2005;352(20):2047-2048.

15. Haupt, A, Kane, TT, Population Handbook, Washington, DC: Population Reference Bureau. 2004.

16. Health Status Statistics: Mortality. Available at: www.who.int/healthinfo/statistics/indneonatalmortality/en/. Accessed June 25, 2006.

17. Haupt, A, Kane, TT, Population Handbook, Washington, DC: Population Reference Bureau. 2004.

18. Human Development Indicators 2003. Available at: http://hdr.undp.org/reports/global/2003/indicator/indic_78_1_1.html. Accessed June 25, 2006.

19. Last JM. *A dictionary of epidemiology*. 4th ed. New York: Oxford University Press; 2001:118.

20. Haupt, A, Kane, TT, Population Handbook, Washington, DC: Population Reference Bureau. 2004.

21. Last JM. *A dictionary of epidemiology*. 4th ed. New York: Oxford University Press; 2001:51.

22. Haupt, A, Kane, TT, Population Handbook, Washington, DC: Population Reference Bureau. 2004.

23. Summary Country Profile for HIV/AIDS Treatment Scale-Up: Botswana. www.who.int/3by5/support/June 2005_bwa.pdf. Accessed June 25, 2006.

24. Haupt, A, Kane, TT, Population Handbook, Washington, DC: Population Reference Bureau. 2004.

25. Country Profile: India. Available at: http://www.stoptb.org/countries/GlobalReport2006/ind.pdf. Accessed June 25, 2006.

26. Last JM. *A dictionary of epidemiology*. 4th ed. New York: Oxford University Press; 2001:35.

27. Lopez AD, Mathers CD, Murray CJL. The Burden of Disease and Mortality by Condition: Data, Methods, and Results for 2001. In: Lopez AD, Mathers CD, Ezzati M, Jamison DT, Murray CJL, eds. *Global burden of disease and risk factors*. New York: Oxford University Press; 2006:126-129.

28. Merson MH, Black RE, Mills AJ. *International public health : diseases, programs, systems, and policies*. Gaithersburg, MD: Aspen Publishers; 2000:28.

29. Health Adjusted Life Expectancy: Statistics Canada. www.statcan.ca/ennglish/fav/hale. Accessed May 25, 2006.

30. Global Burden of Disease. www.who.int/trade/glossary/story036/en/ Accessed May 25, 2006.

31. Jamison DT, Brennan J, Measham A, et al., eds. *Priorities in Health*. New York: Oxford University Press; 2006.

32. World development report 1993. New York: Oxford University Press; 1993:25-29.

33. Lopez AD, Mathers CD, Ezzati M, Jamison DT, Murray CJL. Measuring the Global Burden of Disease and Risk Factors, 1990-2001. In: *Global burden of disease and risk factors*. New York: Oxford University Press; 2006:1-15.

34. Basch P. *Textbook of International Health*. 2nd ed. New York: Oxford University Press; 2001:108-112.

35. Lopez AD, Mathers CD, Ezzati M, Jamison DT, Murray CJL. In: Lopez AD, Mathers CD, Ezzati M, Jamison DT, Murray CJL, eds. *Global burden of disease and risk factors*. New York: Oxford University Press; 2006:8.

36. Lopez AD, Mathers CD, Ezzati M, Jamison DT, Murray CJL. Measuring the Global Burden of Disease and Risk Factors, 1990-2001. In: Lopez AD, Mathers CD, Ezzati M, Jamison DT, Murray CJL, eds. *Global burden of disease and risk factors*. New York: Oxford University Press; 2006:3.

37. Lopez AD, Mathers CD, Murray CJL. The Burden of Disease and Mortality by Condition: Data, Methods, and Results for 2001. In: Lopez AD, Mathers CD, Ezzati M, Jamison DT, Murray CJL, eds. *Global burden of disease and risk factors*. New York: Oxford University Press; 2006:228-231.

38. Lopez A, Begg S, Bos E. Demographic and Epidemiological Characteristics of Major Regions, 1990-2001. In: Lopez A, Mathers C, Ezzati M, Jamison D, Murray C, eds. *Global Burden of Disease and Risk Factors*. New York: Oxford University Press; 2006:15-44.

39. Last JM. *A dictionary of epidemiology*. 4th ed. New York: Oxford University Press; 2001:160.

40. Beaglehole R, Irwin A, Prentice T. The world health report 2004 : changing history. Internet Resource] xvii, 169 p. : ill. ; 126 cm. Available at: http://www.who.int/whr/2004/en/

Materials specified: HTML VERSION http://www.who.int/whr/2004/en/Materials specified: PDF VERSION TO DOWNLOAD http://www.who.int/whr/2004/download/en/print.html

41. Lopez AD, Mathers CD, Ezzati M, Jamison DT, Murray CJL. Measuring the Global Burden of Disease and Risk Factors, 1990-2001. In: Lopez AD, Mathers CD, Ezzati M, Jamison DT, Murray CJL, eds. *Global burden of disease and risk factors*. New York: Oxford University Press; 2006:9.

42. Last JM. *A dictionary of epidemiology*. 4th ed. New York: Oxford University Press; 2001:70.

43. Lee R. The Demographic Transition: Three Centuries of Fundamental Change, Journal of Economic Perspectives. *Journal of Economic Perspectives*. 2003;17(4):167-190.

44. Omran AR. The Epidemiologic Transition: A Theory of the Epidemiology of Population Change. *The Milbank Quarterly*. 2005;83(4):731.

45. Jamison DT. Investing in Health. In: Jamison DT, Breman JG, Measham AR, et al., eds. *Disease Control Priorities in Developing Countries*. New York: Oxford University Press; 2006:3-34.

46. Registrar General & Census Commissioner. *Census of India 2001, Provisional population Totals*. New Delhi: Government of India, New Delhi; 2001.

47. Black JA. Kerala's demographic transition: determinants and consequences. *Bmj.* Jun 26 1999;318(7200):1771.

48. Zachariah K. *The Anomaly of the Fertility Decline in India's Kerala State.* Washington DC 1984.

49. Black JA. Family Planning and Kerala. *National Medical Journal of Kerala.* 1989;3:187-197.

50. Tharakan P, Navaneetham K. *Population Projection and Policy Implications for Education: A Discussion with Reference to Kerala*: Centre for Development Studies (Thiruvananthapuram) 1999.

51. Ratcliffe J. Social justice and the demographic transition: lessons from India's Kerala State. *International Journal of Health Services.* 1978;8(1):123-144.

52. United Nations Development Programme. Kerala—Human Development Fact Sheet. Available at: http://www.undp.org.in/programme/undpini/factsheet/kerala.pdf. Accessed July 21, 2006.

53. UNICEF. *State of the World's Children.* New York: Oxford University Press; 2004.

54. International Institute for Population Sciences and OrcMacro. *National Family Health Survey (NFHS-2) 1998-1999.* Mumbai: International Institute for Population Sciences and OrcMacro; 2000.

55. United Nations Economic and Social Commission for Asia and the Pacific. India: National Population Policy. Available at: http://www.unescap.org/esid/psis/population/database/poplaws/law_india/indiaappend3.htm. Accessed July 21, 2006.

56. Kutty VR. Historical analysis of the development of health care facilities in Kerala State, India. *Health Policy Plan.* Mar 2000;15(1):103-109.

57. Centers for Disease Control and Prevention. Life Expectancy. Available at: http://www.cdc.gov/nchs/fastats/lifexpec.htm. Accessed January 3, 2007.

58. Tsai KS. Debating Decentralized Development: A Reconsideration of the Wenzhou and Kerala Models. *India Journal of Economics & Business, Special Issue China & India*; 2006.

59. Joseph K. *Migration and Economic Development of Kerala.* New Delhi: Mittal Publications; 1988.

CHAPTER 3

Evidence-based Public Health

LEARNING OBJECTIVES

By the end of this chapter the student will be able to:

- explain the steps in the evidence-based public health process.
- describe a public health problem in terms of morbidity and mortality.
- describe the approach used in public health to identify a contributory cause of a disease or other condition and establish the efficacy of an intervention.
- describe the process of grading evidence-based recommendations.
- use an approach to identify options for intervention based on "when, who, and how."
- explain the role that evaluation plays in establishing effectiveness as part of evidence-based public health.

Tobacco was introduced to Europe as a new world crop in the early 1600s. Despite the availability of pipe tobacco and later, cigars, the mass production and consumption of tobacco through cigarette smoking did not begin until the development of the cigarette rolling machine by James Duke in the 1880s. This invention allowed mass production and distribution of cigarettes for the first time. Men were the first mass consumers of cigarettes. During World War I, cigarettes were widely distributed free of charge to American soldiers.

Cigarette smoking first became popular among women in the 1920s—an era noted for changes in the role and attitudes of women—and at this time advertising of cigarettes began to focus on women. The mass consumption of cigarettes by women, however, trailed that of men by at least two decades. By the 1950s, over 50 percent of adult males and approximately 25 percent of adult females were regular cigarette smokers.

The health problems of cigarette smoking were not fully recognized until decades after the habit became widespread. As late as the 1940s, R.J. Reynolds advertised that "more doctors smoke Camels than any other cigarette."

Epidemiologists observed that lung cancer deaths were increasing in frequency in the 1930s and 1940s. The increase in cases did not appear to be due to changes in efforts to recognize the disease, ability to recognize the disease, or the definition of the disease. Even after the increasing average life span and aging of the population was taken into account, it was evident that the rate of death from lung cancer was increasing—and more rapidly for men than women. In addition, it was noted that residents of states with higher rates of smoking had higher rates of lung cancer. In the 1950s, the number of lung cancer deaths in females also began to increase and by the 1960s, the disease had become the most common cause of cancer-related deaths in males and was still rising among women.[1,2]

This type of information was the basis for describing the problems of cigarette smoking and lung cancer and developing ideas or hypotheses about its etiology, or cause. Let us take a look at how the evidence-based public health approach has been used to address the problem of cigarette smoking. There are four basic questions that we need to ask that together make up what we will call the evidence-based public health approach.[3]

1. Problem: What is the health problem?
2. Etiology: What is/are the contributory cause(s)?
3. Recommendations: What works to reduce the health impacts?
4. Implementation: How can we get the job done?

These four questions provide a framework for defining, analyzing, and addressing a wide range of public health issues and can be applied to cigarette smoking for the purposes of this chapter.[4] We will call this framework the **P.E.R.I. process**. This process is really circular as illustrated in Figure 3-1. If the evaluation suggests that more needs to be done, the cycle can and should be repeated. Thus, it is an ongoing process.

Using cigarette smoking as an example, we will illustrate the steps needed to apply the evidence-based public health approach.

HOW CAN WE DESCRIBE A HEALTH PROBLEM?

The first step in addressing a health problem is to describe its impact. That is, we need to begin by understanding the occurrence of disability and death due to a disease, which we call the **burden of disease**. In public heath, disability is often called **morbidity** and death is called **mortality**. We also need to determine whether there has been a recent change in the impact of the disease. Thus, the first question we ask in describing a health problem is: what is the burden of disease in terms of morbidity and mortality and has it changed over time?

The second question we need to ask is: are there differences in the distribution of disease and can these differences generate ideas or hypotheses about the disease's etiology (cause)? That is, we need to examine how the disease is spread out or distributed in a population. We call this the **distribution of disease**. Public health professionals called **epidemiologists** investigate factors known as "person" and "place" to see if they can find patterns or associations in the frequency of a disease. We call these **group associations**. Group associations may suggest ideas or hypotheses about the cause, or etiology of a disease.

FIGURE 3-1 Evidence-based public health: The P.E.R.I. approach

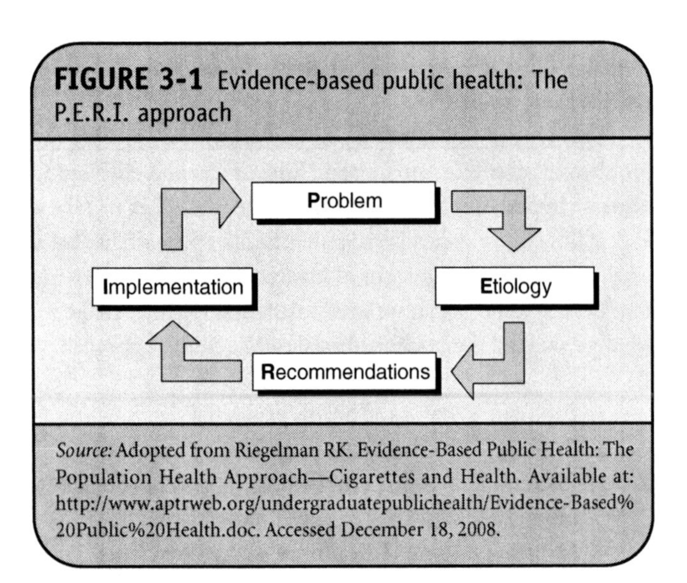

Source: Adopted from Riegelman RK. Evidence-Based Public Health: The Population Health Approach—Cigarettes and Health. Available at: http://www.aptrweb.org/undergraduatepublichealth/Evidence-Based%20Public%20Health.doc. Accessed December 18, 2008.

"Person" includes demographic characteristics which describe people, such as age, gender, race, and socioeconomic factors. It also includes behaviors or exposures, such as cigarette smoking, exercise, radiation exposure, and use of medications. "Place" implies geographic location, such as a city or state, but it also includes connections between people, such as a university community or a shared Internet site. When these types of factors occur more frequently among groups with the disease than among groups without the disease we call them **risk indicators** or **risk markers**.[a]

Finally, epidemiologists take a scientific approach to addressing public health problems. They are often skeptical of initial answers to a question and ask: could there be another explanation for the differences or changes in the distribution of disease? They often ask: are the differences or changes real or are they artifactual? **Artifactual** implies that the apparent association is actually the result of the data collection process.

When trying to determine whether an association is artifactual or real, epidemiologists ask whether, the observed changes or differences may be due to comparing apples to oranges—for example comparing groups of subjects of different average ages. Age is especially important to epidemiologists because it is very strongly related to the occurrence of disease. Thus, the third question that we need to ask in describing a problem is: are the differences or changes used to suggest group associations artifactual or real?

Before we can answer these three questions we need to understand more about the measurements that epidemiologists use to describe a health problem. We need to look carefully at how we measure the changes or differences in disease, disability, and death. In public health, we use **rates** to summarize our measurement. Let us begin by looking at what we mean by rates and then we will return to the three questions that need to be addressed when describing a health problem.

WHAT DO WE NEED TO KNOW ABOUT RATES IN ORDER TO DESCRIBE A HEALTH PROBLEM?

The term "rate" will be used to describe the types of measurements that have a numerator and a denominator where the numerator is a subset of the denominator—that is, the numerator includes only individuals who are also included in the denominator. In a rate, the numerator measures the number of times an event, such as the diagnosis of lung cancer, occurs. The denominator measures the number of times the event

[a] The term risk indicator or risk marker needs to be distinguished from the term risk factor. A risk factor is a candidate for being a contributory cause and implies that at least an association at the individual level has been established as we will discuss later in this chapter. We will also add "time" to "person" and "place" as a basic characteristic for generating hypotheses.

could occur. We often use the entire population in the denominator, but at times we may only use the **at-risk population**. For instance, when measuring the rate of cervical cancer we would only use the population of women in the denominator and when measuring rates of prostate cancer we would only use the population of men in the denominator.[b]

There are two basic types of rates that are key to describing a disease.[5, 6] These are called **incidence** rates and **prevalence**. Incidence rates measure the chances of developing a disease over a period of time—usually one year. That is, incidence rates are the number of new cases of a disease that develop during a year divided by the number of people in the at-risk population, as in the following equation:

$$\textit{Incidence rate} = \frac{\textit{\# of new cases of a disease in a year}}{\textit{\# of people in the at-risk population}}$$

We often express incidence rates as the number of events per 100,000 population in the denominator. For instance, the incidence rate of lung cancer might be 100 per 100,000 per year. In evidence-based public health, comparing incidence rates is often a useful starting point when trying to establish the cause of a problem.

Mortality rates are a special type of incidence rate that measure the incidence of death due to a disease during a particular year. When most people who develop a disease die from the disease, as is the situation with lung cancer, the mortality rate and the incidence rates are very similar. Thus, if the incidence rate of lung cancer is 100 per 100,000 per year, the mortality rate might be 95 per 100,000 per year. When mortality rates and incidence rates are similar and mortality rates are more easily or more reliably obtained, epidemiologists may substitute mortality rates for incidence rates.[c]

The relationship between the incidence rate and the mortality rate is important since it estimates the chances of dying from the disease once it is diagnosed. We call this the **case-fatality**. In our example, the chances of dying from lung cancer—the morality rate divided by the incidence rate—is 95 percent, which indicates that lung cancer results in a very poor prognosis once it is diagnosed.

[b] When talking about the term "rate," many epidemiologists also include a unit of time, such as a day or a year, over which the number of events in the numerator is measured. This may also be called a **true rate**. The term "rate," as used in this book includes true rates, as well as proportions. A **proportion** is a fraction in which the numerator is a subset of the denominator. A time period is not required for a proportion, however, it often reflects the situation at one point in time.

[c] This is an example of the pragmatic approach that is often taken by epidemiologists when they are limited by the available data. The question facing epidemiologists is frequently: is the data good enough to address the question? Thus, epidemiology can be thought of as an approximation science.

Prevalence is the number of individuals who have a disease at a particular time divided by the number of individuals who could potentially have the disease. It can be represented by the following equation:

$$\textit{Prevalence} = \frac{\textit{\# living with a particular disease}}{\textit{\# in the at-risk population}}$$

Thus, prevalence tells us the proportion or percentage of individuals who have the disease.[5, 6]

Despite the fact that lung cancer has become the most common cancer, the prevalence will be low—perhaps one-tenth of one percent or less—because those who develop lung cancer do not generally live for a long period of time. Therefore, you will rarely see people with lung cancer. The prevalence of chronic diseases of prolonged duration, such as asthma or chronic obstructive pulmonary disease (COPD), is often relatively high, hence you will often see people with these diseases.[d]

Prevalence is often useful when trying to assess the total impact or burden of a health problem in a population and can help identify the need for services. For example, knowledge that there is a high prevalence of lung cancer in a certain region may indicate that there is a need for healthcare services in that area. Prevalence is also very useful in clinical medicine as the starting point for screening and diagnosis. Now that we have addressed rates, we can return to the three questions for describing a health problem.

WHAT IS THE BURDEN OF DISEASE IN TERMS OF MORBIDITY AND MORTALITY AND HAS IT CHANGED OVER TIME?

As we have seen, lung cancer is a disease with a very poor prognosis; therefore, the burden of disease is high as measured by its high mortality rate. This was the situation in the past and to a large extent continues to be the situation.

Mortality rates have been obtained from death certificates for many years. The cause of death on death certificates is classified using a standardized coding system known as the International Classification of Diseases (ICD). No equally complete or accurate system has been available for collecting data on the incidence rate of lung cancer. However, as we learned in

[d] The relationship between incidence and prevalence rates is approximately: the incidence rate × average duration of the disease = the prevalence rate. Both the incidence rate and the average duration affect the prevalence of the disease. Together, the incidence, prevalence, and case-fatality rates provide a population-based summary of the course of a disease. Incidence reflects the chance of developing the disease, prevalence indicates the chances of having the disease, and case-fatality indicates the prognosis or chance of dying from the disease.

our discussion of rates, the incidence rates and mortality rates for lung cancer are very similar. Therefore, we can use mortality data as a substitute for incidence data when evaluating the overall burden of lung cancer in a population.

By the 1930s, epidemiologists had concluded from the study of death certificates that lung cancer deaths were rapidly increasing. This increase continued through the 1950s—with cancer occurring two decades or more after the growth in consumption of cigarettes. Therefore, it was not immediately obvious that the two were related. In order to hypothesize that cigarettes were a cause of lung cancer, one needed to conclude that there was a long delay and/or a need for long-term exposure to cigarettes before lung cancer developed. There was a need for more evidence linking cigarettes and lung cancer. Let us turn our attention to the second question to see where this evidence came from.

ARE THERE DIFFERENCES IN THE DISTRIBUTION OF DISEASE AND CAN THESE DIFFERENCES GENERATE IDEAS OR HYPOTHESES ABOUT THEIR ETIOLOGY OR CAUSE?

In looking at the distribution of disease and the potential risk factors, epidemiologists found some important relationships. In terms of "person," the increases in lung cancer mortality observed in the 1930s through 1950s were far more dramatic among men than among women, though by the 1950s the mortality rate among women had begun to increase as well. It was noted that cigarette use had increased first in men and later among women. There appeared to be a delay of several decades between the increase in cigarette smoking and the increase in lung cancer mortality among both men and women. This illustrates that "time" along with "person" and "place" is important in generating hypotheses.

In terms of "place," it was found that the relationship between cigarette smoking and lung cancer mortality was present throughout the United States, but was strongest in those states where cigarette smoking was most common. Therefore, changes over time and the distribution of disease using "person" and "place" led epidemiologists to the conclusion that there was an association between groups of people who smoked more frequently and the group's mortality rates due to lung cancer. These relationships generated the idea that cigarettes might be a cause of lung cancer. Box 3-1 illustrates some other examples of how distributions of disease by "person", "place," and "time" can generate hypotheses about their cause.

Box 3-1 Generating Hypotheses from Distributions of Person and Place.

An increased frequency of disease based upon occupation has often provided the initial evidence of a group association based upon a combination of "person" and "place." The first recognized occupational disease was found among chimney sweeps often exposed for long periods of time to large quantities of coal dust who were found to have a high incidence of testicular cancer.

The Mad Hatter described in *Alice's Adventures in Wonderland* by Lewis Carroll made infamous the 19th century recognition that exposure to mercury fumes was associated with mental changes. Mercury fumes were created when making the felt used for hats, hence the term "mad as a hatter."

The high frequency of asbestosis among those who worked in shipyards suggested a relationship decades before the dangers of asbestos were fully recognized and addressed. A lung disease known as silicosis among those who worked in the mining industry likewise suggested a relationship that led to in-depth investigation and greater control of the risks.

More recently, a rare tumor called angiosarcoma was found to occur among those exposed over long periods to polyvinyl chloride (PVC), a plastic widely used in construction. The initial report of four cases of this unusual cancer among workers in one PVC plant was enough to strongly suggest a cause-and-effect relationship based upon "place" alone.

An important example of the impact that "place" can have on generating ideas or hypotheses about causation is the history of fluoride and cavities. In the early years of the 20th century, children in the town of Colorado Springs, Colorado, were found to have a very high incidence of brown discoloration of the teeth. It was soon recognized that this condition was limited to those who obtained their water from a common source. Ironically, those with brown teeth were also protected from cavities. This clear relationship to "place" was followed by over two decades of research that led to the understanding that fluoride in the water reduces the risk of cavities, while very high levels of the compound also lead to brown teeth. Examination of the levels of fluoride in other water systems eventually led to the establishment of levels of fluoride that could protect against cavities without producing brown teeth.

Such strong and clear-cut relationships are important, but relatively unusual. Often, examinations of the characteristics of "person," "place," and "time" in populations suggests hypotheses that can be followed-up among individuals to establish cause and effect relationships.[5, 6]

It is important to realize that these mortality rates are group rates. This data did not include any information about whether those who died from lung cancer were smokers. It merely indicated that groups who smoked more, such as males, also had higher mortality rates from lung cancer. The most that we can hope to achieve from this data is to generate hypotheses based on associations between groups or group associations. When we try to establish causation or etiology, we will need to go beyond group association and focus on associations at the individual level. However, before addressing etiology, we need to ask our third question:

ARE THE DIFFERENCES OR CHANGES USED TO SUGGEST GROUP ASSOCIATIONS ARTIFACTUAL OR REAL?

As we have seen from the 1930s through the 1950s, a large number of studies established that lung cancer deaths were increasing among men, but not among women. That is, there was a change over time and a difference between groups. When epidemiologists observe these types of changes and differences in rates, they ask: are the changes or differences in rates real or could they be artificial or artifactual? There are three basic reasons that changes in rates may be artifactual rather than real:

- Changes in the interest in identifying the disease
- Changes in the ability to identify the disease
- Changes in the definition of the disease

For some conditions, such as HIV/AIDS, these changes have all occurred. New and effective treatments have increased the interest in detecting the infection. Improved technology has increased the ability to detect HIV infections at an earlier point in time. In addition, there have been a number of modifications of the definition of AIDS based on new opportunistic infections and newly recognized complications. Therefore, with HIV/AIDS we need to be especially attentive to the possibility that artifactual changes have occurred.

With lung cancer, on the other hand, the diagnosis at the time of death has been of great interest for many years. The ability to diagnose the disease has not changed substantially. In addition, the use of ICD codes on death certificates has helped standardize the definition of the disease. Epidemiologists concluded that it was unlikely that changes in interest, ability, or definition explained the changes in the rates of lung cancer observed in males, thus they concluded that the changes were not artifactual, but real.[e]

However, it was still possible that the increased mortality rates from lung cancer were due to the increasing life span that was occurring between 1930 and 1960, along with the subsequent aging of the population. Perhaps older people are more likely to develop lung cancer and the aging of the population itself explains the real increase in the rates. To address this issue, epidemiologists use what is called **age adjustment**. To conduct age adjustment, epidemiologists look at the rates of the disease in each age group and also the **age distribution** or the number of people in each age group in the population. Then, they combine the rates for each age group taking into account or adjusting for the age distribution of a population.[f]

Taking into account the age distribution of the population in 1930 and 1960 did have a modest impact on the changes in the mortality rates from lung cancer, but large differences remained. As a result, epidemiologists concluded that lung cancer mortality rates changed over this period especially among men; the changes in rates were real; and the changes could not be explained simply by the aging of the population. Thus, epidemiologists had established the existence of a group association between groups that smoked more cigarettes and groups that developed lung cancer.

WHAT IS THE IMPLICATION OF A GROUP ASSOCIATION?

Group associations are established by investigations that use information on groups or a population without having information on the specific individuals within the group. These studies have been called **population comparisons** or **ecological studies.** Having established the existence of a group association, we still don't know if the individuals who smoke cigarettes are the same ones who develop lung cancer. We can think of a group association as a hypothesis that requires investigation at the individual level. The group association between cigarettes and lung cancer was the beginning of a long road to establish that cigarettes are a cause of lung cancer.

Not all group associations are also individual associations. Imagine the following situation: the mortality rates from drowning are higher in southern states than northern states. The per capita consumption of ice cream is also higher in southern states than northern states. Thus, a group association was established between ice cream consumption and drowning. In thinking about this relationship, you will soon realize that there is another difference between southern and northern states. The average temperature is higher in southern states and higher temperatures are most likely associated with

[e] There are actually several types of lung cancer defined by the ICD codes. Most, but not all, types of lung cancer are strongly associated with cigarette smoking.

[f] Adjustment for age is often performed by combining the rates in each age group using the age distribution of what is called a standard population. The age distribution of the U.S. population in 2000 is currently used as the standard population. Adjustment is not limited to age and may at times be conducted using other characteristics that may differ among the groups, such as gender or race, which may affect the probability of developing a disease.

more swimming and also more ice cream consumption. Ice cream consumption is therefore related both to swimming and to drowning. We call this type of factor a **confounding variable**. In this situation, there is no evidence that those who drown actually consumed ice cream. That is, there is no evidence of an association at the individual level. Thus group associations can be misleading if they suggest relationships that do not exist at the individual level.

Epidemiology research studies that look at associations at the individual level are key to establishing etiology, or cause. Etiology is the second component of the P.E.R.I. approach. Let us turn our attention to how to establish etiology.

ETIOLOGY: HOW DO WE ESTABLISH CONTRIBUTORY CAUSE?

Understanding the reasons for disease is fundamental to the prevention of disability and death. We call these reasons etiology or causation. In evidence-based public health, we use a very specific definition of causation—**contributory cause**. The evidence-based public health approach relies on epidemiological research studies to establish a contributory cause. This requires that we go beyond group association and establish three definitive requirements.[7]

1. The "cause" is associated with the "effect" at the individual level. That is, the potential "cause" and the potential "effect" occur more frequently in the same individual than would be expected by chance. Therefore, we need to establish that individuals with lung cancer are more frequently smokers than individuals without lung cancer.
2. The "cause" precedes the "effect" in time. That is, the potential "cause" is present at an earlier time than the potential "effect." Therefore, we need to establish that cigarette smoking comes before the development of lung cancer.
3. Altering the "cause" alters the "effect." That is, when the potential "cause" is reduced or eliminated, the potential "effect" is also reduced or eliminated. Therefore, we need to establish that reducing cigarette smoking reduces lung cancer rates.

Box 3-2 illustrates the logic behind using these three criteria to establish a cause-and-effect relationship, as well as what the implications of a contributory cause are.

These three definitive requirements are ideally established using three different types of studies, all of which relate potential "causes" to potential "effects" at the individual level. That is, they investigate whether individuals who smoke cigarettes are the same individuals that develop lung cancer.[6] The three basic types of investigations are called **case-control** or **retrospective studies**, **cohort studies** or **prospective studies**, and **randomized clinical trials** or **experimental studies**.

Case-control studies are most useful for establishing requirement #1 previously, i.e., the "cause" is associated with the "effect" at the individual level. Case-control studies can demonstrate that cigarettes and lung cancer occur together more

Box 3-2 Lightning, Thunder, and Contributory Cause.

The requirements for establishing the type of cause-and-effect relationship known as contributory cause used in evidence-based public health can be illustrated by the cause-and-effect relationship between lightning and thunder that human beings have recognized from the earliest times of civilization.

First, lightning is generally associated with thunder, that is, the two occur together far more often than one would expect if there were no relationship. Second, with careful observation it can be concluded that the lightning is seen a short time before the thunder is heard. That is, the potential "cause" (the lightning) precedes in time the "effect" (the thunder). Finally, when the lightning stops, so does the thunder—thus, altering the "cause" alters the "effect."

Notice that lightning is not always associated with thunder. "Heat lightning" may not produce audible thunder or the lightning may be too far away for the thunder to be heard. Lightning is not sufficient in and of itself to guarantee that our ears will subsequently always hear thunder. Conversely, in recent years it has been found that the sound of thunder does not always require lightning. Other reasons for rapidly expansion of air, such as an explosion, can also create a sound similar or identical to thunder.

The recognition of lightning as a cause of thunder came many centuries before human beings had any understanding of electricity or today's appreciation for the science of light and sounds. Similarly, cause-and-effect relationships established by epidemiological investigations do not always depend on understanding the science behind the relationships.

frequently than would be expected by chance alone. To accomplish this, cases with the disease (lung cancer) are compared to controls without the disease to determine whether the cases and the controls previously were exposed to the potential "cause" (cigarette smoking).

When a factor such as cigarettes has been demonstrated to be associated on an individual basis with an outcome such as lung cancer, we often refer to that factor as a **risk factor.**[g]

During the 1940s and early 1950s, a number of case-control studies established that individuals who developed lung cancer were far more likely to be regular smokers compared to similar individuals who did not smoke cigarettes. These case-control studies established requirement #1—the "cause" is associated with the "effect" at the individual level. They established that cigarettes are a risk factor for lung cancer.

Cohort studies are most useful for establishing requirement #2 previously—the "cause" precedes the "effect." Those with the potential "cause" or risk factor (cigarette smoking) and those without the potential "cause" are followed over time to determine who develops the "effect" (lung cancer).[h]

Several large scale cohort studies were conducted in the late 1950s and early 1960s. One conducted by the American Cancer Society followed nearly 200,000 individuals over three or more years to determine the chances that smokers and nonsmokers would develop lung cancer. Those who smoked regularly at the beginning of the study had a greatly increased chance of developing lung cancer over the course of the study, thus establishing requirement #2, the "cause" precedes the "effect" in time.

Randomized clinical trials are most useful for establishing requirement #3—altering the "cause" alters the "effect." Using a chance process known as **randomization**, individuals are assigned to be exposed or not exposed to the potential "cause" (cigarette smoking). Individuals with and without the potential "cause" are then followed over time to determine who develops the "effect." Conducting a randomized clinical trial of cigarettes and lung cancer would require investigators to randomize individuals to smoke cigarettes or not smoke cigarettes and follow them over many years. This illustrates the obstacles that can occur in seeking to definitively establish contributory cause. Once there was a strong suspicion that cigarettes might cause lung cancer, randomized clinical trials were not practical or ethical as a method for establishing cigarette smoking as a contributory cause of lung cancer. Therefore, we need to look at additional criteria that we can use to help us establish the existence of contributory cause.[i]

Figure 3-2 illustrates the requirements for definitively establishing contributory cause and the types of studies that may be used to satisfy each of the requirements. Notice that the requirements for establishing contributory cause are the same as the requirements for establishing **efficacy**. Efficacy implies that an intervention works, that is, it increases positive outcomes or benefits in the population being investigated.

WHAT CAN WE DO IF WE CANNOT DEMONSTRATE ALL THREE REQUIREMENTS TO DEFINITIVELY ESTABLISH CONTRIBUTORY CAUSE?

When we cannot definitively establish a contributory cause, we often need to look for additional supportive evidence.[7] In evidence-based public health, we often utilize what have been called **supportive** or **ancillary criteria** to make scientific judgments about cause and effect. A large number of these criteria have been used and debated. However, four of them are widely used and pose little controversy. They are:

- Strength of the relationship
- Dose-response relationship
- Consistency of the relationship
- Biological plausibility

Let us examine what we mean by each of these criteria. The **strength of the relationship** implies that we are interested in knowing how closely related the risk factor (cigarette smoking) is to the disease (lung cancer). In other words, we want to know the probability of lung cancer among those who smoke cigarettes compared to the probability of lung cancer among those who do not smoke cigarettes. To measure the strength of the relationship we calculate what we call the **relative risk.** The

[g] A risk factor, as we just discussed, usually implies that the factor is associated with the disease at the individual level. At times it may be used to imply that the factor not only is associated with the disease at the individual level, but that it precedes the disease in time. Despite the multiple uses of the term, a risk factor does not in and of itself imply that a cause-and-effect relationship is present, though it may be considered a possible cause.

[h] It may seem obvious that cigarette smoking precedes the development of lung cancer. However, the sequence of events is not always so clear. For instance, those who have recently quit smoking cigarettes have an increased chance of being diagnosed with lung cancer. This may lead to the erroneous conclusion that stopping cigarette smoking is a cause of lung cancer. It is more likely that early symptoms of lung cancer lead individuals to quit smoking. The conclusion that stopping cigarette smoking causes lung cancer is called **reverse causality**. Thus, it was important that cohort studies followed smokers and nonsmokers for several years to establish that the cigarette smoking came first.

[i] At times, a special form of a cohort study called a **natural experiment** can help establish that altering the cause alters the effect. A natural experiment implies that an investigator studies the results of a change in one group, but not in another similar group that was produced by forces outside the investigator's control. For instance, after the Surgeon General's *1964 Report on Smoking and Health* was released, approximately 100,000 physicians stopped smoking. This did not happen among other professionals. Over the next decade, the rates of lung cancer among physicians dropped dramatically, but not among other professionals. Despite the fact that natural experiments can be very useful, they are not considered as reliable as randomized clinical trials. Randomization, especially in large studies, eliminates differences between groups or potential confounding differences, even when these differences in characteristics are not recognized by the investigators.

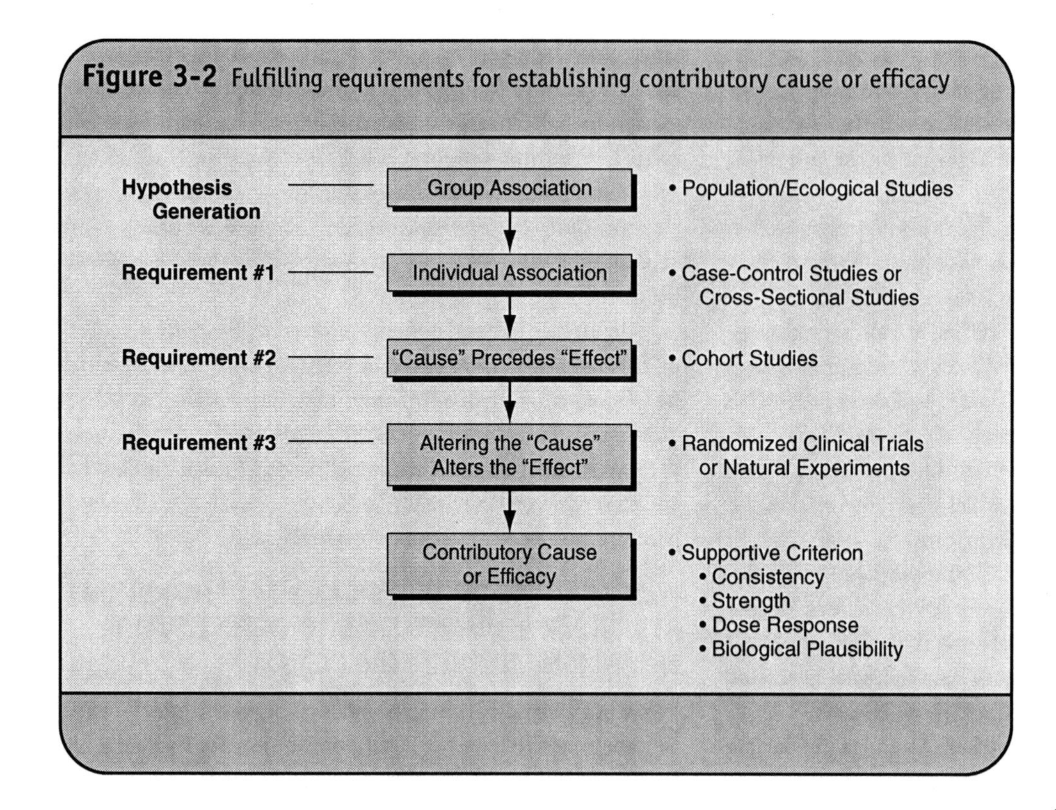

Figure 3-2 Fulfilling requirements for establishing contributory cause or efficacy

relative risk is the probability of developing the disease if the risk factor is present compared to the probability of the disease if the risk factor is not present. Therefore, the relative risk for cigarette smoking is calculated as:

$$\textit{Relative risk} = \frac{\textit{probability of lung cancer for cigarette smokers}}{\textit{probability of lung cancer for nonsmokers}}$$

The relative risk for cigarette smoking and lung cancer is approximately ten. A relative risk of ten is very large. It tells us that the chances or probability of developing lung cancer are ten times as great for the average smoker compared to the average nonsmoker.[j]

In addition to looking at the strength of the overall relationship between smoking cigarettes and lung cancer, we can ask whether smoking more cigarettes is associated with a greater chance of developing lung cancer. If it is, then we say there is a **dose-response relationship**. For instance, smoking one pack of cigarettes per day over many years increases the chances of developing lung cancer compared to smoking half a pack per day. Similarly, smoking two packs per day increases the chances of developing the disease compared to smoking one pack per day. These examples show that a dose-response relationship is present.[k]

Consistency implies that studies in different geographic areas and among a wide range of groups produce similar results. A very large number of studies of cigarettes and lung cancer in many countries and among those of nearly every race and socioeconomic group have consistently demonstrated a strong individual association between cigarette smoking and lung cancer.

The final support criterion is **biological plausibility.** This term implies that we can explain the occurrence of disease based upon known and accepted biological mechanisms. We can explain the occurrence of lung cancer by the fact that cigarette smoke contains a wide range of potentially toxic chemicals which reach the locations in the body where lung cancer occurs.

Thus, the ancillary criteria add support to the argument that cigarette smoking is a contributory cause of lung cancer. Table 3-1 summarizes the use of ancillary or support criteria in making scientific judgments about contributory cause and illustrates these principles using the cigarette smoking and lung cancer scenario. It also cautions to use these criteria carefully because a cause-and-effect relationship may be present even when some or all of these criteria are not fulfilled.[7]

We have now summarized the approach used in evidence-based public health to establish a contributory cause. We

[j] A relative risk of ten does not tell us the **absolute risk**. The absolute risk is the actual chance or probability of developing the disease (lung cancer) in the presence of the risk factor (cigarette smoking), expressed numerically—for example, as 0.03 or 3%. A relative risk of ten might imply an increase from 1 in 1000 individuals to 1 in 100 individuals. Alternatively it might imply an increase from 1 in 100 individuals to 1 in 10 individuals. A relative risk can be calculated whenever we have follow-up data on groups of individuals; therefore, it does not in and of itself imply that a contributory cause is present. We need to be careful not to imply that the risk factor will increase the chances of developing the disease or that reducing or eliminating the risk factor will reduce or eliminate the disease unless we have evidence of contributory cause. For case-control studies, a measure known as the **odds ratio** can be calculated and is often used as an approximation of relative risk.

[k] A dose-response relationship may also imply that greater exposure to a factor is associated with reduced probability of developing the disease, such as with exercise and coronary artery disease. In this case, the factor may be called a **protective factor** rather than a risk factor.

Table 3-1 Ancillary or Supportive Criteria—Cigarettes and Lung Cancer

Criteria	Meaning of the criteria	Evidence for cigarettes and lung cancer	Cautions in using criteria
Strength of the relationship	The relative risk for those with the risk factor is greatly increased compared to those without the risk factor	The relative risk is large or substantial. The relative risk is greater than 10 for the average smoker implying that the average smoker has more than 10 times the probability of developing lung cancer compared to nonsmokers	Even relatively modest relative risks may make important contributions to disease when the risk factor is frequently present. A relative risk of 2 for instance implies a doubling of the probability of developing a disease.
Dose-response relationship	Higher levels of exposure and/or longer duration of exposure to the "cause" is associated with increased probability of the "effect"	Studies of cigarette and lung cancer establish that smoking half a pack a day over an extended period of time increases the risk compared to no smoking. Smoking one pack per day and two packs per day further increases the risk	No dose-response relationship may be evident between no smoking and smoking one cigarette a day or between smoking three and four packs per day
Consistency of the relationship	Studies at the individual level produce similar results in multiple locations among populations of varying socioeconomic and cultural backgrounds	Hundreds of studies in multiple locations and populations consistently establish an individual association between cigarettes and lung cancer	Consistency requires the availability of numerous studies that may not have been conducted
Biological plausibility	Known biological mechanisms can convincingly explain a cause-and-effect relationship	Cigarette smoke directly reaches the areas where lung cancer appears	Exactly which component(s) of cigarette smoking produce lung cancer are just beginning to be understood

started with the development of group associations that generate hypotheses and moved on to look at the definitive requirements for establishing contributory cause. We also looked at the ancillary or supportive criteria that are often needed to make scientific judgments about contributory cause. Table 3-2 summarizes this process and applies it to cigarette smoking and lung cancer.

WHAT DOES CONTRIBUTORY CAUSE IMPLY?

Establishing a contributory cause on the basis of evidence is a complicated, and often a time, consuming job. In practice, our minds often too quickly jump to the conclusion that a cause-and-effect relationship exists. Our language has a large number of words which may subtly imply a cause-and-effect relationship, even in the absence of evidence. Box 3-3 illustrates how we often rapidly draw conclusions about cause and effect.

It is important to understand what the existence of a contributory cause implies and what it does not imply. Despite the convincing evidence that cigarette smoking is a contributory cause of lung cancer, some individuals never smoke and still develop lung cancer. Therefore, cigarettes are not what we call a **necessary cause** of lung cancer. Others smoke cigarettes all their lives and do not develop lung cancer. Thus, cigarettes are not what we call a **sufficient cause** of lung cancer.

Table 3-2 Cigarettes and Lung Cancer—Establishing Cause and Effect

Requirements for contributory cause	Meaning of the requirements	Types of studies that can establish the requirement	Evidence for cigarette smoking and lung cancer
Associated at a population level (Group association)	A group relationship between a "cause" and an "effect."	Ecological study or population comparison study: a comparison of population rates between an exposure and a disease.	Men began mass consumption of cigarettes decades before women and their rates of lung cancer increased decades before those of women.
Individual association: "Requirement #1"	Individuals with a disease ("effect") also have an increased chance of having a potential risk factor ("cause").	Case-control studies: cases with the disease are compared to similar controls without the disease to see who had the exposure.	Lung cancer patients were found to have 10 times or greater chance of smoking cigarettes regularly compared to those without lung cancer.
Prior association: "Requirement #2"	The potential risk factor precedes—in time—the outcome.	Cohort studies: exposed and similar nonexposed individuals are followed over time to determine who develops the disease.	Large cohort studies found that those who smoke cigarettes regularly have a 10 times or greater chance of subsequently developing lung cancer.
Altering the "cause" alters the "effect": "Requirement #3"	Active intervention to expose one group to the risk factor results in a greater chance of the outcome.	Randomized clinical trials allocating individuals by chance to be exposed or not exposed are needed to definitively establish contributory cause. Note: these studies are not always ethical or practical.	Alternatives to randomized clinical trials, such as "natural experiments" established that those who quit smoking have greatly reduced chances of developing lung cancer. In addition, the four supportive criteria also suggest contributory cause.

The fact that not every smoker develops lung cancer implies that there must be factors that protect some individuals from lung cancer. The fact that some nonsmokers develop lung cancer implies that there must be additional contributory causes of lung cancer. Thus, the existence of a contributory cause implies that the "cause" increases the chances that the "effect" will develop. Its presence does not guarantee that the disease will develop. In addition the absence of cigarette smoking does not guarantee that the disease will not develop.

Despite the fact that cigarettes have been established as a contributory cause of lung cancer, they are not a necessary or a sufficient cause of lung cancer. In fact, the use of the concepts of necessary and sufficient cause is not considered useful in the evidence-based public health approach because so few, if any, diseases fulfill the definitions of necessary and sufficient cause. These criteria are too demanding to be used as standards of proof in public health or medicine.

By 1964, the evidence that cigarette smoking was a contributory cause of lung cancer was persuasive enough for the Surgeon General of the United States to produce the first Surgeon General's *Report on Smoking and Health.* The report concluded that cigarettes are an important cause of lung cancer. Over the following decades, the Surgeon General's reports documented the evidence that cigarette smoking not only caused lung cancer, but other cancers—including cancer of the throat and larynx. Cigarette smoking is also a contributory cause of chronic obstructive pulmonary disease (COPD) and coronary artery disease. Smoking during pregnancy poses risks to the unborn child and passive or second-hand smoke creates increased risks to those exposed—especially children.[8] Based on the Surgeon

Box 3-3 Words that Imply Causation.

Often when reading the newspaper or other media you will find that conclusions about cause and effect are made based upon far less rigorous examination of the data than we have indicated are needed to definitively establish cause and effect. In fact, we often draw conclusions about cause and effect without even consciously recognizing we have done so. Our language has a large number of words that imply a cause-and-effect relationship, some of which we use rather casually.

Let's take a look at the many ways that a hypothetical newspaper article might imply the existence of a cause-and-effect relationship or a contributory cause even when the evidence is based only upon a group association or upon speculation about the possible relationships.

Over several decades the mortality rates from breast cancer in the United States were observed to increase each year. This trend was ***due to*** *and can be* ***blamed on*** *a variety of factors including the increased use of estrogens and exposure to estrogens in food. The recent reduction in breast cancer* ***resulted from*** *and can be* ***attributed to*** *the declining use of estrogens for menopausal and postmenopausal women. The declining mortality rate was also* ***produced by*** *the increased use of screening tests for breast cancer that were* ***responsible for*** *early detection and treatment. These trends* ***demonstrate that*** *reduced use of estrogens and increased use of screening tests have* ***contributed to*** *and* ***explain*** *the reduction in breast cancer.*

While these conclusions sound reasonable and may well be cause-and-effect relationships, note that they rely heavily on assertions for which there is no direct evidence provided. For instance, the following words are often used to imply a cause-and-effect relationship when evidence is not or cannot be presented to support the relationship:

- due to
- blamed on
- result from
- attributable to
- produced by
- responsible for
- contributed to
- explained by

It is important to be aware of conscious or unconscious efforts to imply cause-and-effect relationships when the data suggest only group associations and do not meet our more stringent criteria establishing cause and effect.

General's findings, there is clearly overwhelming evidence that cigarette smoking is a contributory cause of lung cancer and a growing list of other diseases. Thus, let us turn our attention to the third component of the P.E.R.I. process: recommendations.

RECOMMENDATIONS: WHAT WORKS TO REDUCE THE HEALTH IMPACT?

The evidence for cigarette smoking as a cause of lung cancer, as well as other diseases, was so strong that it cried out for action. In evidence-based public health, however, action should be grounded in **recommendations** that incorporate evidence. That is, evidence serves not only to establish contributory cause, but is central to determining whether or not specific interventions work.[9, 10] Recommendations are built upon the evidence from studies of interventions. Thus, recommendations are summaries of the evidence of which interventions work to reduce the health impacts and they indicate whether actions should be taken. These studies utilize the same types of investigations we discussed for contributory cause. In fact, the requirements of contributory cause are the same as those for establishing that an intervention works or has efficacy on the particular population that was studied.

In the decades since the Surgeon General's initial report, a long list of interventions have been implemented and evaluated. As we have discussed, the term intervention is a very broad term in public health. Interventions range from individual counseling and prescription of pharmaceutical drugs which aid smoking cessation; to group efforts, such as peer support groups; to social interventions, such as cigarette taxes and legal restriction on smoking in restaurants.

Recommendations for action have been part of public health and medicine for many years. Evidence-based recommendations, however, are relatively new. They have been contrasted with the traditional *eminence-based* recommendation, which uses the opinion of a respected authority as its foundation. Evidence-based recommendations ask about the research evidence supporting the benefits and harms of potential interventions. In evidence-based recommendations the opinions of experts are most important when research evidence does not or cannot provide answers.

Before looking at the evidence-based recommendations on cigarette smoking made by the Centers for Disease Control and Prevention (CDC), let us look at how they are often made and can be graded. Evidence-based recommendations are based upon two types of criteria—the quality of the evidence and the magnitude of the impact. Each of these criteria is given what is called a **score.**[9, 10] The quality of the evidence is scored based in large part upon the types of investigations and how well the investigation was conducted. Well-conducted randomized clinical trials that fully address the health problem are considered the highest quality evidence. Often, however, cohort and case control studies are needed and are used as part of the recommendation.

Expert opinion, though lowest on the hierarchy of evidence, is often essential to fill in the holes in the research evidence.[9, 10] The quality of the evidence also determines whether the data collected during an intervention is relevant to its use in a particular population or setting. Data from young adults may not be relevant to children or the elderly. Data from severely ill patients may not be relevant to mildly ill patients. Thus, high quality evidence needs to be based not only on the research which can establish efficacy in one particular population, but on the **effectiveness** of the intervention in the specific population in which it will be used.

In evidence-based public health the quality of the evidence is often scored as good, fair, or poor. Good quality implies that the evidence fulfills all the criteria for quality. Poor quality evidence implies that there are fatal flaws in the evidence and recommendations cannot be made. Fair quality lies in between having no fatal flaws.[l]

In addition to looking at the quality of the evidence, it is also important to look at the magnitude of the impact of the intervention. The magnitude of the impact asks the question: how much of the disability and/or death due to the disease can be potentially removed by the intervention? In measuring the magnitude of the impact, evidence-based recommendations take into account the potential benefits of an intervention, as well as the potential harms. Therefore, we can regard the magnitude of the impact as the benefits minus the harms, or the "net benefits."[m]

The magnitude of the impact, like the quality of the evidence, is scored based upon a limited number of potential categories. In one commonly-used system, the magnitude of the impact is scored as substantial, moderate, small, and zero/negative.[9] A substantial impact may imply that the intervention works extremely well for a small number of people, such as a drug treatment for cigarette cessation. These are the types of interventions that are often the focus of individual clinical care. A substantial impact may also imply that the intervention has a modest net benefit for any one individual, but can be applied to large numbers of people, such as in the form of media advertising or taxes on cigarettes. These are the types of interventions that are most often the focus of traditional public health and social policy.

Evidence-based recommendations combine the score for the quality of the evidence with the score for the impact of the intervention.[9] Table 3-3 summarizes how these aspects can be combined to produce a classification of the strength of the recommendation—graded as A, B, C, D, and I.

It may be useful to think of these grades as indicating the following:

A = Must—A strong recommendation
B = Should—In general, the intervention should be used unless there are good reasons or contraindications for not doing so.
C = May—The use of judgment is often needed on an individual-by-individual basis. Individual recommendations depend on the specifics of an individual's situation, risk-taking attitudes, and values.
D = Don't—There is enough evidence to recommend against using the intervention.
I = Indeterminant, insufficient or I don't know—The evidence is inadequate to make a recommendation for or against the use of the intervention at the present time.

Notice that evidence-based public health and medicine rely primarily on considerations of benefits and harms.

[l] To fulfill the criteria for good quality data, evidence is also needed to show that the outcome being measured is a clinically important outcome. Short-term outcomes called **surrogate outcomes**, such as changes in laboratory tests, may not reliably indicate longer term or clinically important outcomes.

[m] The magnitude of the impact can be measured using the relative risk calculation. When dealing with interventions, the people who receive the intervention are often placed in the numerator. Thus, an intervention that reduces the bad outcomes by half would have a relative risk of 0.5. The smaller the relative risk is, the greater the measured impact of the intervention. If the relative risk is 0.20, then those with the intervention have only 20 percent of the risk remaining. Their risk of a bad outcome has been reduced by 80 percent. The reduction in bad outcome is called the **attributable risk percentage** or the **percent efficacy**. The intervention can only be expected to accomplish this potential reduction in risk when a contributory cause is present and the impact of the "cause" can be immediately and completely eliminated.

Table 3-3 Classification of Recommendations

	Magnitude of the impact			
	Net benefit: substantial	Net benefit: moderate	Net benefit: small	Net benefit: zero/negative
Quality of the evidence				
Good	A	B	C	D
Fair	B	B	C	D
Poor (insufficient evidence)	I	I	I	I

Source: Agency for Healthcare Research and Quality, U.S. Preventive Services Task Force Guide to Clinical Preventive Services Vol 1, AHRQ Pub. No.02-500.

However, recently issues of financial cost have begun to be integrated into evidence-based recommendations. At this point, however, cost considerations are generally only taken into account for "close calls." Close calls are often situations where the net benefits are small to moderate and the costs are large.

The evidence-based public health approach increasingly relies on the use of evidence-based recommendations that are graded based on the quality of the evidence and the expected impact of the intervention. The recommendations are made by a wide array of organizations as discussed in Box 3-4. It is important to appreciate the source of the recommendations, as well as the methods used to develop them.[7]

Let us take a look at some examples of how interventions to prevent smoking, detect lung cancer early, or cure lung cancer have been graded. The CDC publishes *The Guide to Community Prevention Services.*[10] This guide indicates that the following interventions are recommended, implying a grade of A or B:

- Clean indoor air legislation prohibiting tobacco use in indoor public and private workplaces
- Federal, state, and local efforts to increase taxes on tobacco products as an effective public health intervention to promote tobacco use cessation and to reduce the initiation of tobacco use among youths
- The funding and implementation of long-term, high-intensity mass media campaigns using paid broadcast times and media messages developed through formative research

Box 3-4 Who Develops Evidence-Based Recommendations?

Evidence-based recommendations may be developed by a range of groups including government, practitioner-oriented organizations, consumer-oriented organizations, organized health care systems, and even for-profit organizations. Organizations developing evidence-based recommendations, however, are expected to acknowledge their authorship and identify the individuals who participated in the process, as well as their potential conflicts of interest. In addition, regardless of the organization, the evidence-based recommendations should include a description of the process used to collect the data and make the recommendations.

For-profit organizations may make evidence-based recommendations. However, their obvious conflicts of interest often lead them to fund other groups to make recommendations. Thus, the funding source(s) supporting the development of evidence-based recommendations should also be acknowledged as part of the report.

One well-regarded model for development of evidence-based recommendations is the task force model used by the United States Preventive Services Task Force of the Agency for Healthcare Research and Quality (AHRQ), as well as by the Task Force on Community Preventive Services of the Centers for Disease Control and Prevention (CDC).[9, 10] The task force model aims to balance potential conflicts of interest and ensures a range of expertise by selecting a variety of experts, as well as community participants based upon a public nomination process. Once the task force members are appointed, their recommendations are made by a vote of the task force and do not require approval by the government agency.

Thus, as a reader of evidence-based recommendations, it is important that you begin by looking at which group developed the recommendations, whether they have disclosed their membership including potential conflicts of interest, and the groups' procedures for developing the recommendations.

- Proactive telephone cessation support services (quit lines)
- Reduced or eliminated copayments for effective cessation therapies
- Reminder systems for healthcare providers (encouraging them to reinforce the importance of cigarette cessation)
- Efforts to mobilize communities to identify and reduce the commercial availability of tobacco products to youths

Additional recommendations encourage clinicians to specifically counsel patients against smoking, prescribe medications for adults, encourage support groups for smoking cessation, and treat lung cancer with the best available treatments when detected.

Of interest is the grade of D for recommending against screening for early detection of lung cancer using traditional chest X-rays. The evidence strongly suggests that screening using this method may detect cancer at a slightly earlier stage, but not early enough to alter the course of the disease. Therefore early detection does not alter the outcome of the diseases. Research continues to find better screening methods to detect lung cancer in time to make a difference.

Recommendations are not the end of the process. There may be a large number of recommendations among which we may need to choose. In addition, we need to decide the best way(s) to put the recommendations into practice. Thus, implementation is not an automatic process. Issue of ethics, culture, politics, and risk-taking attitudes can and should have major impacts on implementation. A fourth step in the evidence-base public health approach requires us to look at the options for implementation and to develop a strategy for getting the job done.

IMPLEMENTATION: HOW DO WE GET THE JOB DONE?

Strong recommendations based upon the evidence are ideally the basis of implementation. At times, however, it may not be practical or ethical to obtain the evidence needed to establish contributory cause and develop evidence-based recommendations. Naturally-occurring implementation itself may be part of the process of establishing causation, as it was for cigarette smoking in the 1960s when 100,000 physicians stopped smoking and their rates of lung cancer declined rapidly, as compared to other similar professionals who did not stop smoking.

Today, there are often a large number of interventions with adequate data to consider implementation. Many of the interventions have potential harms, as well as potential benefits. The large and growing array of possible interventions means that health decisions require a systematic method for deciding which interventions to use and how to combine them in the most effective and efficient ways. One method for examining the options for implementation uses a structure we will call the "When-Who-How" approach.

"When" asks about the timing in the course of disease in which an intervention occurs. This timing allows us to categorize interventions as **primary**, **secondary**, and **tertiary**. Primary interventions take place before the onset of the disease. They aim to prevent the disease from occurring. Secondary interventions occur after the development of a disease or risk factor, but before symptoms appear. They are aimed at early detection of disease or reducing risk factors while the patient is asymptomatic. Tertiary interventions occur after the initial occurrence of symptoms, but before irreversible disability. They aim to prevent irreversible consequences of the disease. In the cigarette smoking and lung cancer scenario, primary interventions aim to prevent cigarette smoking. Secondary interventions aim to reverse the course of disease by smoking cessation efforts or screening to detect early disease. Tertiary interventions diagnose and treat diseases caused by smoking in order to prevent permanent disability and death.

"Who" asks: at whom should we direct the intervention? Should it be directed at individuals one at a time as part of clinical care? Alternatively, should it be directed at groups of people, such as vulnerable populations, or should it be directed at everyone in a community or population?[n]

Finally, we need to ask: how should we implement interventions? There are three basic types of interventions when addressing the need for behavioral change. These interventions can be classified as: information (education), motivation (incentives), and obligation (requirements).[o]

An information or education strategy aims to change be-

---

[n] The CDC defines four levels of intervention: the individual, the relationship (e.g., the family), the community, and society or the population as a whole. This framework has the advantage of separating immediate family interventions from community interventions. The group or at-risk group relationship used here may at times refer to the family unit or geographic communities. It may also refer to institutions or at-risk vulnerable groups within the community. The use of group or at-risk group relationship provides greater flexibility allowing application to a wider range of situations. In addition, the three levels used here correlate with the measurements of relative risk, attributable risk percentage, and population attributable percentage, which are the fundamental epidemiological measurements applied to the magnitude of the impact of an intervention.[7]

[o] An additional option is innovation. Innovation implies a technical or engineering solution. The development of a safer cigarette might be an innovation. A distinct advantage of technical or engineering solutions is that they often require far less behavior change. Changing human behavior is frequently difficult. Nonetheless, it is an essential component of most, if not all, successful public health interventions. Certainly, that is the case with cigarette smoking.

Table 3-4 Framework of Options for Implementation

	When	Who	How
Levels	1) Primary—Prior to disease or condition 2) Secondary—Prior to symptoms 3) Tertiary—Prior to irreversible complications	1) Individual 2) At-risk group 3) General population/ community	1) Information (education) 2) Motivation (incentives) 3) Obligation (requirement)
Meaning of levels	1) Primary—Remove underlying cause, increase resistance, or reduce exposure 2) Secondary—Post-exposure intervention, identify and treat risk factors or screen for asymptomatic disease 3) Tertiary—Reverse the course of disease (cure), prevent complications, restore function	1) Individual often equals patient care 2) At-risk implies groups with common risk factors 3) General population includes defined populations with and without the risk factor	1) Information—Efforts to communicate information and change behavior on basis of information 2) Motivation—Rewards to encourage or discourage without legal requirement 3) Obligation—Required by law or institutional sanction
Cigarette smoking example	1) Primary—Prevention of smoking, reduction in second-hand exposure 2) Secondary—Assistance in quitting, screening for cancer if recommended 3) Tertiary—Health care to minimize disease impact	1) Individual smoker 2) At-risk—Groups at risk of smoking or disease caused by smoking, e.g., adolescents as well as current and ex-smokers 3) Population—Entire population including those who never have or never will smoke	1) Information—Stop smoking campaigns, advertising, warning on package, clinician advice 2) Motivation—Taxes on cigarettes, increased cost of insurance 3) Obligation—Prohibition on sales to minors, exclusion from athletic eligibility, legal restrictions on indoor public smoking

havior through individual encounters, group interactions, or the mass media. Motivation implies use of incentives for changing or maintaining behavior. It implies more than strong or enthusiastic encouragement, it implies tangible reward. Obligation relies on law and regulations requiring specific behaviors. Table 3-4 illustrates how options for intervention for cigarettes might be organized using the "When-Who-How" approach. To better understand the "who" and "how" of the options for intervention when behavior change is needed, refer to Table 3-5, which outlines nine different options.

Deciding when, who, and how to intervene depends in large part upon the available options and the evidence that they work. They also depend in part on our attitudes toward different types of interventions. In American society, we prefer to rely on information or educational strategies. These approaches preserve freedom of choice which we value in public, as well as private, decisions. Use of mass media informational strategies may be quite economically efficient relative to the large number of individuals they reach though messages often need to be tailored to different audiences. However, information is often ineffective in accomplishing behavioral change—at least on its own.

Strategies based upon motivation, such as taxation and other incentives, may at times be more effective than information alone, though educational strategies are still critical to justify and reinforce motivational interventions. Motivational interventions

Table 3-5 Examples of "Who" and "How" Related to Cigarette Smoking

	Information	Motivation	Obligation
Individual	Clinician provides patient with information explaining reasons for changing behavior	Clinician encourages patient to change behavior in order to qualify for a service or gain a benefit, e.g., status or financial	Clinician denies patient a service unless patient changes behavior
	Example: Clinician distributes educational packet to a smoker and discusses his or her own smoking habit	*Example: Clinician suggests that the financial savings from not buying cigarettes be used to buy a luxury item*	*Example: Clinician implements recommendation to refuse birth control pills to women over 35 who smoke cigarettes*
High-risk group	Information is made available to all those who engage in a behavior	Those who engage in a behavior are required to pay a higher price	Those who engage in a behavior are barred from an activity or job
	Example: Warning labels on cigarette packages	*Examples: Taxes on cigarettes*	*Example: Smokers banned from jobs that will expose them to fumes that may damage their lungs*
Population	Information is made available to the entire population, including those who do not engage in the behavior	Incentives are provided for those not at risk to discourage the behavior in those at risk	An activity is required or prohibited for those at risk and also for those not at risk of the condition
	Example: Media information on the dangers of smoking	*Example: Lower health care costs for everyone results from reduced percentage of smokers*	*Example: Cigarettes sales banned for those under 18*

should be carefully constructed and judiciously used or they may result in what has been called **victim blaming**. For example, victim blaming in the case of cigarette smoking implies that we regard the consequences of smoking as the smokers' own fault.

The use of obligation or legally-required action can be quite effective if clear-cut behavior and relatively simple enforcement, such as restrictions on indoor public smoking, are used. These types of efforts may be regarded by some as a last resort, but others may see them as a key to effective use of other strategies. Obligation inevitably removes freedom of choice and if not effectively implemented with regard for individual rights, the strategy may undermine respect for the law. Enforcement may become invasive and expensive, thus obligation requires careful consideration before use as a strategy.

Understanding the advantages and disadvantages of each type of approach is key to deciphering many of the controversies we face in deciding how to implement programs to address public health problems; however, implementation is not the end of the evidence-based public health process.

WHAT HAPPENS AFTER IMPLEMENTATION?

Public health problems are rarely completely eliminated with one intervention—there are few magic bullets in this field. Therefore, it is important to evaluate whether an intervention or combination of interventions has been successful in reducing the problem. It is also critical to measure how much of the problem has been eliminated by the intervention(s).

For instance, studies of cigarette smoking between the mid-1960s and the late 1990s demonstrated that there was nearly a 50 percent reduction in cigarette smoking in the United States and that the rates of lung cancer were beginning to fall—at least among males. However, much of the problem still existed because the rates among adolescent males and females remained high and smoking among adults was preceded by smoking as adolescents nearly 90 percent of the time. Thus, an evaluation of the success of cigarette smoking interventions led to a new cycle of the P.E.R.I. process. It focused on how to address the issue of adolescent smoking and nicotine addiction among adults. Many of the interventions being used today grew out of this effort to cycle once again through the evidence-based public health process and look for a new understanding of the problem, its etiology, evidence-based recommendations, and options for implementation as illustrated in Figure 3-3.

Figure 3-3 Evidence-based public health: The complete P.E.R.I. approach

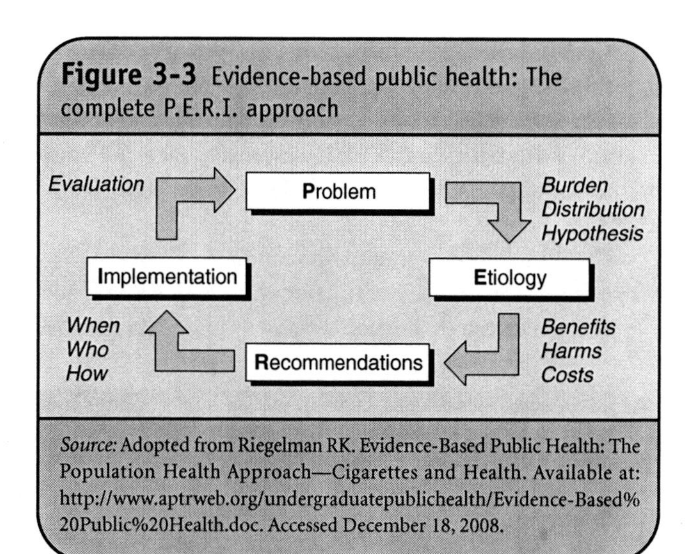

Source: Adopted from Riegelman RK. Evidence-Based Public Health: The Population Health Approach—Cigarettes and Health. Available at: http://www.aptrweb.org/undergraduatepublichealth/Evidence-Based%20Public%20Health.doc. Accessed December 18, 2008.

Deciding the best combination of approaches to address a public health problem remains an important part of the judgment needed for the practice of public health. In general, multiple approaches are often needed to effectively address a complex problem like cigarette smoking. Population and high risk group approaches, often used by public health professionals, and individual approaches, often used in as part of health care, should be seen as complementary. Often using both types of interventions is more effective than either approach alone. Social interventions, such as cigarette taxes and restrictions on public smoking are also important interventions to consider when asking how to intervene.

The scope of public health problems and the options for intervention are expanding rapidly and now include global, as well as local and national efforts. In China, for instance, 75 percent of adult males are reported to be smokers making China—with its large population—number one in terms of the number of smokers, as well as the number of deaths caused by smoking. An important example of a social intervention is global collaboration to address smoking and health. World Health Organization's (WHO) efforts have led to what the WHO calls the Framework Convention on Tobacco Control (WHO FCTC).[11]

Today, an enormous body of evidence exists on the relationship between tobacco and health. Understanding the nature of the problems, the etiology or cause-and-effect relationships,

Table 3-6 Questions to Ask—Evidence-Based Public Health Approach

1. **Problem**—What is the health problem?
   - What is the burden of disease and has it changed over time?
   - Are there differences in the distribution of disease and can these differences generate ideas or hypotheses about their etiology?
   - Are the differences or changes used to suggest group associations artifactual or real?
2. **Etiology**—What are the contributory cause(s)?
   - Has an association been established at the individual level?
   - Does the "cause" precede the "effect"?
   - Has altering the "cause" been shown to alter the "effect" (if not use ancillary criteria)?
3. **Recommendations**—What works to reduce the health impacts?
   - What is the quality of the evidence for the intervention?
   - What is the impact of the intervention in terms of benefits and harms?
   - What grade should be given indicating the strength of the recommendation?
4. **Implementations**—How can we get the job done?
   - When should the implementation occur?
   - At whom should the implementation be directed?
   - How should the intervention(s) be implemented?

Source: Adapted from Riegelman RK. Evidence-Based Public Health: The Population Health Approach—Cigarettes and Health. Available at: http://www.aptrweb.org/undergraduatepublichealth/Evidence-Based%20Public%20Health.doc. Accessed December 18, 2008.

the evidence-based recommendations, and the approaches for implementing and evaluating the options for interventions, remain key to the public health approach to smoking and health.[4] Figure 3-3 diagrams the full P.E.R.I approach. Table 3-6 summarizes the questions to ask in the evidence-based public health approach.

The P.E.R.I. process summarizes as a mneumonic the steps in evidence-based public health. It emphasizes the need to understand the nature of the problem and its underlying causes. It also helps structure the use of evidence to make recommendations and decide on which options to put into practice. Finally the circular nature of the P.E.R.I. process reminds us that the job of improving health goes on often requiring multiple efforts to understand and address the problem.[12]

Now that we have an understanding of the basic approach of evidence-based public health let us turn our attention in Section II to the fundamental tools at our disposal for addressing public health problems.

Key Words

- P.E.R.I. process
- Burden of disease
- Morbidity
- Mortality
- Distribution of disease
- Epidemiologists
- Group associations
- Risk indicators (or risk markers)
- Artifactual
- Rate
- At-risk population
- True rate
- Incidence rate
- Prevalence rate
- Case-fatality
- Age adjustment
- Age distribution
- Standard population
- Population comparisons
- Ecological studies
- Confounding variable
- Contributory cause
- Case-control or retrospective studies
- Cohort or prospective studies
- Randomized clinical trials or experimental studies
- Risk factor
- Reverse causality
- Randomization
- Natural experiment
- Efficacy
- Supportive criteria
- Ancillary criteria
- Relative risk
- Absolute risk
- Odds ratio
- Dose-response relationship
- Protective factor
- Biological plausibility
- Necessary cause
- Sufficient cause
- Effectiveness
- Surrogate outcomes
- Attributable risk percentage (or the percent efficacy)
- Primary, secondary, and tertiary interventions
- Victim blaming
- Proportion
- Consistency
- Recommendation
- Evidence

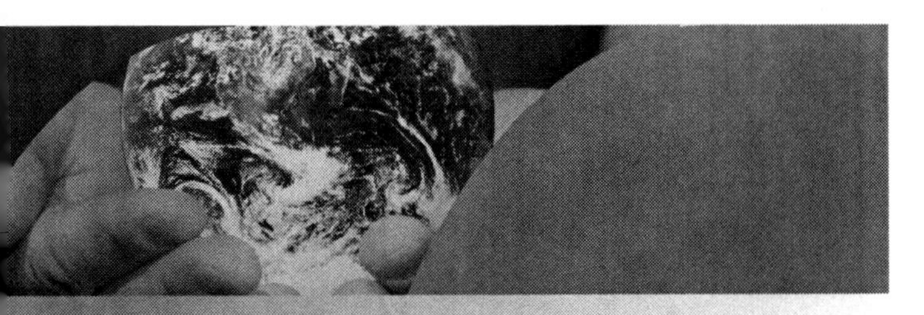

Discussion Questions

1. Use the P.E.R.I. framework and the list of questions to outline how each step in the P.E.R.I. process was accomplished for cigarette smoking.
2. How would you use the P.E.R.I. process to address the remaining issues of cigarette smoking?

REFERENCES

1. Cable News Network. Focus: Tobacco Under Attack. Available at: http://www.cnn.com/US/9705/tobacco/history/#cigars.htm. Accessed December 20, 2008.

2. Johnson, Dr. G. A Long Trail of Evidence Links Cigarette Smoking to Lung Cancer. ON SCIENCE column. Available at: http://www.txtwriter.com/Onscience/Articles/smokingcancer2.html. Accessed March 12, 2009.

3. Centers for Disease Control and Prevention. The Public Health Approach to Violence Prevention. Available at: http://www.cdc.gov/ncipc/dvp/PublicHealthApproachTo_ViolencePrevention.htm. Accessed March 12, 2009.

4. Riegelman RK. The Population Health Approach—Cigarettes and Health. Available at: http://www.teachprevention.org/. Accessed March 12, 2009.

5. Gordis L. *Epidemiology*, 4th ed. Philadelphia: Elsevier Saunders; 2009.

6. Friis RH, Sellers TA. *Epidemiology for Public Health Practice*, 4th ed. Sudbury, MA: Jones and Bartlett Publishers; 2009.

7. Riegelman RK. *Studying a Study and Testing a Test: How to Read the Medical Evidence*, 5th ed. Philadelphia: Lippincott, Williams & Wilkins; 2005.

8. United States Department of Health and Human Services. Surgeon General's Reports on Smoking and Tobacco Use. Available at: http://www.cdc.gov/tobacco/data_statistics/sgr/index.htm. Accessed March 12, 2009.

9. Agency for Healthcare Research and Quality, *U.S. Preventive Services Task Force Guide to Clinical Preventive Services.* 2002; Vols. 1 and 2, AHRQ Pub. No. 02-500.

10. Centers for Disease Control and Prevention. The Community Guide. Available at: http://www.thecommunityguide.org/. Accessed March 12, 2009.

11. World Health Organization. Global tobacco treaty enters into force with 57 countries already committed. Available at: http://www.who.int/mediacentre/news/releases/2005/pr09/en/index.html. Accessed March 12, 2009.

12. Centers for Disease Control and Prevention. The Social-Ecological Model: A Framework for Prevention. Available at: http://www.cdc.gov/ncipc/dvp/social-ecological-model_dvp.htm. Accessed March 12, 2009.

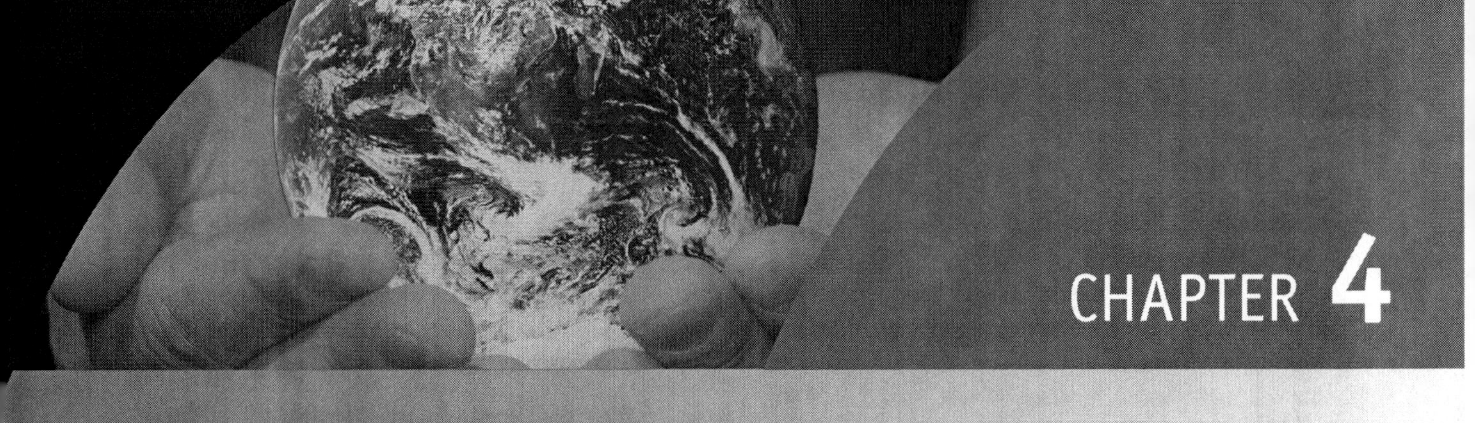

Public Health Institutions and Systems

Learning Objectives

By the end of this chapter, the student will be able to:

- identify goals of governmental public health.
- identify the ten essential services of public health.
- describe basic features of local, state, and federal public health agencies in the United States.
- identify global public health organizations and agencies and describe their basic roles.
- identify roles in public health for federal agencies not identified as health agencies.
- illustrate the need for collaboration by governmental public health agencies with other governmental and nongovernmental organizations.
- describe approaches to connecting public health and the health-care system.

A young man in your dormitory is diagnosed with tuberculosis. The health department works with the student health service to test everyone in the dorm, as well as in his classes, with a TB skin test. Those who are positive for the first time are advised to take a course of a medicine called INH. You ask: is this standard operating procedure?

You go to a public health meeting and learn that many of the speakers are not from public health agencies, but from the Departments of Labor, Commerce, Housing, and Education. You ask: what do these departments have to do with health?

You hear that a new childhood vaccine was developed by the NIH, approved by the FDA, endorsed for federal payment by the CDC and recommended for use by the American Academy of Pediatrics. You ask: do all these agencies and organizations always work so well together?

A major flood in Asia leads to disease and starvation. Some say it is due to global warming, others to bad luck. Coordinated efforts by global health agencies, assisted by nongovernmental organizations (NGOs) and outside governmental donors, help get the country back on its feet. You ask: what types of cooperation are needed to make all of this happen?

A local community health center identifies childhood obesity as a problem in their community. They collect data demonstrating that the problem begins as early as elementary school. They develop a plan that includes clinical interventions at the health center and also at the elementary school. They ask the health department to help them organize an educational campaign and assist in evaluating the results. Working together, they are able to reduce the obesity rate among elementary school children by one-half. This seems like a new way to practice public health, you conclude. What type of approach is this?

These cases all reflect the responsibilities of public health agencies at the local, federal, and global levels. They illustrate public health working the way it is supposed to work. Of course, this is not always the case. Let us start by taking a look at the goals and roles of public health agencies.

WHAT ARE THE GOALS AND ROLES OF GOVERNMENTAL PUBLIC HEALTH AGENCIES?

Public health is often equated with the work of governmental agencies. The role of government is only a portion of what we mean by public health, but it is an important component. So important, in fact, that we often define the roles of other components in terms of how they relate to the work of governmental public health agencies.

In 1994, the United States Public Health Service put forth the "Public Health in America Statement," which provided the framework that continues to define the goals and services of governmental public health agencies.[1] These goals should already be familiar to you. They are:

- to prevent epidemics and the spread of disease
- to protect against environmental hazards
- to prevent injuries
- to promote and encourage healthy behaviors
- to respond to disasters and assist communities in recovery
- to ensure the quality and accessibility of health services

These are ambitious and complicated goals to achieve. To be able to successfully achieve them, it is important to further define the roles that governmental public health agencies themselves play, and by implication, the roles that other governmental agencies and nongovernmental organizations need to play.

The Public Health in America Statement built upon the Institute of Medicine's (IOM) 1988 report called The Future of Public Health.[2] The IOM defined three **core public health functions** that governmental public health agencies need to perform. The concept of "core function" implies that the job cannot be delegated to other agencies or to nongovernmental organizations. It also implies that the governmental public health agencies will work together to accomplish these functions because as a group they are responsible for public health as a whole—no one agency at the local, state, or federal level is specifically or exclusively responsible for accomplishing the essential public health services.[a]

The core functions defined by the IOM are: 1) assessment, 2) policy development, and 3) assurance.[2]

- **Assessment** includes obtaining data that defines the health of the overall population and specific groups within the population, including defining the nature of new and persisting health problems.
- **Assurance** includes governmental public health's oversight responsibility for ensuring that key components of an effective health system, including health care and public health, are in place even though the implementation will often be performed by others.
- **Policy development** includes developing evidence-based recommendations and other analyses of options, such as health policy analysis, to guide implementation including efforts to educate and mobilize community partnerships.

The three core functions, while useful in providing a delineation of responsibilities and an intellectual framework for the work of governmental public health agencies, were not tangible enough to provide a clear understanding or definition of the work of public health agencies. Thus, in addition to the goals of public health, the Public Health in America Statement defined a series of **ten essential public health services** that build upon the IOM's core functions, guide day-to-day responsibilities, and provide a mechanism for evaluating whether the core functions are fulfilled. These ten services have come to define the responsibilities of the combined local, state, and federal governmental public health system.

WHAT ARE THE TEN ESSENTIAL PUBLIC HEALTH SERVICES?

Table 4-1 outlines the ten essential public health services and organizes them according to which IOM core function they aim to fulfill.[1] A description of each service is presented in column two and examples of these essential services are listed in column three.

We have now looked at the core public health functions and the ten essential services of public health agencies. Figure 4-1 puts these together to allow you to see the connections.

These public health services are delivered through a complex web of local and federal agencies, as well as via increasing involvement of global organizations. Let us take a look at the work of public health agencies at each of these levels.

Figure 4-2 provides a framework to guide our review of the delivery of public health services. It diagrams the central role of governmental public health agencies and the complicated connections required to accomplish their responsibilities. We will begin by taking at look at the structure and function of governmental public health agencies at the local/state, federal, and global levels. Then, we will examine the key connections with other governmental agencies, community, and private organizations, and finally with the healthcare delivery system as a whole.

WHAT ARE THE ROLES OF LOCAL AND STATE PUBLIC HEALTH AGENCIES?

The United States Constitution does not mention public health. Thus, public health is first and foremost a state responsibility. States may retain the authority, voluntarily request or

[a] This does not imply that components of the work cannot be contracted to nongovernmental organizations. This activity is increasingly occurring. The concept of core function, however, implies that public health agencies remain responsible for these functions even when the day-to-day work is conducted through contracts with an outside organization.

TABLE 4-1 Ten Essential Public Health Services

Essential service	Meaning of essential service	Example
ASSESSMENT—Core function		
1. Monitor health status to identify and solve community health problems	This service includes accurate diagnosis of the community's health status; identification of threats to health and assessment of health service needs; timely collection, analysis, and publication of information on access, utilization, costs, and outcomes of personal health services; attention to the vital statistics and health status of specific groups that are at a higher risk than the total population; and collaboration to manage integrated information systems with private providers and health benefit plans.	Vital Statistics Health Surveys Surveillance, including reportable diseases
2. Diagnose and investigate health problems and health hazards in the community	This service includes epidemiologic identification of emerging health threats; public health laboratory capability using modern technology to conduct rapid screening and high-volume testing; active infectious disease epidemiology programs; and technical capacity for epidemiologic investigation of disease outbreaks and patterns of chronic disease and injury.	Epidemic investigations CDC–Epidemiology Intelligence Service State Public Health Laboratories
POLICY DEVELOPMENT—Core function		
3. Inform, educate, and empower people about health issues	This service includes social marketing and media communications; providing accessible health information resources at community levels; active collaboration with personal health care providers to reinforce health promotion messages and programs; and joint health education programs with schools, churches, and worksites.	Health education campaigns, such as comprehensive state tobacco programs
4. Mobilize community partnerships and action to identify and solve health problems	This service includes convening and facilitating community groups and associations, including those not typically considered to be health-related, in undertaking defined preventive, screening, rehabilitation, and support programs; and skilled coalition-building to draw upon the full range of potential human and material resources in the case of community health.	Lead control programs: testing and follow-up of children, reduction of lead exposure, educational follow-up, and addressing underlying causes
5. Develop policies and plans that support individual and community health efforts	This service requires leadership development at all levels of public health; systematic community and state-level planning for health improvement in all jurisdictions; tracking of measurable health objectives as a part of continuous quality improvement strategies; joint evaluation with the medical health care system to define consistent policy regarding prevention and treatment services; and development of codes, regulations, and legislation to guide public health practice.	Newborn screening program for PKU and other genetic and congenital diseases

continues

TABLE 4-1 Ten Essential Public Health Services (continued)

Essential service	Meaning of essential service	Example
ASSURANCE—Core function		
6. Enforce laws and regulations that protect health and ensure safety	This service involves full enforcement of sanitary codes, especially in the food industry; full protection of drinking water supplies; enforcement of clean air standards; timely follow-up of hazards, preventable injuries, and exposure-related diseases identified in occupational and community settings; monitoring quality of medical services (e.g. laboratory, nursing home, and home health care); and timely review of new drug, biological, and medical device applications.	Local: Fluoridation and chlorination of water State: Regulation of nursing homes Federal: FDA drug approval and food safety
7. Link people to needed personal health services and ensure the provision of health care when otherwise unavailable	This service (often referred to as "outreach" or "enabling" service) includes ensuring effective entry for socially disadvantaged people into a coordinated system of clinical care; culturally- and linguistically-appropriate materials and staff to ensure linkage to services for special population groups; ongoing "care management"; and transportation.	Community Health Centers
8. Ensure the provision of a competent public and personal health care workforce	This service includes education and training for personnel to meet the needs for public and personal health services; efficient processes for licensure of professionals and certification of facilities with regular verification and inspection follow-up; adoption of continuous quality improvement and lifelong learning within all licensure and certification programs; active partnerships with professional training programs to ensure community-relevant learning experiences for all students; and continuing education in management and leadership development programs for those charged with administrative/executive roles.	Licensure of physicians, nurses, and other health professionals
9. Evaluate effectiveness, accessibility, and quality of personal and population-based health services	This service calls for ongoing evaluation of health programs, based on analysis of health status and service utilization data, to assess program effectiveness and to provide information necessary for allocating resources and reshaping programs.	Development of evidence-based recommendations
ALL THREE IOM—Core function		
10. Research for new insights and innovative solutions to health problems	This service includes continuous linkage with appropriate institutions of higher learning and research and an internal capacity to mount timely epidemiologic and economic analyses and conduct needed health services research.	NIH, CDC, AHRQ other federal agencies

Source: Data from Public Health in America. Essential Public Health Services. Available at http://www.health.gov/phfunctions/public.htm. Accessed November 8, 2008.

FIGURE 4-1 Essential public health services and IOM core functions

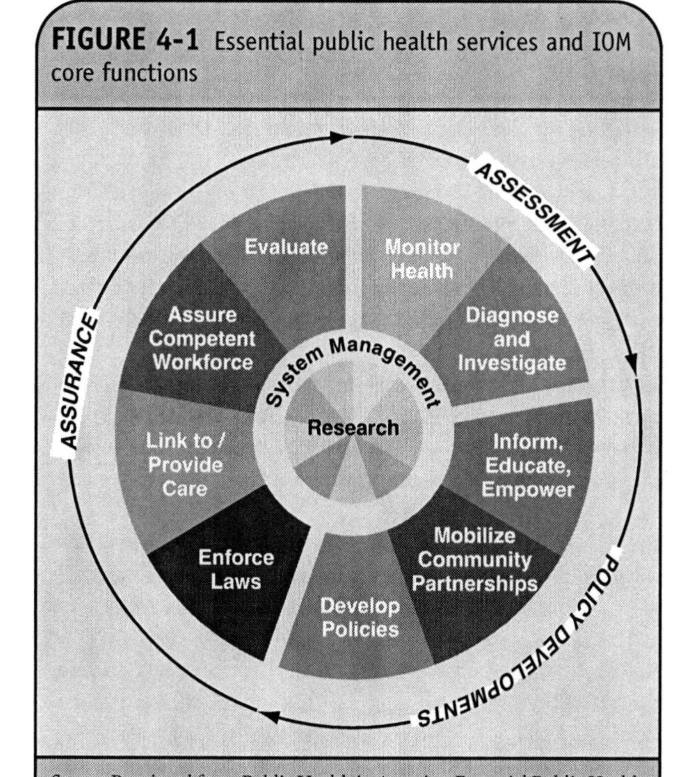

Source: Reprinted from Public Health in America. Essential Public Health Services. Available at http://www.health.gov/phfunctions/public.htm. Accessed November 8, 2008.

FIGURE 4-2 Framework for viewing governmental public health agencies and their complicated connections

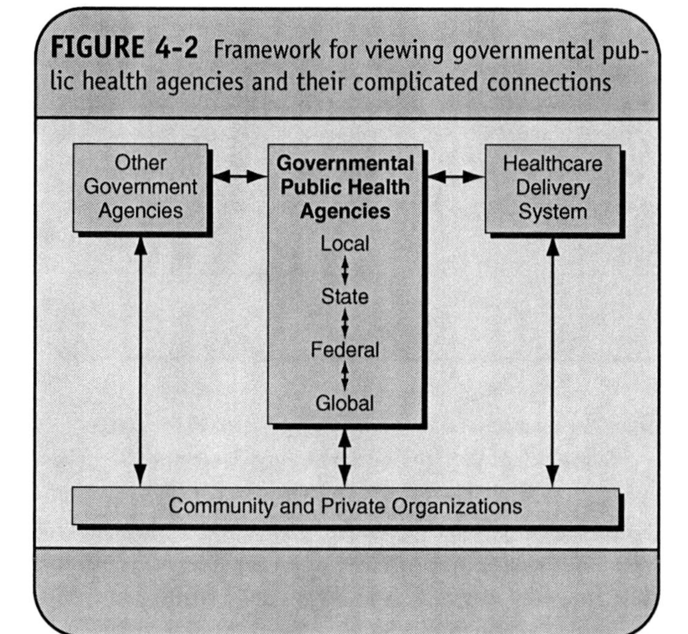

accept help from the federal government, or delegate their responsibility and/or authority to local agencies at the city, county, or other local levels.[b]

Box 4-1 describes a brief history of public health agencies in the United States. It is a complex history and has resulted in more structures than there are states—more because large cities often have their own public health systems.[3] In addition, the District of Columbia and several U.S. territories have their own systems and often have authority to make public health system decisions as if they were states.

To understand the role of local health departments, it is useful to think of two models.[4] In the first model, which we will call the home rule or local autonomy model, authority is delegated from the state to the local health department. The local health department, or the local government, has a great deal of autonomy in setting its own structure and function and often raising its own funding.

In the second model, which we will call the branch office model, the local health department can be viewed as a branch office of the state agency with little or no independent authority or funding. Most health departments lie somewhere in between these two extreme models, however these models provide a framework for understanding the many varieties of department structures. Thus, when we speak of local public health, we may be speaking of a state agency with branch offices or a relatively independent local agency. Regardless of which model a state uses, many public health responsibilities of local public health departments are quite similar and they usually have authority and responsibility for at least the following:[4]

- immunizations for those not covered by the private system
- communicable disease surveillance and initial investigation of outbreaks
- communicable disease control, often including at a minimum tuberculosis and syphilis case finding and treatment
- inspection and licensing of restaurants
- environmental health surveillance
- coordinating public health screening programs, including newborn and lead screenings
- tobacco control programs
- public health preparedness and response to disasters

Health departments in many parts of the United States have also served as the healthcare provider for those without

[b] This delegation may occur at the discretion of the state government or it may be included in the state's constitution providing what is called **home rule authority** to local jurisdictions. In general, jurisdictions with home rule authority exercise substantially more autonomy.

BOX 4-1 Brief History of American Public Health Agencies.

An understanding of the history of American public health institutions requires an understanding of the response of local, state, and federal governments to public health crises and the complex interactions between these levels of government.

The colonial period in America saw repeated epidemics of smallpox, cholera, and yellow fever focused in the port cities. These epidemics brought fear and disruption of commerce, along with accompanying disease and death. One epidemic in Philadelphia in 1793 in what was then the nation's capital nearly shut down the federal government. These early public health crises brought about the first municipal Boards of Health, made up of respected citizens authorized to act in the community's interest to implement quarantine, evacuation, and other public health interventions of the day. The federal government's early role in combating epidemics led to the establishment in 1798 of what later became known as the U.S. Public Health Service.

Major changes in public health awaited the last half of the 19th century with the great expansion of understanding of disease and the ability to control it through community actions. The Shattuck Commission in Massachusetts in 1850 outlined the roles of state health departments as responsible for: sanitary inspections, communicable disease control, food sanitation, vital statistics, and services for infants and children. Over the next 50 years, the states gradually took the lead in developing public health institutions based upon delivery of these services.

Local health departments outside of the largest cities did not exist until the 20th century. The Rockefeller Foundation stimulated and helped fund early local health departments and campaigns in part to combat specific diseases, such as hookworm. There was no standard model for local health departments. Local health departments developed in at least 50 different ways in the 50 states and were chronically underfunded.

The federal government played a very small role in public health throughout the 1800s and well into the 20th century. An occasional public health crisis stimulated in part by media attention did bring about federal action. The founding of the Food and Drug Administration in 1906 resulted in large part from the journalistic activity known as "muckraking," which exposed the status of food and drug safety. The early years of the 20th century set the stage for expansion of the federal government's role in public health through the passage of the 16th Amendment to the Constitution authorizing federal income tax as a major source of federal government funding.

The Great Depression, in general, and the Social Security Act of 1935, in particular, brought about a new era in which federal funding became a major source of financial resources for state and local public health departments and nongovernmental organizations. The founding of the what was then called the Communicable Disease Centers (CDC) in 1946 led to a national and eventually international leadership role for the CDC which attempts to connect and hold together the complex local, state, and federal public health efforts and integrate them into global public health efforts.

The Johnson Administration's War on Poverty, as well as the Medicare and Medicaid programs, brought about greatly expanded funding for health care services and led many health departments to provide direct healthcare services especially for those without other sources of care. The late 1980s and 1990s saw a redefinition of the roles of governmental public health including the Institute of Medicine's definition of core functions and the development of the 10 Essential Public Health Services. These documents have guided the development of a broad population focus for public health and a move away from the direct provision of healthcare services.

The terrorism of 9/11 and the subsequent anthrax scare moved public health institutions to the center of efforts to protect the public's health through emergency and disaster preparedness. The development of flexible efforts to respond to expected and unexpected hazards is now a central feature of public health institutions' roles and funding. The success of these efforts requires new levels of coordination of local, state, federal, and global public health agencies utilizing state-of-the-art surveillance, laboratory technology, and communications systems.

other sources of health care. This has been called the **healthcare safety net**. In recent years, many health departments have reduced or discontinued these services often transferring them to the healthcare system or integrating their efforts into community health centers. The concept of core functions holds that while these activities can be performed by other organizations or agencies, the public health agencies still retain responsibility for ensuring access to and the quality of these services.

The work of local public health agencies cannot be viewed in isolation. The State Health Department usually retains important roles even in those states where the local departments have home rule authority. These responsibilities often include: collecting vital statistics, running a public health laboratory, licensing of health professionals, administering nutrition programs, and regulation of health facilities, such as nursing homes. In addition, drinking water regulation, administration of the state Medicaid program, and the office of the medical examiner may also fall under the authority of the State Health Department.

Today, the federal government has a great deal of involvement in national and global issues of public health and often works closely with local agencies. Let us take a look at the structure and role of the federal government in public health.

WHAT ARE THE ROLES OF FEDERAL PUBLIC HEALTH AGENCIES?

The federal government's role in public health does not explicitly appear in the United States Constitution. It has been justified largely by the Interstate Commerce clause, which provides federal government authority to regulate commerce between the states. Federal public health authority often rests on the voluntary acceptance by the states of funding provided by the federal government. This funding may come with requirements for state action in order to qualify for the funding.

The Department of Health and Human Services (HHS) is the central public health agency of the federal government. It includes operating agencies each of which report directly to the cabinet-level Secretary of HHS. Table 4-2 outlines most of these agencies, their roles and authority, and their basic public health structure and activities.[5]

The National Institutes of Health (NIH) is far and away the largest agency within HHS with a budget of over $30 billion—as much as all the other six agencies' budgets combined. However, most of its efforts are devoted to basic science research and the translation of research into clinical practice. Some of the federal agencies, such as the Health Services and Resources Administration (HRSA), Substance Abuse and Mental Health Services Administration (SAMHSA), and the Indian Health Service, provide or fund individually-oriented health services in addition to population-oriented preventive services. The Indian Health Service is unique because it is responsible for both public health and healthcare services for a defined population.

The Centers for Disease Control and Prevention (CDC) is perhaps the agency most closely identified with public health at the federal level. Box 4-2 describes its first 50 years from 1946 to 1996 in a reprint of its official history first published in the *Morbidity and Mortality Weekly Report* (MMWR), a weekly publication of agency.[6]

Today, the CDC's role in connecting federal, state, and local governmental public health efforts is central to the success of the system. Approximately half of the CDC's current approximately $10 billion budget is channeled to state and local health departments. A key function of the CDC is to provide national leadership and to coordinate the efforts of local/state and federal public health agencies.

To understand the local/state and federal public health system, it is important to appreciate that only five percent of all health-related funding goes to public health and of that, less than half goes to population-based prevention as opposed to providing healthcare services as a safety net for individuals. In addition, the role of governmental public health is limited by social attitudes toward government. For instance, we have seen that there are constitutional limitations on the authority of public health and other government agencies to impose actions on individuals. These may limit public health agencies' abilities to address issues ranging from tuberculosis and HIV control to responses to emergencies. The social attitudes of Americans may also limit the authority and resources provided to public health agencies. Americans often favor individual or private efforts over governmental interventions when they believe that individuals and private organizations are capable of success. For instance, some Americans resist active efforts in the schools to provide information and access to contraceptives, while others resist the type of case-finding efforts for HIV/AIDS that have been used successfully in investigating and controlling other communicable diseases.

Today, governmental public health is a global enterprise. Let us take a look at the roles of global health organizations and agencies.

WHAT ARE THE ROLES OF GLOBAL HEALTH ORGANIZATIONS AND AGENCIES?

Public health is increasingly becoming a global enterprise. Global governmental efforts have grown dramatically in recent years. The World Health Organization (WHO) was created in 1948. Its impact has become more prominent in the 21st century with the increasing importance of global health issues. The WHO is a part of the United Nations organizations, which also include the United Nations Infant and Child Emergency Fund (UNICEF) and the Joint United Nations Programme on AIDS/HIV (UNAIDS).[7]

Today, the World Bank and other multilateral financial institutions are the largest funding source for global health efforts.[8] National governmental aid programs, including the United States Agency for International Development (USAID), also play an important role in public health. Table 4-3 outlines the structure/governance, roles, and limitations of global public health agencies.

The complexity of local, state, federal, and global public health agencies raises the question of whether or not these

TABLE 4-2 Key Federal Health Agencies of the Department of Health and Human Services

Agency	Roles/Authority	Examples of Structures/Activities
Centers for Disease Control and Prevention (CDC) and Agency for Toxic Substances and Disease Registry (ATSDR)	CDC is the lead agency for prevention, health data, epidemic investigation, and public health measures aimed at disease control and prevention The CDC administers ATSDR, which works with the Environmental Protection Agency to provide guidance on health hazards of toxic exposures.	The CDC and ATSDR work extensively with state and local health departments. The CDC's Epidemiology Intelligence Service (EIS) functions domestically and internationally at the request of governments.
National Institutes of Health (NIH)	Lead research agency. Also funds training programs and communication of health information to the professional community and the public.	17 institutes in all—the largest being the National Cancer Institute. The National Library of Medicine is part of NIH Centers. The Centers include the John E. Fogarty International Center for Advanced Study in the Health Sciences. NIH is the world's largest biomedical research enterprise with intramural research at NIH and extramural research grants throughout the world.
Food and Drug Administration (FDA)	Consumer protection agency with authority for safety of foods and safety and efficacy of drugs, vaccines and other medical and public health interventions	Divisions responsible for food safety, medical devices, drug efficacy and safety pre- and post- approval
Health Resources and Services Administration (HRSA)	Seeks to ensure equitable access to comprehensive quality health care	Funds community health centers, HIV/AIDS services, scholarships for health professional students
Agency for Healthcare Research and Quality (AHRQ)	Research agenda to improve the outcomes and quality of health care, including patient safety and access to services	Supports U.S. Preventive Services Task Force, Evidence-based medicine research, and Guidelines Clearinghouse
Substance Abuse and Mental Health Services Administration (SAMHSA)	Works to improve quality and availability of prevention, treatment, and rehabilitation for substance abuse and mental illness	Research, data collection and funding of local services
Indian Health Service (IHS)	Provides direct health care and public health services to federally-recognized tribes	Services provided to 550 federally-recognized tribes in 35 states Only comprehensive federal responsibility for health care, plus public health services

BOX 4-2 History of the CDC.

The Communicable Disease Center was organized in Atlanta, Georgia on July 1, 1946; its founder, Dr. Joseph W. Mountin, was a visionary public health leader who had high hopes for this small and comparatively insignificant branch of the Public Health Service (PHS). It occupied only one floor of the Volunteer Building on Peachtree Street and had fewer than 400 employees, most of whom were engineers and entomologists. Until the previous day, they had worked for Malaria Control in War Areas, the predecessor of CDC, which had successfully kept the southeastern states malaria-free during World War II and, for approximately 1 year, from murine typhus fever. The new institution would expand its interests to include all communicable diseases and would be the servant of the states, providing practical help whenever called.

Distinguished scientists soon filled CDC's laboratories, and many states and foreign countries sent their public health staffs to Atlanta for training....Medical epidemiologists were scarce, and it was not until 1949 that Dr. Alexander Langmuir arrived to head the epidemiology branch. Within months, he launched the first-ever disease surveillance program, which confirmed his suspicion that malaria, on which CDC spent the largest portion of its budget, had long since disappeared. Subsequently, disease surveillance became the cornerstone on which CDC's mission of service to the states was built and, in time, changed the practice of public health.

The outbreak of the Korean War in 1950 was the impetus for creating CDC's Epidemiological Intelligence Service (EIS). The threat of biological warfare loomed, and Dr. Langmuir, the most knowledgeable person in PHS about this arcane subject, saw an opportunity to train epidemiologists who would guard against ordinary threats to public health while watching out for alien germs. The first class of EIS officers arrived in Atlanta for training in 1951 and pledged to go wherever they were called for the next 2 years. These "disease detectives" quickly gained fame for "shoe-leather epidemiology" through which they ferreted out the cause of disease outbreaks.

The survival of CDC as an institution was not at all certain in the 1950s. In 1947, Emory University gave land on Clifton Road for a headquarters, but construction did not begin for more than a decade. PHS was so intent on research and the rapid growth of the National Institutes of Health that it showed little interest in what happened in Atlanta. Congress, despite the long delay in appropriating money for new buildings, was much more receptive to CDC's pleas for support than either PHS or the Bureau of the Budget.

Two major health crises in the mid-1950s established CDC's credibility and ensured its survival. In 1955, when poliomyelitis appeared in children who had received the recently approved Salk vaccine, the national inoculation program was stopped. The cases were traced to contaminated vaccine from a laboratory in California; the problem was corrected, and the inoculation program, at least for first and second graders, was resumed. The resistance of these 6- and 7-year-olds to polio, compared with that of older children, proved the effectiveness of the vaccine. Two years later, surveillance was used again to trace the course of a massive influenza epidemic. From the data gathered in 1957 and subsequent years, the national guidelines for influenza vaccine were developed.

CDC grew by acquisition....When CDC joined the international malaria-eradication program and accepted responsibility for protecting the earth from moon germs and vice versa, CDC's mission stretched overseas and into space.

CDC played a key role in one of the greatest triumphs of public health, the eradication of smallpox. In 1962 it established a smallpox surveillance unit, and a year later tested a newly developed jet gun and vaccine in the Pacific island nation of Tonga....CDC also achieved notable success at home tracking new and mysterious disease outbreaks. In the mid-1970s and early 1980s, it found the cause of Legionnaires disease and toxic-shock syndrome. A fatal disease, subsequently named acquired immunodeficiency syndrome (AIDS), was first mentioned in the June 5, 1981, issue of *MMWR*.

Although CDC succeeded more often than it failed, it did not escape criticism. For example, television and press reports about the Tuskegee study on long-term effects of untreated syphilis in black men created a storm of protest in 1972. This study had been initiated by PHS and other organizations in 1932 and was transferred to CDC in 1957. Although the effectiveness of penicillin as a therapy for syphilis had been established during the late 1940s, participants in this study remained untreated until the study was brought to public attention. CDC was also criticized because of the 1976 effort to vaccinate the U.S. population against swine flu, the infamous killer of 1918–1919. When some vaccinees developed Guillain-Barre syndrome, the campaign was stopped immediately; the epidemic never occurred.

As the scope of CDC's activities expanded far beyond communicable diseases, its name had to be changed. In 1970 it became the Center for Disease Control and in 1981, after extensive reorganization, Center became Centers. The words "and Prevention" were added in 1992, but, by law, the well-known three-letter acronym was retained. In health emergencies CDC means an answer to SOS calls from anywhere in the world, such as the recent one from Zaire where Ebola fever raged.

Fifty years ago CDC's agenda was non-controversial (hardly anyone objected to the pursuit of germs), and Atlanta was a backwater. In 1996, CDC's programs are often tied to economic, political, and social issues, and Atlanta is as near Washington as the tap of a keyboard.

Source: Reprinted from Centers for Disease Control and Prevention, MMWR 1996;45: 526–528.

TABLE 4-3 Global Public Health Organizations

Type of agency	Structure/Governance	Role(s)	Limitations
World Health Organization	United Nations Organization Seven "regional" semi-independent components, e.g., Pan American Health Organization covers North and South America	Policy development, e.g., tobacco treaty, epidemic control policies Coordination of services, e.g., SARS control, vaccine development Data collection and standardization, e.g., measures of health care quality, measures of health status	Limited ability to enforce global recommendations, limited funding and complex international administration
International organizations with focused agenda	UNICEF UNAIDS	Focus on childhood vaccinations Focus on AIDS	Limited agendas and limited financing
International financing organizations	The World Bank Other multilateral regional banks, e.g., InterAmerican and Asian Development Banks	World Bank is largest international funder. Increasingly supports "human capital" projects and reform of health care delivery systems and population and nutrition efforts Provides funding and technical assistance primarily as loans	Criticized for standardized approach with few local modifications
Bilateral governmental aid organizations	USAID Many other developed countries have their own organizations and contribute a higher percentage of their gross domestic product to those agencies than does the United States	Often focused on specific countries and specific types of programs, such as the United States' focus on HIV/AIDS, and maternal and child health	May be tied to domestic politics and global economic, political, or military agendas

agencies can and do work together. It should not surprise you that close collaboration, while the goal, is often difficult to achieve with so many organizations involved. Thus, it is important to ask: how can public health agencies work together?

HOW CAN PUBLIC HEALTH AGENCIES WORK TOGETHER?

Coordination among public health agencies has been a major challenge that is built into our local, state, and federal system of governance. Increasingly, coordination also requires a global aspect as well. Efforts on all levels have a long way to go. There are signs of hope with the recent progress in such fields as tobacco control, food safety, and most notably, the response to SARS. Box 4-3 discusses the dramatic events of the 2003 SARS epidemic, providing an example of what can be done and what needs to be done to address future public health emergencies.[9]

Collaboration needs to be an everyday effort, and not just a requirement for emergencies or epidemics. Let us look at the relationships and needed collaboration among governmental public health and other governemental agencies, nongovernmental organizations, and the healthcare delivery system.

BOX 4-3 SARS and the Public Health Response.

The SARS epidemic of 2003 began with little notice, most likely somewhere in the heartland of China and then spread to other areas of Asia. The world took notice after television screens filled with reports of public health researchers sent to Asia to investigate the illness subsequently contracting and dying from the disease. Not an easily transmissible disease except for those in very close contact, such as investigators, family members, and healthcare providers, the disease spread slowly but steadily through areas of China. Among those infected, the case-fatality rate was very high especially without the benefits of modern intensive care facilities.

The disease did not respond to antibiotics and was thought to be a viral disease by its epidemiological pattern of spread and transmission, but at first no cause was known. The outside world soon felt the impact of the brewing epidemic when cases appeared in Hong Kong that could be traced to a traveler from mainland China. Fear spread when cases were recognized that could not be explained by close personal contact with a SARS victim.

The epidemic continued to spread jumping thousands of miles to Toronto, Canada, where the second greatest concentration of disease appeared. Soon, the whole world was on high alert, if not quite on the verge of panic. At least 8000 people worldwide became sick and almost 10 percent of them died. Fortunately, progress came quite quickly. Researchers coordinated by the World Health Organization (WHO) were able to put together the epidemiological information and laboratory data and establish a presumed cause, a new form of the coronavirus never before seen in humans leading to the rapid introduction of testing.

The WHO and the CDC put forth recommendations for isolation, travel restrictions, and intensive monitoring that rapidly controlled the disease even in the absence of an effective treatment aimed at a cure. SARS disappeared as rapidly as it emerged, especially after systematic efforts to control spread were put in place in China. Not eliminated, but no longer a worldwide threat, SARS left a lasting global impact. The WHO established new approaches for reporting and responding to epidemics—these now have the widespread formal acceptance of most governments.

Once the world could step back and evaluate what happened, it was recognized that the potential burden of disease posed by the SARS epidemic had worldwide implications and raised the threat of interruption of travel and trade. Local, national, and global public health agencies collaborated quickly and effectively. Infection control recommendations made at the global level were rapidly translated into efforts to identify disease at the local level and manage individual patients in hospitals throughout the world. It is a model of communicable disease control that will be needed in the future.

WHAT OTHER GOVERNMENT AGENCIES ARE INVOLVED IN HEALTH ISSUES?

To address health issues, it is important to recognize the important roles that government agencies not designated as health agencies play in public health. Such agencies exist at the local/state, federal, and global levels. To illustrate the involvement of these agencies in health issues, let's begin with the roles of nonhealth agencies at the federal level.

A number of federal agencies serve public health functions even though they are not defined as health agencies. The roles they play are important especially when we take the population health perspective that includes the totality of efforts to promote and protect health and prevent disease, disability, and death.

Environmental health issues are an important part of the role of the Environmental Protection Agency (EPA). Reducing injury and hazardous exposures in the workplace are key goals of the Occupational Safety and Health Administration (OSHA), which is part of the Department of Labor.

Protecting health as part of preparation and response to disasters and terrorism is central to the role of the Department of Homeland Security. The Department of Agriculture shares with the FDA the role of protecting the nation's food supply. The Department of Housing and Urban Development influences the built environment and its impacts on health. The Department of Energy plays important roles in setting radiation safety standards for nuclear power plants and other sources of energy.

The multiple federal agencies involved in health-related matters often means that coordination and collaboration are required across agencies. This is certainly the case with food safety and disaster planning and response. It is true as well for efforts to address problems that cut across agencies, such as lead exposure or efforts to reduce the environmental causes of asthma.

WHAT ROLES DO NONGOVERNMENTAL ORGANIZATIONS PLAY IN PUBLIC HEALTH?

Nongovernmental organizations play increasingly important roles in public health in the United States and around the world. The United States has a long tradition of private groups organizing to advocate for public health causes, delivering public health services, and providing funding to support public health efforts. In recent years, these efforts have been expanding globally as well.

The American Red Cross and its network of international affiliates represent a major international effort to provide public health services. The organization plays a central role in obtaining volunteers for blood donations and ensuring the safety and effectiveness of the U.S. and world supply of blood products in collaboration with the U.S. Food and Drug Administration. The ability of the Red Cross to obtain donations, mobilize volunteers, and publicize the need for disaster assistance has allowed it to play a central role in providing lifesaving public health services.

Many private organizations provide public health education, support research, develop evidence-based recommendations, and provide other public health services. Many of these are organized around specific diseases or types of disease, such as the American Cancer Association, the American Heart Association, the American Lung Association and the March of Dimes, which focuses on birth defects. Other private organizations focus primarily on advocacy for individuals with specific diseases, but these organizations also may advocate for specific public health interventions. For instance, Mothers Against Drunk Driving (MADD) has had a major impact on the passage and enforcement of drunk driving laws. HIV/AIDS advocacy groups have influenced policies on confidentiality, funding, and public education.

Globally, nongovernmental organizations (NGOs) increasingly play a key role in providing services and advocating for public health policies. CARE and OXFAM are examples of the types of organizations involved in global health-related crises. Physician groups, including Physicians for Social Responsibility and Doctors without Borders, have been active in advocating for public health efforts, seeking funding for public health needs, and addressing the ethical implementation of public health programs.

New combinations of governmental and nongovernmental organizations are increasingly developing to fill in the gaps. At the global level, the Global Fund to Fight AIDS, Tuberculosis and Malaria, a public-private effort, provides funding for evidence-based interventions to address these diseases. It is funded not only by governments, but also by private foundations, such as the Bill and Melinda Gates Foundation.

Private foundations have played major roles in funding public health efforts and also stimulating governmental funding. The Rockefeller Foundation's efforts were instrumental in developing local health departments and initiating Schools of Public Health in the United States during the early years of the 20th century. The Kellogg Foundation, the Robert Wood Johnson Foundation, and most recently the Gates Foundation have all played key roles in advancing public health efforts in areas ranging from nutrition to tobacco control to advancing new public health technologies.

Foundation funding has been the catalyst in initiating new funding efforts and sustaining those that are not adequately funded by governments. They cannot be expected, however, to provide long-term support for basic public health services. Thus, additional strategies are required. One key strategy is to link public health efforts with the efforts of healthcare professionals and the healthcare system.

HOW CAN PUBLIC HEALTH AGENCIES PARTNER WITH HEALTH CARE TO IMPROVE THE RESPONSE TO HEALTH PROBLEMS?

We have already seen a number of traditional connections between public health and health care. Clinicians and public health professionals increasingly share a common commitment to evidence-based thinking, cost-effective delivery of services, and computerized and confidential data systems. They also increasingly share a commitment to provide quality services to the entire population and eliminate health disparities. The potential for successful collaboration between public health and health care is illustrated by the National Vaccine Plan, which is discussed in Box 4-4.[10]

In the mid-1990s, a Medicine-Public Health Initiative was initiated to investigate better ways to connect public health with medicine, in particular, and health care, in general. Connecting these two fields has not always had easy or successful results. Additional structures are needed to formalize effective and efficient bonds. Models do exist and new ideas are being put forth to connect clinical care and public health. Box 4-5 discusses one such model called **community-oriented primary care (COPC).**[11]

Despite efforts in the healthcare system to reach out to the community and address public health issues (such as COPC), it remains the primary responsibility of public health to organize and mobilize community-based efforts. Working with nongovernmental organizations and healthcare professionals and organizations is imperative to effectively and efficiently accomplish the goals of public health. But, how exactly can public health agencies accomplish these goals?

BOX 4-4 National Vaccine Plan.

In 1994, a National Vaccine Plan was developed as part of a coordinated effort to accomplish the following goals:

1. Develop new and improved vaccines.
2. Ensure the optimal safety and effectiveness of vaccines and immunizations.
3. Better educate the public and members of the health profession on the benefits and risks of immunizations.

A recent Institute of Medicine (IOM) report evaluated progress since 1994 on achieving the above goals and made recommendations for the development of a revised National Vaccine Plan.[10] The IOM highlighted a number of successes since 1994 in achieving each of the goals of the Plan. These successes illustrate the potential for improved collaboration between public health systems and healthcare systems.

In terms of the development of new and improved vaccines since 1994, over 20 new vaccine products resulting from the collaborative efforts of the National Institutes of Health (NIH), academic, and industry researchers were approved by the Food and Drug Administration (FDA). Novel vaccines introduced include vaccines against pediatric pneumococcal disease, meningococcal disease, and the human papillomavirus (HPV)—a cause of cervical cancer.

In terms of safety, vaccines and vaccination approaches with improved safety have been developed since 1994, including those directed against rotavirus, pertussis (whooping cough), and polio. The FDA Center for Biologics Evaluation and Research (CBER), which regulates vaccines, now has an expanded array of regulatory tools to facilitate the review and approval of safe and efficacious vaccines. The FDA and the Centers for Disease Control and Prevention (CDC) have collaborated on surveillance for and evaluation of adverse events. Efforts have also been made to increase collaboration with the Centers for Medicare and Medicaid, the Department of Defense, and the Department of Veterans Affairs to improve surveillance and reporting of adverse events following immunization in the adult populations these agencies serve.

In terms of better education of health professionals and the public, progress has also been made. The American Academy of Pediatrics (AAP) collaborates with the CDC for its Childhood Immunization Support. The American Medical Association (AMA) cosponsors the annual National Influenza Vaccine Summit, a group that represents 100 public and private organizations interested in preventing influenza.

Despite the growing collaboration and success in vaccine development and use, new issues have appeared in recent years. Vaccines are now correctly viewed by the health professionals and the public as having both benefits and harms. In recent years, the public has grown more concerned about the safety of vaccines, including the issue of the use of large numbers of vaccines in children. The limitations of vaccines to address problems, such as HIV/AIDS, have also been increasingly recognized. Hopefully, the new National Vaccine Plan will build upon these recent successes and address the new realities and opportunities.

HOW CAN PUBLIC HEALTH TAKE THE LEAD IN MOBILIZING COMMUNITY PARTNERSHIPS TO IDENTIFY AND SOLVE HEALTH PROBLEMS?

An essential service of public health is the mobilization of community partnerships and action to identify and solve health problems. These efforts by public health agencies are critical to putting the pieces of the health system together to protect and promote health and prevent disability and death.

Examples of successful collaboration include state tobacco control programs that have been led by public health agencies, but rely heavily on nongovernmental organizations, healthcare professionals and other governmental agencies. These efforts have been able to substantially reduce statewide cigarette smoking rates.

Efforts to organize coordinated programs for lead control have also met with some success. Collaborative efforts between public health and health care have identified and treated children with elevated lead levels. Cooperation with other agencies has provided for the removal of lead paint from homes and testing and control of lead in playgrounds, water, and most recently, toys.

It is possible to view the coordinated mobilization of public and private efforts as **community-oriented public health (COPH)**. We can see this as a parallel to COPC. In COPC, healthcare efforts are expanded to take on additional public health roles. In COPH, public health efforts are expanded to collaborate with healthcare delivery institutions, as well as other community and governmental efforts. Child oral health, an example of COPH, is illustrated in Box 4-6.[12]

Developing community partnerships is a time-consuming and highly political process that requires great leadership and diplomatic skills. Central authority and command and con-

BOX 4-5 Community Oriented Primary Care (COPC).

Community-oriented primary care (COPC) is a structured effort to expand the delivery of health services from a focus on the individual to also include an additional focus on the needs of communities. Serving the needs of communities brings healthcare and public health efforts together. COPC can be seen as an effort on the part of healthcare delivery sites, such as community health centers, to reach out to their community and to governmental public health institutions.

Table 4-4 outlines the six steps in the COPC process and presents a question to ask when addressing each of these steps. Notice the parallels between COPC and the evidence-based approach that we have outlined. In both cases, the process is actually circular because evaluation efforts often lead to recycling to move the process ahead.

TABLE 4-4 The Six Sequential Steps of Community-Oriented Primary Care (COPC)

Steps in the COPC process	Questions to ask
1. Community definition	How is the community defined based upon geography, institutional affiliation, or other common characteristics, e.g., use of an Internet site?
2. Community characterization	What are the demographic and health characteristics of the community and what are its health issues?
3. Prioritization	What are the most important health issues facing the community and how should they be prioritized based upon objective data and perceived need?
4. Detailed assessment of the selected health problem	What are the most effective and efficient interventions for addressing the selected health problem based upon an evidence-based assessment?
5. Intervention	What strategies will be used to implement the intervention?
6. Evaluation	How can the success of the intervention be evaluated?

Source: Data from District of Columbia Area Health Education Center. The Conceptual Framework for COPC. Available at: http://dcahec.gwumc.edu/education/session4/index.html. Accessed November 8, 2008.

A series of principles underlies COPC including:

- Healthcare needs are defined by examining the community as a whole, not just those who seek care.
- Needed healthcare services are provided to everyone within a defined population or community.
- Preventive, curative, and rehabilitative care are integrated within a coordinated delivery system.
- Members of the community directly participate in all stages of the COPC process.

The concept of COPC, if not the specific structure, has been widely accepted as an approach for connecting the organized delivery of primary health care with public health. It implies that public health issues can and should be addressed when possible at the level of the community with the involvement of healthcare providers and the community members themselves.

trol approaches are generally not effective in the complex organizational structures of the United States. New approaches and new strategies are needed to bring together the organizations and individuals who can get the job done.

We have now looked at the organization of the public health system and the challenges it faces in accomplishing its

BOX 4-6 Child Oral Health and Community Oriented Public Health (COPH).

The problem of childhood dental disease illustrates the potential for community-oriented public health (COPH). A lack of regular dental care remains a major problem for children in developed, as well as developing countries. The need for this type of care is often high on the agenda of parents, teachers, and even the children themselves.

Public health efforts to improve oral health go back to the late 19th- and early 20th centuries when toothbrushing and toothpaste were new and improved technologies. The public health campaigns of the early 20th century were very instrumental in making toothbrushing a routine part of American life. The history of public health interventions in childhood oral health is a story of great hope and partial success. The benefits of the fluoridation of drinking water were well grounded in evidence. The American Dental Association and the American Medical Association have supported this intervention for over half a century. Resistance from those who view it as an intrusion of governmental authority, however, has prevented universal use of fluoridation in the United States. After over a half century of effort, fluoridation has reached less than two-thirds of Americans through the water supply.

Today, new technologies from dental sealants to more cost-effective methods for treating cavities have again made oral health a public health priority. However, the number of dentists has not grown in recent years to keep up with the growing population. In addition, dental care for those without the resources to pay for it is often inadequate and inaccessible. Thus, a new approach is needed to bringing dental care to those in need. Perhaps a new strategy of COPH can make this happen.

Community-oriented public health can reach beyond the institutional and geographical constraints that COPC faces when based in a community health center or other institutions serving a geographically defined population or community. COPH as a governmentally led effort allows a greater range of options for intervention includes those that require changes in laws, incentives and governmental procedures. These might include: authorizing new types of clinicians, providing services in nontraditional settings such as schools, funding innovations to put new technologies into practice, and addressing the regulatory barriers to rapid and cost-effective delivery of services.

core functions and providing its essential services. The role of public health cannot be viewed only in its current form. Understanding public health also requires considering its future and how we can plan for the expected and the unexpected.

Key Words

- Core public health functions
- Assessment
- Assurance
- Policy development
- Ten essential public health services
- Home rule authority
- Healthcare safety net
- Community-oriented primary care (COPC)
- Community-oriented public health (COPH)

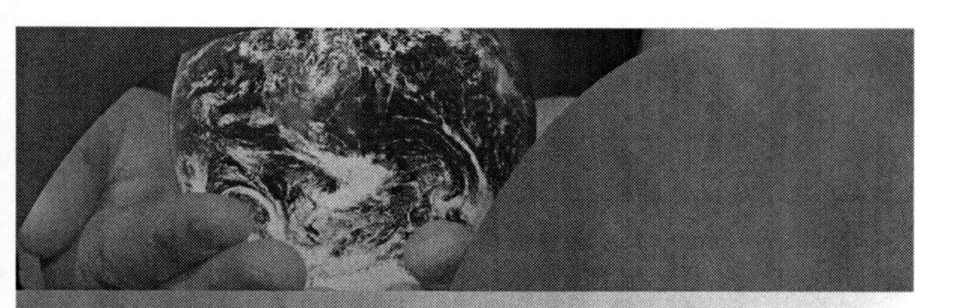

Discussion Question

Take a look at the questions posed in the following scenarios which were presented at the beginning of this chapter. See now whether you can answer them.

1. *A young man in your dormitory is diagnosed with tuberculosis. The health department works with the student health service to test everyone in the dorm, as well as in his classes, with a TB skin test. Those who are positive for the first time are advised to take a course of a medicine called INH. You ask: is this standard operating procedure?*
2. *You go to a public health meeting and learn that many of the speakers are not from public health agencies, but from the Departments of Labor, Commerce, Housing, and Education. You ask: what do these departments have to do with health?*
3. *You hear that a new childhood vaccine was developed by the NIH, approved by the FDA, endorsed for federal payment by the CDC and recommended for use by the American Academy of Pediatrics. You ask: do all these agencies and organizations always work so well together?*
4. *A major flood in Asia leads to disease and starvation. Some say it is due to global warming, others to bad luck. Coordinated efforts by global health agencies, assisted by nongovernmental organizations (NGOs) and outside governmental donors, help get the country back on its feet. You ask: what types of cooperation are needed to make all of this happen?*
5. *A local community health center identifies childhood obesity as a problem in their community. They collect data demonstrating that the problem begins as early as elementary school. They develop a plan that includes clinical interventions at the health center and also at the elementary school. They ask the health department to help them organize an educational campaign and assist in evaluating the results. Working together, they are able to reduce the obesity rate among elementary school children by one half. This seems like a new way to practice public health, you conclude. What type of approach is this?*

REFERENCES

1. Public Health in America. Essential Public Health Services. Available at: http://www.health.gov/phfunctions/public.htm. Accessed April 3, 2009.
2. Institute of Medicine. *The Future of Public Health.* Washington, DC: National Academies Press; 1988.
3. Turnock BJ. *Public Health: What It Is and How It Works.* 4th ed. Sudbury, MA: Jones and Bartlett Publishers; 2009.
4. Turnock BJ. *Essentials of Public Health.* Sudbury, MA: Jones and Bartlett Publishers; 2007.
5. United States Department of Health and Human Services. Organizational Chart. Available at: http://www.hhs.gov/about/orgchart/. Accessed April 3, 2009.
6. Centers for Disease Control and Prevention. History of CDC. *Morbidity and Mortality Weekly Report.* 1996;45: 526–528.
7. World Health Organization. About WHO. Available at: http://www.who.int/about/en/. Accessed April 3, 2009.
8. The World Bank. Health, Nutrition and Population. Available at: http://web.worldbank.org/WBSITE/EXTERNAL/TOPICS/EXTHEALTH NUTRITIONANDPOPULATION/0,,menuPK:282516~pagePK:149018~piPK:149093~theSitePK:282511,00.html. Accessed April 3, 2009.
9. Duffin J, Sweetman A. *SARS in Context: Memory, History, Policy.* Montreal: McGill-Queen's University Press; 2006.
10. Institute of Medicine. Initial Guidance for an Update of the National Vaccine Plan: A Letter Report to the National Vaccine Program Office. Available at: http://www.nap.edu/catalog/12257.html. Accessed April 3, 2009.
11. District of Columbia Area Health Education Center. The Conceptual Framework for COPC. Available at: http://dcahec.gwumc.edu/education/session4/index.html. Accessed April 3, 2009.
12. Pfizer Global Pharmaceuticals. *Milestones in Public Health: Accomplishments in Public Health over the Last 100 Years.* New York: Pfizer Global Pharmaceuticals; 2006.

CHAPTER 5

Ethical and Human Rights Concerns in Global Health

Learning Objectives

By the end of this chapter the reader will be able to:

- Discuss some of the key treaties and conventions related to human rights
- Discuss the meaning of a "human rights" approach to health
- Review selected ethical and human rights concerns as they relate to global health
- Review the most important ethical guidelines for research on human subjects
- Discuss some of the most historically significant cases in human subjects research

VIGNETTES

Suraiya was a 21-year-old woman in Kabul, Afghanistan. Her sister recently died in childbirth at the age of 16 years. She had taken her sister to a health center when she was having trouble with her labor. However, the health center was 50 miles away from their house. In addition, partly because of the neglect of the last government and its discrimination against women, the health center was dilapidated. It had no equipment and the midwife there was unable to save Suraiya's sister. The baby died a few days later.

John Williams was a 21-year-old office clerk in a small country in Africa. For 3 months, he had experienced weight loss, continuous fever, and chronic fatigue. He finally got up the strength to visit the local hospital. When he got there, the staff was not welcoming. They did not treat him kindly. They did not offer to help him. They did not arrange for him to be seen by a doctor. They knew that he had HIV and did not want to treat him in their hospital.

Nandita, like many newborns, died in her first week of life in a small village in the highlands of Nepal. She had been born to a poor family in an area that was very underdeveloped and dominated by large landlords. The area around their home had almost no health workers. Her mother had no formal education, had received no prenatal care or counseling about the birth, and could not get medical help when the baby fell ill. There are international agreements about "the right to health" to which Nepal is a signator. Therefore, it is important to ask questions, such as: Was Nepal unable to provide the health services needed to save lives like Nandita's or were the political and social forces in Nepal unwilling to make such services a priority? Is this failure a matter of health policy, human rights, or both?

A potential microbicide against HIV was being tested on women in 10 cities in Africa. The women were to apply the microbicide before any sexual encounter. The developers of the microbicide were hopeful that it would be at least partially effective in stopping the transmission of HIV. However, there was still a risk that some of the women using the microbicide would become HIV positive while participating in the study. There was an important debate among those working on the microbicide about their ethical obligations to anyone who became HIV positive. Did they have to provide them with AIDS drugs for the remainder of their life, as some were suggesting?

THE IMPORTANCE OF ETHICAL AND HUMAN RIGHTS ISSUES IN GLOBAL HEALTH

Ethical and human rights issues are extremely important in global health because they cut across many areas of both human endeavor and government responsibility. In addition, there is a strong complementarity between good ethical and human rights practices on the one hand and good health outcomes on the other.[1] The previous vignettes touch only a very small sample of the many areas in global health that relate to ethical and human rights matters.

The importance of human rights issues to global health is highlighted by the fact that there are international conventions and treaties that recognize access to health services and health information, among other health areas, as human rights. Yet, there are remarkable gaps in many countries in access to health services. In addition, the poor and the disenfranchised suffer from those gaps the most.

Moreover, the failure to respect human rights is often associated with harm to human health. This has often been the case, for example, concerning diseases that are highly stigmatized, such as leprosy, TB, and HIV. If leprosy patients are not provided with the best standards of care because some health workers are afraid to work with them, the leprosy patients cannot stop the progression of their disease. If TB patients are shunned by health workers, they will die, after infecting many other people. There are many examples, such as in the vignettes about Suraiya and John, that show how the failure to respect the right to health of women or of HIV positive people can lead to poor health outcomes.

There are also a number of critical ethical issues that relate to global health. Some concern ensuring that decisions about health investments are fair, are made in fair ways, and take sufficient account of equity across groups. Another set of ethical matters is associated with appropriate ways to carry out research on human subjects.

Finally, efforts to maintain public health while dealing with new and emerging diseases, such as SARS or a potential avian influenza, raise an array of ethical and human rights issues. When we face a potential health threat, for example, what are the rights of individuals compared to the rights of society to protect itself from illness? Is it acceptable to quarantine a city? It is fair to ban travel to and from certain places? Should patients with TB who refuse to take their medicines be kept in a hospital and forced to take them? These are real issues with which health practitioners and policy makers must wrestle.

This chapter will provide an overview of some of the most critical links between human rights and global health. It will also examine how some of those links have evolved. It will briefly review the most important charters and conventions that set the foundation for the health and human rights concerns we have today. It will also touch upon a number of ethical issues that are central to global health. The chapter will conclude with comments on key challenges to enhancing ethical and human rights interests in global health activities.

The chapter is meant to be introductory. Nonetheless, it is very important as you review this chapter that you get a sense of key concerns about ethics and human rights as they relate to global health. It is also critical that you keep these concerns in mind both as you read this book and as you do further reading, writing, or working in the field of global health. More detailed information can be found in the materials that are referenced in this chapter.

THE FOUNDATIONS FOR HEALTH AND HUMAN RIGHTS

There are a number of treaties and conventions that set the foundation for human rights concerns. The most significant international declaration which focuses on human rights is the Universal Declaration of Human Rights (UDHR), which was promulgated in 1948. The UDHR is generally regarded as the cornerstone on which most of the later treaties and documents pertaining to human rights are based. The UDHR is also considered to set the standard for human rights globally, despite the fact that it does not have the force of law.

With respect to health, the UDHR states in Article 25:

> (1) Everyone has the right to a standard of living adequate for the health and well-being of himself and of his family, including food, clothing, housing and medical care and necessary social services, and the right to security in the event of unemployment, sickness, disability, widowhood, old age or other lack of livelihood in circumstances beyond his control.
>
> (2) Motherhood and childhood are entitled to special care and assistance. All children, whether born in or out of wedlock, shall enjoy the same social protection.[2]

Since 1948, more than 20 multilateral treaties that relate to health have been formulated which are legally binding on the countries that sign them. The European Convention on the Protection of Human Rights was signed in 1950. In 1966, two important treaties were adopted, The International Covenant on Economic, Social, and Cultural Rights (ICESR) and The International Covenant on Civil and Political Rights (ICCPR).[2–4] The ICESR has been ratified and signed by 155 countries and the ICCPR by 160 countries.[5,6] The ICESCR focuses on the well-being of individuals, including their right to work in safe conditions, receive fair wages, be free from hunger, get an education, and enjoy the highest attainable standard of physical and mental health. The ICCPR discusses rights of equality, liberty, security, and "freedom of movement, religion, expression, and association."[2–4]

In addition, under the auspices of the United Nations, a number of other important international conventions have been written, especially on specialized topics. The Convention on the Elimination of all Forms of Discrimination Against Women, for example, was adopted in 1979 by the United Nations General Assembly. It has been ratified by 83 countries. The Convention commits states to legally promote equality between men and women, ensure effective protection against discrimination against women, and to eliminate discriminatory practices aganst women. The Convention also affirms the reproductive rights of women.[7] A number of regional treaty arrangements on human rights, the most extensive of which are European and Latin American, are complementary to the UN human rights treaty system.

Many international human rights documents, including the ICCPR, have specific clauses for protecting the rights of children. Most articles in the general human rights instruments also apply equally to both adults and children. The Convention on the Rights of the Child (CRC), however, which was agreed upon in 1989, is the first human rights document which focuses specifically on the rights of children.[8] This document, which defines a child as "every human being below the age of 18 years," accords rights to be free of discrimination due to ethnicity, disability, or any other cause. It also grants the right to health and education. In addition, it includes the premise that children must have a say in decisions affecting their lives. The CRC also puts the rights of children on the same plane as the rights of adults.[8]

In its own words, the Convention on the Rights of the Child says the following, among other things, concerning health and education:

> States Parties recognize the right of the child to the enjoyment of the highest attainable standard of health and to facilities for the treatment of illness and rehabilitation of health. States Parties shall strive to ensure that no child is deprived of his or her right of access to such health care services.
>
> States Parties recognize the right of the child to education, and with a view to achieving this right progressively and on the basis of equal opportunity, they shall, in particular:
>
> (a) Make primary education compulsory and available free to all;
>
> (b) Encourage the development of different forms of secondary education, including general and vocational education, make them available and accessible to every child, and take appropriate measures such as the introduction of free education and offering financial assistance in case of need;
>
> (c) Make higher education accessible to all on the basis of capacity by every appropriate means;
>
> (d) Make educational and vocational information and guidance available and accessible to all children;
>
> (e) Take measures to encourage regular attendance at schools and the reduction of drop out rates.[8]

THE "RIGHTS BASED APPROACH"

"Human rights" is a term with which most people are familiar but which many people find difficult to define. It *is* generally accepted, however, that the "International Bill of Rights" is made up of the Universal Declaration of Human Rights, the International Covenant on Civil and Political Rights, and the International Covenant on Economic, Social, and Cultural Rights. It is also accepted that governments have an obligation to respect these rights, take measures to enforce them, and take steps to prevent others from violating them.[9]

In simple terms, if we were to apply the human rights concepts discussed above to global health, this would mean, among other things that we would:

- assess the impact of health policies, programs, and practices on human rights
- take account of the health impacts resulting from violations of human rights
- see health and human rights as inextricably linked and bring this notion to consideration of the determinants of health and ways in which health issues may be addressed.[1]

If we took this perspective, it would also cause us to pay particular attention in the design and implementation of global health efforts to:

- the participation in program design and planning of affected parties and communities
- equity across groups

- the empowerment of individuals over their own lives
- holding people accountable for engaging in health efforts in a manner that respects human rights.[10]

In addition, this approach to work in health would cause us to ask the following questions about different health interventions:

- Who is being served?
- How are they being served?
- Are they being served fairly?
- Are they being served with dignity and respect for their culture?
- Are they participating in decisions about these services?
- Are decisions made in open and transparent ways, in conjunction with the community?
- Who is not being served, and why are they not being served?
- Is there clear accountability for the services being rendered appropriately or not?[10]

SELECTED HUMAN RIGHTS ISSUES

There are a variety of human rights issues that relate to health that could be discussed here. In the section that follows, however, four selected topics are examined briefly because they are indicative of some of these human rights issues. These include: health as a human right, HIV/AIDS and human rights, some matters related to patents and access to medicines, and the extent to which human rights in health are absolute.

Health as a Human Right

The preamble to the constitution of the World Health Organization, which was formulated in 1946, states, "The enjoyment of the highest attainable standard of health is one of the fundamental rights of every human being."[11] In addition, as noted above, a number of treaties signed after 1946 have further promoted the principle that health is a fundamental human right. One very important question, however, is the extent to which countries are able or willing to honor this right.

The simplest answer to this question is that, while there is increasing attention globally to the links between health and human rights, there is no mechanism for holding countries accountable for ensuring that they honor or even try to honor the right to health. The international mechanism now in place for reviewing compliance with treaties and conventions that include the right to health is voluntary reporting by countries. In addition, there are provisions in human rights treaties and conventions that recognize that resource poor countries will not be able to help all of their people to "achieve the highest standard of health possible."[9] There is also no clear definition of the meaning of the right to health or indicators agreed among countries for measuring progress against that goal.[12] Although there is considerable attention to the MDGs and the progress of meeting them, the discussion that surrounds the MDGs globally frequently does not explicitly take human rights issues into account.

Nonetheless, several countries, including Brazil, Thailand, and South Africa have recently incorporated human rights important to health into national legislation and new constitutions.[13] In addition, a 1999 court case in Venezuela has interesting relevance to the matter of health and human rights. In this case, the court held that the Venezuelan government violated the constitutional right of its people to health by failing to guarantee people living with HIV/AIDS access to antiretroviral therapy. The court ruled that this right is both part of the Venezuelan constitution and also a part of the ICESCR, to which Venezuela is party.[14]

Human Rights and HIV/AIDS

As much as any health condition in history, HIV/AIDS raises a host of human rights issues. These issues arise partly from the fact that HIV/AIDS is a health condition that is associated in most cultures with significant amounts of stigma and discrimination. Many people see HIV/AIDS, for example, as a disease that people bring on themselves by engaging in what they consider to be promiscuous behavior. This could include engaging in homosexual sex, injecting drug use, having multiple sex partners, or participating in commercial sex work. In addition, in places that are not familiar with how the disease is spread, there is often great fear of catching the disease. Although an entire book could be written about this subject, some brief comments are given on a small number of the human rights issues related to HIV/AIDS.

An important question that has arisen in many societies is how to protect the rights of people who are HIV positive to employment, schooling, and full participation in social activities. When the epidemic was first recognized in a number of developed countries, there was considerable discrimination against people who are HIV positive, some of whom lost their jobs or were not allowed to enroll in school. Such discrimination continues in many places, which raises fundamental questions of the rights of people who are living with HIV/AIDS.

Another matter that has arisen, as suggested earlier, is the access of people with HIV to health care. At least at the early stages of an HIV epidemic in a country, most health workers are poorly informed about HIV, not aware of how it is spread, and have serious fears about caring for people who are HIV positive. There are examples of many settings in which people living with HIV/AIDs have been denied care or treated with discrimination and stigma when they did receive care.

There are also a number of questions concerning HIV testing. For many years, a cardinal principle of work on HIV has been that testing for it should be voluntary and confidential. This is to ensure that people are not forced against their will to get tested and then discriminated against if people find out that they are HIV-positive. More recently, however, an increasing number of people involved in HIV activities have come to believe that in settings with high rates of prevalence of HIV, every adult should be tested for it. People promoting this approach want to encourage much greater testing for HIV because it is spread largely by people who are HIV positive, do not know their status, and have unprotected sex with multiple partners.

In line with this, Botswana has become the first country to have a policy of testing for HIV that is based on "opting out" of testing, rather than volunteering to get tested. In this case, any adult having contact with the health system is asked to take an HIV test. They have to opt out and ask not to get a test or one will be given. Despite the increasing calls for this type of approach, there remains considerable concern among a substantial number of those involved in HIV efforts that even a well-organized country like Botswana will not be able to implement such a program without *de facto* coercion of people to get tested.[15]

Other human rights issues that relate to HIV/AIDS concern the issue of patient confidentiality. For many years, there has been widespread agreement that HIV information about patients needed to be kept confidential to ensure that those who are HIV positive would not be discriminated against. Yet, the healthcare settings in many resource-poor countries that have high rates of HIV are poorly organized, do not operate very efficiently, and are not accustomed to treating patients and patient records confidentially. They also may not have the physical space to treat their patients privately and confidentially.

In addition, and also related to concerns about privacy, there are important questions about disclosure of HIV status. Should the healthcare system notify spouses or sexual partners of the HIV status of patients? Should the patients do that? What are the risks, for example, if a husband is notified about the status of his wife that he may harm her, reject her, or that his family will throw her out of the house?

Those issues are just a small sample of the many rights related questions that arise in relation to HIV/AIDS. While these questions may be more prominent when thinking about HIV/AIDS, many of them are relevant to health more generally, such as treating people with respect, treating patients and their records confidentially, not discriminating against people because of their health conditions, and being sensitive to the social and cultural milieus within which patients live.

Human Rights Are Not Always Absolute

The importance of protecting human rights related to health is widely acknowledged. Yet, it is also widely understood that there are exceptional circumstances under which these rights may be temporarily suspended, such as to protect the interest of the public during an influenza epidemic when governments might suspend for a certain time the right of people to leave their homes, to go to work, to travel, or to participate in mass gatherings, such as sporting events. Few people would deny the obligation of governments to have laws that govern public health actions. However, most of those working in public health also believe that any suspension of rights must be carried out with due process. They also believe that it is very important to monitor rights during the suspension period and make all efforts to reinstate rights as soon as possible.[16]

Intellectual Property Rights and Global Health

Any discussion of global health and human rights brings up the question of access to medicines and how this is affected by patent rights. This has become an especially important and contentious matter in the last decade, as the World Trade Organization has been formed and agreements concerning patents have been negotiated, as part of the TRIPS Agreement (Trade-Related Aspects of Intellectual Property Rights). This question has also come to the forefront because of the high costs of drugs to treat AIDS, the inability of most HIV-affected people in low-income countries to pay for those drugs, and the concern of many people that it is not ethical or just to allow so many people to die of AIDS in developing countries when medicines are available to treat them. The challenge with respect to patents for medicines needed by the poor in the developing world is how to encourage scientific discovery of diagnostics, drugs, and vaccines while ensuring the affordability of medicines by poor people in poor countries.

The basic principle behind granting intellectual property rights is to provide incentives for research, development, and use of new technologies. Patents give the inventor the right to exclude others from making, selling, or importing his invention for a fixed time period. The quasi-monopoly granted to the patent holder allows the setting of prices without regard to ordinary market forces and, therefore, allows higher prices than would be the case in the event of competition.

Many people believe that the possibility of getting a patent on a discovery, such as a drug, is essential to ensuring the continued search for new drugs. This is certainly the position of the major pharmaceutical manufacturers and is embedded in international trade agreements to a large extent. On the other hand, WHO has pointed out that in spite of the incentives of patents, only 11 out of the 1223 chemicals developed between 1975 and 1996 were to treat some of the most important diseases that affect poor people in low- and middle-income countries.[17] In fact, a recent WHO commission on intellectual property rights and innovation concluded that patents are only one of a number of factors that encourage innovation of pharmaceutical products and that financial and other incentives are also important. The commission also said that it was important that mechanisms be adopted to ensure access to pharmaceutical products when they are developed.[18]

Some countries have historically refused to grant patents or have granted only process patents on what they regard as "essential drugs," because they believe that their people have a right to these drugs at affordable prices. In principle, the human rights approach to health does not reject the concept of intellectual property rights. However, it does focus on the effect that granting such rights has on the more marginalized and disadvantaged sections of people. It is with this in mind that those advocating a human rights approach to health, as well as others concerned about the price of medicines, insist on safeguard mechanisms to ensure access to medicines by all who need them, and on special exceptions to intellectual property rights for least developed countries.[19]

TABLE 5-1 The Standards of the Nuremburg Code

- Those who participate in the study must freely give their consent to do so. They must be given information on the "nature, duration, and purpose of the experiment." They should know how it will be conducted. They must not be forced or coerced in any way to participate in the experiment.
- The experiment must produce valuable benefits that can not be gotten in other ways.
- The experiment should be based on animal studies and a knowledge of the natural history of the disease or condition being studied.
- The conduct of the research should avoid all unnecessary physical and mental suffering and injury.
- The degree of risk of the research should never exceed that related to the nature of the problem to be addressed.
- The research should be conducted in appropriate facilities that can protect research subjects from harm.
- The research must be conducted by a qualified team of researchers.
- The research subject should be able to end participation at any time.
- The study will be promptly stopped if adverse effects are seen.

Source: Data from Regulations and Ethical Guidelines—Directives for Human Experimentation—Nuremberg Code. Available at: http://ohsr.od.nih.gov/guidelines/nuremberg.html. Accessed August 3, 2006.

THE FOUNDATIONS FOR RESEARCH ON HUMAN SUBJECTS

The foundations for research on human subjects developed out of concerns about unethical and inhumane Nazi experiementation on human subjects during World War II. These concerns grew as people learned more about the medical experiments that the Nazis conducted on prisoners during the war. The first set of guidelines for the ethical conduct of research on human subjects was issued in 1948 and others have followed since then.

The Nuremberg Code

The Nuremberg Code was formulated in 1948, following the verdict of an American military war crimes tribunal that conducted proceedings against 23 Nazi physicians and administrators for their willing participation in what were deemed to be war crimes and crimes against humanity. This group had conducted research studies and experiments on concentration camp prisoners that resulted in death or permanent deformity. The Nuremberg Code sets specific requirements which physicians are supposed to follow when conducting experiments on human subjects.[20] (See Table 5-1.)

The Declaration of Helsinki

In 1964, the World Medical Association developed a set of ethical principles for biomedical research with human subjects. The main purpose of the Declaration of Helsinki was to ensure adequate protection of the rights of individuals who participated in such research. The Declaration of Helsinki was revised in 1975, 1983, 1989, 1996, and 2000.[21]

The basic principles of the Declaration of Helsinki are noted in Table 5-2.

On July 12, 1974, the U.S. National Commission for the Protection of Human Subjects of Biomedical and Behavioral Research was created via the United States National Research Act. The mandate of the Commission was to help identify basic ethical principles for the conduct of biomedical and behavioral research in human subjects and to develop guidelines that researchers would be required to follow so that all human research is in line with the ethical principles identified. The Commission prepared what has come to be known as the Belmont Report. The research principles in that report are outlined in Table 5-3.

These principles are to be put into practice by getting informed consent from any study participant, ensuring that the research is grounded in a rigorous assessment of risks and benefits, and being certain that participants are selected fairly.[22]

TABLE 5-2 The Declaration of Helsinki—Basic Principles

- A physician's duty in research is to protect the life, health, privacy, and dignity of the human participant.
- Research involving humans must conform to generally accepted scientific principles and be based on a thorough knowledge of scientific literature and methods.
- Such research must be governed by research protocols and those protocols should be reviewed by an independent committee.
- Research should be conducted by medically/scientifically qualified individuals.
- The risks and burdens to the participants should not outweigh benefits.
- A researcher should stop a study if risks are found to outweigh potential benefits.
- Research is justified only if there is a reasonable likelihood that the population participating in the study will benefit from the results.
- Participants must be volunteers and give their informed consent to such participation.
- Every precaution must be taken to respect privacy, confidentiality, and participant's physical and mental integrity.
- Tests of medicines must be against the best available medicine that already exists.
- Study participants should get access to any diagnostics or medicines that are developed as a result of the study.
- Investigators are obliged to preserve the accuracy of results; negative and positive results should be publicly available.

Source: Data from World Medical Association, Declaration of Helsinki. Available at: http://www.wma.net/e/policy/b3.htm. Accessed August 12, 2006.

KEY HUMAN RESEARCH CASES

There are a number of cases of research on human subjects historically which have helped to raise ethical concerns about such research and encouraged the development of guidelines for such research, as well. Among the best known of these is the Tuskegee Study that took place in the United States. Several other U.S. cases have also been instrumental in establishing guidance on carrying out research on human subjects. These are discussed briefly below. It is important to note that these took place at times when guidelines for such research were not nearly as developed as they are today.

The Tuskegee Study

In 1932, the United States Public Health Service, in collaboration with the Tuskegee Institute, began a study in Macon County, Alabama, to record the natural history of syphilis. One of the aims of this study was to justify syphilis treatment programs for African Americans, at a time of considerable discrimination against such people and the lack of such programs. This study was called the "Tuskegee Study of Untreated Syphilis in the Negro Male."[23]

Six hundred African-American men took part in the study, 399 with syphilis and 201 who did not have the disease. The men were told by researchers that they were being treated for "bad blood," a term that was used locally to describe a number of ailments, including syphilis, anemia, and fatigue. Those participating in the study received free medical exams, meals, and burial insurance. The study was originally projected to last 6 months but went on for 40 years.[23]

In July 1972, a front-page story appeared in the New York Times about the Tuskegee study. This article caused immense public concern and led the Assistant Secretary for Health and Scientific Affairs to appoint an advisory panel to review the study. The panel found that the men had never been properly informed of the real purpose of the study, that they had been misled, and that they lacked the information needed to give informed consent to participate in the study. In addition, the panel found that the men were never given adequate treatment for their disease even when penicillin became the drug of choice for syphilis in 1947. The panel further found that the participants were never given the choice

TABLE 5-3 The Belmont Report

Basic Ethical Principles
- Respect for Persons: The autonomy of individuals must always be respected and persons with diminished autonomy are entitled to protection.
- Beneficence: Research subjects should be protected from harm at all times. Efforts must also be made to maximize possible benefits and minimize possible harms.
- Justice: The benefits and risks of research must be distributed fairly.

Applications of the Principles
- Informed Consent—Persons must be given an opportunity to choose what shall or shall not happen to them. This must be based on the disclosure to them of sufficient information, in a manner that they can thoroughly understand. This consent must also be given completely voluntarily.
- Assessment of Risks and Benefits—There must be a careful and data based assessment of the magnitude of possible harm and anticipated benefits. This assessment must take account of many possible types of harms and benefits. Inhumane treatment of research subjects is never allowed. Risks must be reduced as far as possible. Special attention should be paid if vulnerable populations will be involved in the research.
- Selection of Subjects—There must be fair procedures and outcomes in the selection of those participating in the research.

Source: Data from Regulations and Ethical Guidelines—The Belmont Report Ethical Principles and Guidelines for the Protection of Human Subjects of Research. Available at: http://ohsr.od.nih.gov/guidelines/belmont.html. Accessed Auguust 3, 2006.

of quitting the study, even when this new, highly effective treatment became widely used.[23]

These findings led the advisory panel to conclude that the knowledge gained from the study was limited when compared to the risks to the study participants and that the study was, therefore, "ethically unjustified." The panel advised that the study immediately be stopped and in November 1972, the Assistant Secretary for Health and Scientific Affairs ended the Tuskegee study.[23]

In the summer of 1973, the study participants received more than $9 million as part of a settlement to a class-action lawsuit filed by the National Association for the Advancement of Colored People (NAACP). As part of the settlement, the U.S. government promised to give free medical and burial services to all living participants, as well as health services for wives, widows, and children who had been infected because of the study.[23]

The manner in which the Tuskegee study was carried out and the important ethical questions it raised are known to almost all researchers who conduct research on human subjects. It has had a profound impact on the carrying out of human subjects research in the future.

The Willowbrook School Study

The Willowbrook State School, situated in New York state in the United States, was an institution for mentally handicapped children. Physicians associated with the institution wanted to do a study of hepatitis, which was rampant at the school. From 1956 to 1972, as part of the study, children were intentionally infected with the hepatitis virus. The study leaders believed that this was ethical because almost all children at the school were likely to become infected within 6 to 12 months after entry to the school and the study leaders did ask the parents of the children to give informed consent for their children's participation in the study. The study design was approved by the funding agency and the Executive Faculty of the New York University School of Medicine. The study was started, however, before there was an appropriate review committee for human experimentation related to the school, but when such a committee was established, it also approved the study design.

The study was halted after public concern about the manner in which it was being conducted. There were two main criticisms of the study. The first concern was that there was no real gain to be had from intentionally infecting the children with hepatitis. Rather, they could have studied the disease in children who became naturally infected. In addition, the school was short on space and it appeared that the only space available was on a ward in which the research was being carried out, which suggested that unless parents consented to their children participating in the study, they could not be admitted to the school. This was thought by critics of the study to be unethical because it essentially coerced parents to participate in the study so that they could get their severely handicapped children into the school.[24,25]

Jewish Chronic Disease Hospital

Studies were conducted at the Jewish Chronic Disease Hospital in New York City in 1963 to better understand the processes involved when the body rejected human transplants. This was done by injecting chronically ill patients who did not have cancer with live human cancer cells. The physicians who managed the study did not inform the patients that they would be injected with live cancer cells. Their rationale in not doing this was that they could safely assume that the patients would reject the cells, and if they were informed they would not have given consent for the live cancer cells to be injected in them. Later review of the study led to the censure of the study investigators, but this was later dropped.[26]

Milgram Obedience Study

Stanley Milgram, a social psychology researcher at Yale University, designed studies to learn about conditions of obedience and disobedience. He asked a group of "teachers," paired to a group of "learners," to give electric shocks of increasing intensity to the learners when the learners made mistakes. Milgram told those serving as teachers that he was studying the effect of punishment on learning behaviors. In fact, he was studying the willingness of the teachers to follow his instructions about shocking the learners. In fact, the learners were not being shocked at all.

In carrying out this experiment, Milgram wanted to understand better what could drive people to be willing to exert pain on others, as was done in World War II during the genocide, when many participants said they harmed others because they were just following orders. Milgram did not reveal the true study design to the teachers, because he wanted to see if they would really give 450 volts of shock to the learners.

Milgram's study was criticized as unethical because it caused great stress to those who thought they were administering the shocks. This raised questions about the extent to which study participants should be subjected to stresses, especially when they were not really told the true design of the study.[27–29]

Institutional Review Boards and Human Subjects Research Today

It is important to reiterate that the studies indicated above were conducted at a time when approaches to research on human subjects were not nearly as well developed as they are today. There are now committees within various organizations that conduct research that review all proposed research on human subjects. These are called Institutional Review Boards (IRBs). As they review proposed research today, they bring to their reviews the lessons and experience that have been generated from research done earlier and some of the problems with such research, such as those indicated above. Individual countries also have organizations that oversee the work of IRBs and help to disseminate knowledge about best practices for their work.

ETHICAL ISSUES IN MAKING INVESTMENT CHOICES IN HEALTH

As noted earlier, one central issue in global health is the need to make choices among investments that can enhance the health of the population. This is necessary, especially in low- and middle-income countries, because resources will always be less than needed to meet all health needs. We have also discussed earlier how cost-effectiveness analysis is one important tool for making such choices. In addition to the issues raised by the application of **cost-effectiveness analysis**, such analysis also raises some interesting ethical issues. A number of these are noted hereafter.

First is the question of the priority that should be given in cost-effectiveness analysis to the worst-off members of society. Many of those who work on health take a view that "benefiting people has greater moral value, the worse off those people are."[30] However, especially in developing countries, there are so many poor people that those carrying out the analysis of health investments and making policies in health will have to consider carefully how much priority they attach to the worse off. Related to this is the question of how such people are defined. Are these people, for example, those who are in ill health today, or are they people who are the most vulnerable to being in ill health in general?[30]

Another interesting question is how one makes choices between providing a small benefit to a large number of people or a large benefit to a small number of people. One case cited in the literature that occurred in the state of Oregon in the United States was an analysis that showed that society would get greater health gains by investing in capping the teeth of 100 people, compared to carrying out the removal of one appendix that was needed because of acute appendicitis. In the end, the state decided that it would have to choose the appendectomy, given that this is life threatening. Consideration of this type of issue caused the state to change its overall approach to the analysis of potential investments in health.[30]

Another ethical issue concerns the choice between "fair chances and best outcomes."[30] Let us say that one has a choice between screening two groups of women for breast cancer. In one group are poor women in a city. In the other group are better-off women in the suburbs. The best outcomes might be achieved by focusing on the better-off women, because they are much more likely to go for follow-up on any findings and have successful outcomes than the poorer women. However, would that be fair? Would it be fairer to give each group an equal chance to get screened? Would it be most fair to focus on the poorer women, given the priority one wants to accord to the disadvantaged? Even if one agreed to put a priority on fair chances, should they be organized by equal proportion, by lottery, or by another method?[30]

There are also interesting questions that arise over the extent to which societal resources should be used to address the health needs of people whose health problems may relate to their own health behaviors. Would you want tax money that you pay to help take care of the health needs of people who smoke? Would you be willing to use your tax money to help meet the health needs of people addicted to heroin? What about someone injured on a motorcycle while not wearing a helmet?[30]

The medical profession provides care only on the basis of need and not on the basis of the actions that have led to that need. Generally, those considering the ethical issues involved in these decisions believe that it would be fair to deny care or give a lower priority to the care of individuals whose behaviors appear to have caused the need for care only if "the needs must have been caused by the behavior; the behavior must have been voluntary; the persons must have known that the behavior would cause the health needs and that if they engaged in it their health needs would receive lower priority."[31] These are rarely, if ever, the case, even when dealing with cigarette smoking, both because it is addictive and because it is usually begun by adolescents who are not well-informed.[31]

There are other questions that arise when considering investment choices in health and the use of cost-effectiveness analysis. These might include decisions about the cut-off value of investments one would be willing to make or the manner in which one should consider people with disabilities, because the methodology for DALYs inherently values a condition of disability less highly than a condition of good health. One could thoughtfully consider these and other related issues at great length. The important point of this section, however, is that it is critical, when considering investment choices and the tools that one will use to make decisions about them, that one should explicitly identify and assess ethical choices and how they relate to the aim of social justice that is at the core of public health work.

KEY CHALLENGES FOR THE FUTURE

Efforts to incorporate ethical and human rights concerns into global health work face a number of challenges. Some of these are briefly indicated here.

One very important point is that many students of public health and global health get insufficient exposure in their training to ethical and human rights issues. Normally, they do have to understand the core concepts of research on human subjects and how an IRB functions. However, they may have few opportunities to take courses that cover broader issues of human rights and health or give them fuller opportunities to cover ethical issues in research and in policy making. This chapter is a small attempt to correct that gap.

Second, as indicated earlier, there are enormous gaps in holding countries accountable for meeting their obligations under international conventions that refer to the right to health. On the one hand, there has been increasing pressure, largely brought on by HIV/AIDS, to hold countries accountable for providing AIDS drugs to their people. On the other hand, as indicated earlier, compliance with human rights norms is self-reported by countries. There are really no indicators for measuring such compliance, and there are really no enforcement mechanisms either. Perhaps the movement to focus attention on global health needs can serve as a platform for having civil society increasingly holding countries accountable for enhancing the right of their people to health, particularly their poorest people.

Third, there is also a lack of explicit review of the fairness of many of the investment choices that are being made, both by countries and by the development assistance agencies with which they work. If one reviews the documents that relate to investments in health in low- and middle-income countries, one will generally see that particular attention is paid to ensuring that project benefits go to disadvantaged people. However, it is rare that there will be explicit reviews or articulation of how investment choices are made, the ethical choices that were a part of them, and the basis for the investment decisions. With respect to HIV/AIDS, for example, what criteria will be used to allocate drugs if there are more people clinically eligible for drugs than the amount of drugs available? Will it be access to the health center, so that there is a greater likelihood that the person will comply with treatment? Will it be pregnancy, so that one can reduce maternal to child transmission?[32] If there were a greater need to articulate these choices more openly, then these decisions might be made more fairly.

In addition, though there has been important progress in establishing IRBs and ensuring that proposed research on human subjects is reviewed before being carried out, there is little review of how the IRBs themselves have been functioning. Such a review and the strengthening of IRBs in relatively weaker or less well endowed settings is important to ensuring that research on human subjects is done properly.[33]

There are also some interesting issues on the agenda of human subjects research that are still being wrestled with internationally. One concerns the standard of care. The Declaration of Helsinki says that vaccines, diagnostics, and therapeutics, for example, must be tested against the best available standard of care that already exists. We may wish to ensure that there is no deviation, even in developing countries, from such standards. However, does this requirement prohibit the development of new drugs, diagnostics, or vaccines that might not be as effective as the existing standard of care but which, nonetheless, might be more cost-effective than that standard in some developing countries?[34]

In addition, considerable attention is being paid to the rights of communities that are participating in research. Some people have suggested that such communities should be given compensation for their participation. Such compensation might include training or cash. It has also been proposed that communities should have access to the products that the study eventually leads to. Thus, if they participated in a study on the effectiveness of AIDS drugs, for example, they would be entitled to such drugs in the future at the expense of those managing the study. There is no clear outcome to such discussions as of yet.[34]

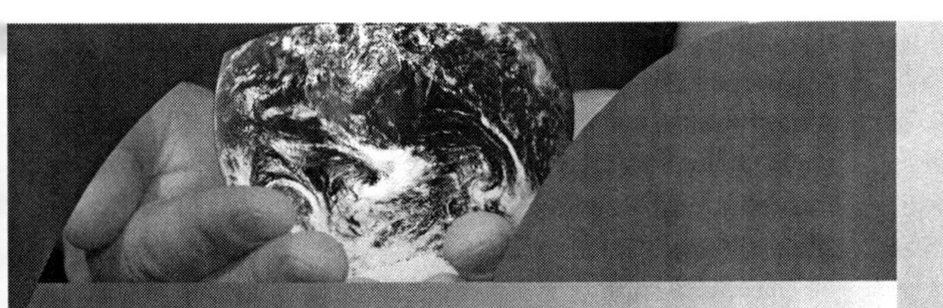

Discussion Questions

1. What is meant by "the right to health?"
2. What are the key features concerning health of the Universal Declaration of Human Rights?
3. What are the most important points of the Convention on the Rights of the Child?
4. How might one carry out a "human rights approach" to health in global health efforts?
5. What are some of the concerns with the impact of patents on the availability of affordable medicines in the developing world?
6. What steps might be taken internationally to encourage the development of drugs, while ensuring their affordability in developing countries?
7. What are some of the key ethical concerns in carrying out research on human subjects?
8. What are some of the most important ethical issues that deserve attention when choices are being made about investments in health?
9. How could one encourage countries and their development partners to pay greater attention to human rights issues in health?
10. What rights and compensation do you think should be given to communities that participate in research on human subjects that is trying to find new drugs?

REFERENCES

1. Mann J, Gostin L, Gruskin S, Brennan T, Lazzarini Z, Fineberg H. Health and Human Rights. *Health and Human Rights.* Fall 1994 1994;1(1):6–23.

2. United Nations General Assembly. Universal Declaration of Human Rights. Available at: http://www.un.org/Overview/rights.html. Accessed September 10, 2006.

3. International Covenant on Economic SaCRI. Unofficial Summary. Available at: http://www.cehat.org/rthc/summary.htm. Accessed September 10, 2006.

4. Office of the United Nations High Commissioner for Human Rights. International Covenant on Civil and Political Rights. Available at: http://www.ohchr.org/english/law/ccpr.htm. Accessed September 10, 2006.

5. Office of the United Nations High Commissioner for Human Rights. International Covenant on Economic, Social and Cultural Rights New York 16 December 1966. Available at: http://www.ohchr.org/english/countries/ratification/3.htm. Accessed January 18, 2007.

6. Office of the United Nations High Commisioner for Human Rights. International Covenant on Civil and Political Rights New York, 16 December 1966. Available at: http://www.ohchr.org/english/countries/ratification/4.htm. Accessed January 18, 2007.

7. United Nations. Convention on the Elimination of All Forms of Discrimination Against Women. Available at: http://www.un.org/womenwatch/daw/cedaw/text/econvention.htm. Accessed January 14, 2007.

8. Office of the United Nations High Commisioner for Human Rights. Convention on the Rights of the Child. Available at: http://www.unhchr.ch/html/menu3/b/k2crc.htm. Accessed August 14, 2006, 2006.

9. Gruskin S, Tarantola D. Health and human rights. In: Gruskin S, Grodin MA, Annas GJ, Marks SP, eds. *Perspectives on Health and Human Rights.* New York: Routledge; 2005:3–58.

10. Gruskin S, Grodin MA, Annas GJ, Marks SP. Introduction: approaches, methods and strategies in health and human rights. In: Gruskin S, Grodin MA, Annas GJ, Marks SP, eds. *Perspectives on Health and Human Rights.* New York: Routledge; 2005:xiii–xx.

11. World Health Organization. Constitution of the World Health Organization. Available at: http://policy.who.int/cgi-bin/om_isapi.dll?hitsperheading=on&infobase=basicdoc&jump=Constitution&softpage=Document42#JUMPDEST_Constitution. Accessed September 15, 2006.

12. Mokhiber CG. Toward a measure of dignity: indicators for rights-based development. In: Gruskin S, Grodin MA, Annas GJ, Marks SP, eds. *Perspectives on Health and Human Rights.* New York: Routledge; 2005:383–392.

13. Gruskin S, Tarantola D. Health and human rights. In: Gruskin S, Grodin MA, Annas GJ, Marks SP, eds. *Perspectives on Health and Human Rights.* New York: Routledge; 2005:23.

14. Torres MA. The human right to health, national courts, and access to HIV/AIDS treatment: a case study from Venezuela. In: Gruskin S, Grodin MA, Annas GJ, Marks SP, eds. *Perspectives on Health and Human Rights.* New York: Routledge; 2005:507–516.

15. Steinbrook R. The AIDS epidemic in 2004. *N Engl J Med.* 2004;351(2):115–117.

16. Easley CE, Marks SP, Morgan Jr. RE. The challenge and place of international human rights in public health. In: Gruskin S, Grodin MA, Annas GJ, Marks SP, eds. *Perspectives on Health and Human Rights.* New York: Routledge; 2005:519–526.

17. Cullet P. Patents and medicines: the relationship between TRIPS and the human right to health. In: Gruskin S, Grodin MA, Annas GJ, Marks SP, eds. *Perspectives on Health and Human Rights.* New York: Routledge; 2005:181.

18. World Health Organization. Public Health, Innovation, and Intellectual Property Rights. Available at: http://www.who.int/intellectualproperty/documents/thereport/ENPublicHealthReport.pdf. Accessed January 13, 2007.

19. Cullet P. Patents and medicines: the relationship between TRIPS and the human right to health. In: Gruskin S, Grodin MA, Annas GJ, Marks SP, eds. *Perspectives on Health and Human Rights.* New York: Routledge; 2005:179-202.

20. National Institutes of Health Office of Human Subjects Research. The Nuremberg Code. Available at: http://ohsr.od.nih.gov/guidelines/nuremberg.html. Accessed August 14, 2006.

21. World Medical Association. Declaration of Helenski. Available at: http://www.wma.net/e/approvedhelsinki.html. Accessed August 5, 2006.

22. U.S. National Institutes of Health Office of Human Subjects Research. The Belmont Report. Available at: http://ohsr.od.nih.gov/guidelines/belmont.html. Accessed August 13, 2006.

23. Centers for Disease Control and Prevention. The Tuskegee Timeline. Available at: http://www.cdc.gov/nchstp/od/tuskegee/time.htm. Accessed January 18, 2007.

24. Texas A&M Philosophy Department. Professional Ethics The Willowbrook Hepatitis Study. Available at: http://falcon.tamucc.edu/~philosophy/pmwiki/pmwiki.php?n=PhilosophyFaculty.WillB. Accessed September 9, 2006.

25. United States Department of Energy. The Development of Human Subject Research at DHEW. Available at: www.eh.doe.gov/ohre/roadmap/achre/chap3_2.html Accessed September 9, 2006.

26. Stanford University. History: The Jewish Chronic Disease Hospital Study. Available at: http://www.stanford.edu/dept/DoR/hs/History/his06.html. Accessed September 9, 2006.

27. Milgram S. The Perils of Obedience. Available at: http://home.swbell.net/revscat/perilsOfObedience.html. Accessed January 18, 2007.

28. University of Rhode Island. Stanley Milgram's Experiment. Available at: http://www.cba.uri.edu/Faculty/dellabitta/mr415s98/EthicEtcLinks/Milgram.htm. Accessed September 9, 2006.

29. Blass A. *The Man Who Shocked the World: The Life and Legacy of Stanley Milgram.* New York: Basic Books; 2004.

30. Brock D, Wikler D. Ethical issues in research allocation, research and new product development. In: Jamison DT, Breman JG, Measham AR, et al., eds. *Disease Control Priorities in Developing Countries.* 2nd ed. New York: Oxford University Press; 2006:259–270.

31. Brock D, Wikler D. Ethical issues in research allocation, research and new product development. In: Jamison DT, Breman JG, Measham AR, et al., eds. *Disease Control Priorities in Developing Countries.* 2nd ed. New York: Oxford University Press; 2006:265.

32. Rosen S, Sanne I, Collier A, Simon JL. Rationing antiretroviral therapy for HIV/AIDS in Africa: choices and consequences. *Public Library of Science.* 2005;2(303).

33. Brock D, Wikler D. Ethical issues in research allocation, research and new product development. In: Jamison DT, Breman JG, Measham AR, et al., eds. *Disease Control Priorities in Developing Countries.* 2nd ed. New York: Oxford University Press; 2006:267.

34. Brock D, Wikler D. Ethical issues in research allocation, research and new product development. In: Jamison DT, Breman JG, Measham AR, et al., eds. *Disease Control Priorities in Developing Countries.* 2nd ed. New York: Oxford University Press; 2006:267–269.

CHAPTER 6

The Public Health Workforce

Learning Objectives

By the end of this chapter, learners will be proficient in identifying and explaining how various occupations, positions, and roles in the public health workforce contribute to carrying out public health's core functions and essential services. Key aspects of this competency expectation include

- Describing the size, composition, and distribution of the current public health workforce
- Identifying and discussing competency frameworks for routine and emergency public health practice
- Describing approaches to strengthening the public health workforce
- Identifying information sources for examining key dimensions of the current and future public health workforce
- Identifying three or more issues that will impact the future public health workforce in terms of its size, composition, and distribution

Public health is important work, and the people who carry out that work contribute substantially to the health status and quality of life of the individuals, families, and communities they serve. Yet public health is not among the best-known or most highly respected careers, in part because when public health efforts are successful, nothing happens. Events that don't occur don't attract attention. For example, the remarkable record of declining mortality rates and ever-increasing spans of healthy life, due in large part to public health efforts, draws little public attention. Indeed, the vast majority of those who will ultimately benefit from the efforts of past and present public health workers are yet to be born. With public health workers not recognized and valued for their accomplishments and contributions, it should not be surprising that careers in public health are among the least understood and appreciated in the health sector.

However, even if the public views public health as poorly defined and abstract, public health workers are real and tangible. These workers make up a **public health workforce** that can be defined and described in several important dimensions, including its size, distribution, composition, skills, and career pathways. Unfortunately, there is less information on these vital statistics of the public health workforce than for many other professional and occupational categories working in the health sector today.

For too long, too little attention has been directed to the public health workforce and its needs. Despite ample warnings in the 1988 Institute of Medicine (IOM) report,[1] there were few efforts between 1980, when Health Resources and Services Administration (HRSA) produced crude estimates of the size and composition for the U.S. Congress,[2] and 2000, when Kristine Gebbie and colleagues completed their landmark enumeration report on the public health workforce at the turn of the century for HRSA.[3] Two decades of inattention provide eloquent testimony to the low priority given to the public health system's most important asset—its workforce.

Beginning in the year 2002, funding for workforce preparedness and training increased dramatically. This influx of funding also brought increased expectations for positive change and greater accountability for results. As a result, the public health system is now under the microscope, with federal, state, and local governments needing to show that the vital signs of the public health infrastructure, including its workforce, are improving. But decades of inattention left little information to serve as a basis for comparison.

A central challenge for public health workforce development efforts over the next decade is to provide more and better information about key dimensions of the public health workforce in terms of its size, distribution, composition, and competency, as well as its impact on public health goals and community health. This chapter, like the *Public Health*

Workforce Enumeration 2000, seeks to advance this important agenda.

This chapter sets the stage for an appreciation of what public health workers do and how they contribute to societal well-being in the 21st century in examining the following questions:

- What is the public health workforce?
- How large is this workforce and how it is distributed?
- What professions and occupations are included?
- How does the public health workforce impact the health of populations?
- Will the public health workforce continue to grow? What trends in the overall economy, the health sector, or the public sector will impact public health jobs and career opportunities in the future?

PUBLIC HEALTH WORK AND PUBLIC HEALTH WORKERS

From a functional perspective, it is the individuals involved in carrying out the core functions and essential services of public health who constitute the public health workforce. Critical to an understanding of this characterization of the public health workforce are the terms **core functions** and **essential public health services**. The practice of public health is described in terms of both its ends (vision, mission, and six broad responsibilities) and how it accomplishes those ends (10 essential public health services). These constitute an aggregate job description for the entire public health workforce, with the workload divided among the many different professional and occupational categories comprising the total public health workforce.

This functional perspective clearly links public health workers to **public health practice**. Unfortunately, this does not simplify the practical task of determining who is, and who is not, part of the public health workforce. There has never been any specific academic degree, even the Master's of Public Health (MPH) degree, or unique set of experiences that distinguish public health's workers from those in other fields. Many public health workers have a primary professional discipline in addition to their attachment to public health. Physicians, nurses, dentists, social workers, nutritionists, health educators, anthropologists, psychologists, architects, sanitarians, economists, political scientists, engineers, epidemiologists, biostatisticians, managers, lawyers, and dozens of other professions and disciplines carry out the work of public health. This multidisciplinary workforce, with somewhat divided loyalties to multiple professions, blurs the distinctiveness of public health as a unified profession. At the same time, however, it facilitates the interdisciplinary approaches to community problem identification and problem solving, which are hallmarks of public health practice.

SIZE AND DISTRIBUTION OF THE PUBLIC HEALTH WORKFORCE

There is little agreement as to the size of the public health workforce in the United States today except that it is only a small subset of the 15 million persons employed in the health sector of the American economy. Enumerations and estimates of public health workers in general, and public health professionals in particular, suffer from several limitations—the definition of a public health worker is unclear; public health workers employed outside governmental public health agencies are difficult to identify; and not all employees of governmental public health agencies have public health responsibilities associated with their jobs. Enumerating specific types of public health workers is also difficult, because many have other professional affiliations.

Because of these limitations, a clear picture of the public health workforce is not available. But it is clear that efforts to identify and categorize public health workers must take into account three important aspects of public health practice[5]:

- Work setting: Public health workers work for organizations actively engaged in promoting, protecting, and preserving the health of a defined population group. The organization may be public or private, and its public health objectives may be secondary or subsidiary to its principal objectives. In addition to governmental public health agencies, other public and private organizations employ public health workers. For example, school health nurses working for the local school district and health educators employed by the local Red Cross chapter are part of the public health workforce.
- Work content: Public health workers perform work addressing one or more of the essential public health services. Many job descriptions for public health workers are tailored from the essential public health services, and the scope of tasks can be very broad. A focus on populations, as opposed to individuals, is often a distinguishing characteristic of these job descriptions. For example, an individual trained as a health educator who works for a community-based teen pregnancy prevention program is clearly a public health worker. But the same can't be said of a health educator working for a commercial advertising firm promoting cosmetics.
- Worker: The individual must occupy a position that conventionally requires at least 1 year of postsecondary specialized public health training and that is (or can be)

assigned a professional, administrative, or technical occupational title (to be defined later in this chapter). This distinction may seem artificial but rests on the notion that public health practice relies on a foundation of knowledge, skills, and attitudes that, in most circumstances, cannot be imparted through work experiences alone.

If public health workers cannot be counted from the ground up, maybe they can be approximated from the top down. Estimates for public health activity expenditures, including both clinical and population-based services, fall in the range of 3–5% of all health expenditures.[1] If public health workers composed a similar percentage of the 15 million health workers in the United States, the number of public health workers would be between 450,000 and 750,000. Because expenditures for some public health activities, such as those for many environmental and occupational health services, are not captured in the total for health expenditures, the actual number of public health workers may range as high as 500,000 to 800,000.

That range is consistent with a crude enumeration of the public health workforce conducted in the year 2000, which identified 450,000 public health workers.[3] The year 2000 enumeration missed most public health workers employed by nongovernmental agencies as well as many public health workers employed by government agencies other than official public health agencies. As a result, the actual total exceeds the 450,000 workers identified in the enumeration.

Data from another source, the ongoing employment census of federal, state, and local health agencies, indicated that there were 586,000 full-time equivalent (FTE) governmental public health workers in 2008.[6] There were nearly 446,000 workers in state and local governments, and another 140,000 were employed by federal agencies (see Table 6–1). Adding in even the admittedly low estimate of 64,000 nongovernmental public health workers from the year 2000 enumeration study, the size of the public health workforce in 2008, using these figures, was nearly 650,000 FTE positions.

The overall workforce in the health sector of the American economy has more than doubled in size since 1975 and has increased by more than 30% since 1990.[7] Table 6–1 indicates that the number of public health workers employed by federal, state, and local health agencies has also been steadily increasing, largely among workers of **local public health agencies**. Unquestionably, the number of public health workers employed by nongovernmental agencies also grew during this period. The number of FTE employees working for governmental health agencies was 487,000 FTEs in 1994 (140,000 federal, 186,000 state, 260,000 local). By 2008, the total was 586,000 (140,000 federal, 186,000 state,

TABLE 6–1 Full Time Equivalent (FTE) Workers of Federal, State, and Local Governmental Health* Agencies, 1994–2005, United States

Year	Federal Health FTE	State Health FTE	Local Health FTE	State + Local FTE	Total (F+S+L) FTE
1994	126,292	157,962	202,732	360,694	486,986
1995	125,048	160,031	208,588	368,619	493,667
1997	119,921	162,605	214,824	377,429	497,350
1998	119,846	166,930	219,655	386,585	506,431
1999	121,033	169,213	223,999	393,212	514,245
2000	120,362	172,678	236,496	409,174	529,536
2001	122,999	172,414	251,399	423,813	546,812
2002	124,979	176,345	252,326	428,671	553,650
2003	124,828	176,868	253,888	430,756	555,584
2004	127,933	174,301	249,857	424,128	552,061
2005	125,163	178,465	246,300	424,765	549,918
2006	126,775	182,694	250,163	432,857	559,632
2007	130,952	183,227	251,207	434,760	565,712
2008	140,026	185,667	260,404	446,071	586,097

*Health: public health services, emergency medical services, mental health, alcohol and drug abuse, outpatient clinics, visiting nurses, food and sanitary inspections, animal control, other environmental health activities (e.g., pollution control), etc.

Source: Data from U.S. Bureau of the Census. Federal, state, and local governments, and public employment and payroll data. http://www.census.gov/govs/www/apes. Accessed June 15, 2010.

260,000 local). Figure 6–1 demonstrates that the ratio of public health workers to population has also increased during this period, although there is evidence that it may be declining somewhat since reaching its highest level (15.1 per 10,000) in 2001. Any downward trend after 2003 and before 2009 would be surprising in view of the substantial influx of federal funding for state and local public health agencies since 2002. The severe economic recession in 2009 did, however, impact the number of governmental health agency workers.

Like most health sector workers, public health workers are more likely to be found in urban and suburban settings rather than rural communities. The public health worker to population ratio, however, is often higher in rural areas than in urban areas. States show significant variation as well, with higher ratios in many of the smaller and less urban states in the East and West and lower ratios in the Central states. Table 6–2 provides the number of FTE workers of state and local governmental health agencies in 2003 and 2008.

In 1980, Health Resources and Services Administration (HRSA) estimated the size of the public health workforce at 500,000 workers including a primary public health workforce of 250,000 professional workers, most working in governmental public health agencies.[2] More than 50,000 occupational health physicians, nurses, and specialists working in the private sector, as well as 20,000 health educators working in schools and 45,000 administrators working in nursing homes, hospitals, and medical group practices were included in the 250,000 professionals characterized by HRSA as the primary public health workforce at the time. If only those working for governmental public health agencies had been included, the number would have been closer to 140,000. The year 2000 public health enumeration identified 40,000 fewer occupational health professionals and did not seek to include health educators working in schools or administrators in nongovernmental clinical settings.

Comparing the overall 1980 estimate (500,000 workers) with the year 2000 public health workforce enumeration suggests that the public health workforce is shrinking. Comparing the 1980 HRSA estimate with current employment census data, on the other hand, suggests that the public health workforce is growing. Because the methods used for the 1980 estimation were considerably different from those in the more recent studies, direct comparison of the results is of questionable value.

The national public health workforce enumeration study completed in 2000 identified one third of the public health workforce employed by state agencies and another one third employed by local governmental agencies.[3] This study also reported that 20% worked for federal agencies and 14% worked for nongovernmental organizations in the voluntary and private sectors. Government employment census data, which excludes nongovernmental workers, also classify one third as state workers but 44% as employees of local government and 24% as working for federal agencies. Some of these differences can be attributed to state public health systems in which state employees work at the local level and may be counted as state employees in the employment census data and as local health department employees in the public health enumeration study. These differences may also be partly attributed to the inclusion of workers in state and local governmental agencies other than the local public health agency in the government employment census data but not in the year 2000 public health enumeration study. For example, substance abuse and mental health

FIGURE 6–1 Full-time equivalent (FTE) workers for state and local health* agencies per 10,000 population, selected years 1998–2008, United States

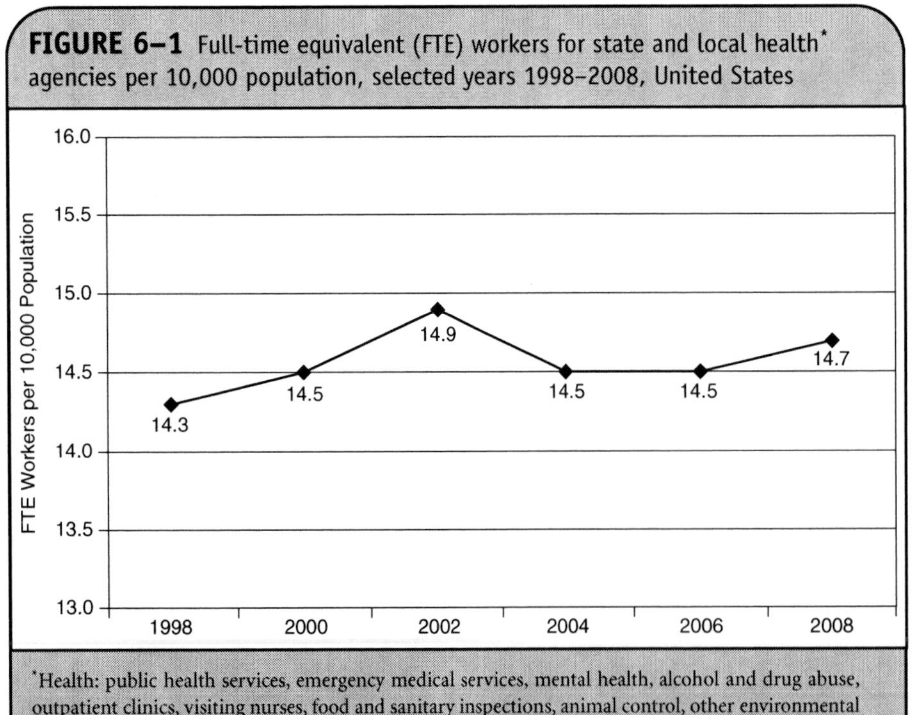

*Health: public health services, emergency medical services, mental health, alcohol and drug abuse, outpatient clinics, visiting nurses, food and sanitary inspections, animal control, other environmental health activities (e.g., pollution control), etc.

Source: Data from U.S. Bureau of the Census. Federal, state, and local governments, and public employment and payroll data. www.census.gov/govs/www/apes. Accessed June 15, 2010.

prevention services, school health services, or restaurant inspections may operate from local mental health agencies, school districts, or consumer affairs agencies rather than from the local health department. The National Association of County and City Health Officials (NACCHO) estimated that LHDs employed 155,000 workers in 2008.

Although recent decades have witnessed an increase in the number of public health workers employed by nongovernmental agencies due to expanded partnerships for public health priorities, governmental public health workers are often considered the primary public health workforce. Their number, composition, distribution, and competence are issues of public concern. The government employment census data provide useful insights into overall trends at the national level and among the various levels of government. The year 2000 public health enumeration study, however, provides richer information on the composition of the public health workforce, such as the proportion and types of professional occupational categories within that workforce. Both sources enrich understanding of the size and composition of the public health workforce today.

COMPOSITION OF THE PUBLIC HEALTH WORKFORCE

Public health is multidisciplinary, with many different professions and occupations involved in its work. In recent years, there has been an effort to identify standard occupational classifications for public health workers resulting in nearly 30 different job categories. Because the total number of public health workers is not clear, the precise proportion of the various subgroups cannot be determined. It is clear that nurses and environmental health practitioners constitute the largest subgroups of public health workers. Managers, epidemiologists, health educators, and laboratory workers are also significant subgroups. Table 6–3 provides information on occupational categories and titles for the public health workforce enumeration completed in 2000. Specific categories and titles were not reported for one fourth of the workers in the study, necessitating the use of an adjustment process to allow for better estimates for public health worker categories and occupational titles.

Despite the lack of precise information, it appears that professional occupational categories comprise more than 300,000, or one half, of the estimated 620,000 workers in the public health workforce. For comparison purposes, there were approximately 2.3 million nurses, 800,000 physicians, 200,000 pharmacists, 170,000 dentists, and 90,000 dieticians/nutritionists working in the United States at the turn of the 21st century.[7]

Studies of local public health agencies document that three positions are found in more than 80% of all LHDs—public health nurse, administrator, and sanitarian/environmental health specialist.[8,9] These positions are present in large and small agencies alike. The next most frequent positions (emergency preparedness coordinators, health

TABLE 6–2 FTE Workers of State and Local Health Agencies by State, 2003 and 2008

State	State + Local FTE in 2003	State + Local FTE in 2008
AL	9,764	11,398
AK	1,180	1,003
AZ	4,971	7,447
AR	4,972	5,240
CA	55,311	60,568
CO	4,937	5,412
CT	3,728	3,445
DE	2,205	2,633
DC	2,021	949
FL	27,139	33,006
GA	17,357	15,854
HI	2,656	2,574
ID	2,117	2,308
IL	10,599	10,597
IN	5,157	5,440
IA	2,674	2,462
KS	3,994	4,545
KY	7,038	7,562
LA	5,401	5,735
ME	1,604	1,481
MD	11,423	11,365
MA	10,704	10,884
MI	13,029	10,943
MN	5,946	6,336
MS	3,258	3,136
MO	7,420	7,130
MT	1,713	1,736
NE	1,426	1,426

(continued)

TABLE 6–2 FTE Workers of State and Local Health Agencies by State, 2003 and 2008 (*continued*)

State	State + Local FTE in 2003	State + Local FTE in 2008
NV	2,105	2,089
NH	1,226	1,160
NJ	7,308	8,829
NM	2,851	2,887
NY	27,734	30,124
NC	24,211	20,602
ND	1,843	1,852
OH	21,659	21,434
OK	8,429	7,305
OR	6,904	5,762
PA	7,319	6,907
RI	1,364	1,289
SC	9,137	8,609
SD	856	896
TN	6,916	9,570
TX	36,106	38,126
UT	3,396	3,150
VT	758	714
VA	11,159	11,451
WA	8,914	9,483
WV	2,117	1,980
WI	7,752	8,033
WY	948	1,216
US Total	430,756	446,083

Source: Data from U.S. Bureau of the Census. Federal, state, and local Governments, and public employment and payroll data. www.census.gov/govs/apes/. Accessed June 2010.

educators, nutritionists, and physicians) are found in 40–60% of LHDs. There is considerable variation in the proportion of LHDs with these positions, associated with agency size (Table 6–4). For example, health educators are employed in only 25% of LHDs serving populations under 10,000 persons but in 97% of agencies serving 500,000 or more.

Two general patterns of LHD staffing exist around a core set of employees. One pattern focuses on clinical services, the other on more population-based programs.[10] The core employees consist of dietitian/nutritionists, sanitarians/environmental specialists, administrators, lab specialists, and health educators. The clinical pattern adds physicians, nurses, and dental health workers. The population-based pattern includes epidemiologists, public health nurses, social workers, and program specialists.

The availability of information on public health workers at the state and local level varies from state to state and is often inconsistent and incomplete. Detailed information from the official state health departments has not been available since the late 1980s and even then did not include public health workers employed by state agencies other than the official state health department. The periodic profiles of LHDs completed by the NACCHO before 2005 provide only general data on the proportion of responding agencies that employ specific public health job titles, either directly or through contracted services. The national profile of LHDs completed in 2008 is the source of estimates for the number of workers in key job titles presented in Table 6–5.

The lack of information on the public health workforce extends to some of the most basic and important characteristics of that workforce. For example, there is very little information available on the racial and ethnic characteristics of the overall public health workforce. Although important, information on cultural competency is also lacking.

PUBLIC HEALTH WORKER ETHICS AND SKILLS

Public health workers may come from different academic, professional, and experiential backgrounds, but they share a common bond. All are committed to a common mission and share common ethical principles, as exemplified by the following list advanced by the American Public Health Association[11]:

- Public health should address principally the fundamental causes of disease and requirements for health, aiming to prevent adverse health outcomes.
- Public health should achieve community health in a way that respects the rights of individuals in the community.
- Public health policies, programs, and priorities should be developed and evaluated through processes that ensure an opportunity for input from community members.
- Public health should advocate and work for the empowerment of disenfranchised community members, aiming to ensure that the basic resources and conditions necessary for health are accessible to all.
- Public health should seek the information needed to implement effective policies and programs that protect and promote health.

TABLE 6–3 Number of Public Health Workers in Selected Occupational Categories and Titles, United States, 2000

Gov PH Workers		Reported #		Adjusted #
Administrators		15,920		21,247
Professionals		176,980		236,202
Technicians		61,088		81,530
Other support		59,085		69,283
Unreported		104,763		
	TOTAL	417,836	TOTAL	417,836
Occupational Categories				
Health administrators		15,920		21,247
Admin support staff		37,805		62,981
Admin/business prof		4,725		7,306
Attorney/hearing officer		601		929
Biostatistician		1,164		1,800
Environmental engineer		4,549		7,034
Environmental specialist		14,882		23,013
Epidemiologist		927		1,433
Policy analyst/plan/econ		3,678		5,687
Disease investigator		783		1,211
License/inspection spec		13,780		21,309
Social, behavioral, mental		3,762		5,817
Occ. health and safety spec		5,593		8,649
PH dental worker		2,032		3,142
PH educator		2,230		3,448
PH lab professional		14,088		21,785
PH nurse		41,232		63,759
PH nutritionist		6,680		10,330
PH pharmacist		1,496		2,313
PH physician		6,008		9,290
PH program specialist		7,820		12,092
PH veterinarian/animal cont spec		2,037		3,150
Public relations/public info		563		871
Other PH professional		14,119		21,833
Computer specialist		4,326		6,210
Environmental eng technician		414		594
En health technician		501		719
Health info system/data analyst		605		868
Occ health and safety technician		95		136
PH laboratory technician		5,700		8,182
Other PH technician (LPN, etc.)		26,953		38,690
Community outreach/field worker		676		902
Other paraprofessional		18,902		25,227

Source: Data from Health Resources and Services Administration, Bureau of Health Professions, National Center for Health Workforce Information and Analysis and Center for Health Policy, Columbia School of Nursing. *The Public Health Workforce Enumeration 2000.* Washington, DC: HRSA; 2000.

- Public health institutions should provide communities with the information they have that is needed for decisions on policies or programs and should obtain the community's consent for their implementation.
- Public health institutions should act in a timely manner on the information they have within the resources and the mandate given to them by the public.

TABLE 6–4 Local Health Departments with Employees in Selected Occupations, by Size of Population Serviced, United States, 2008

	All LHDs	Under 10,000	10,000 to 24,999	25,000 to 49,999	50,000 to 99,999	100,000 to 249,999	250,000 to 499,999	500,000 to 999,999	1 million +
Clerical staff	95%	85%	95%	97%	97%	100%	99%	100%	100%
Nurse	94%	82%	94%	96%	97%	98%	100%	97%	100%
Manager/director	91%	79%	89%	94%	96%	97%	100%	97%	100%
Environmental health specialist (sanitarian)	80%	54%	78%	86%	90%	92%	93%	88%	88%
Emergency preparedness coordinator	57%	38%	43%	52%	66%	77%	94%	96%	100%
Health Educator	56%	25%	40%	57%	70%	78%	87%	96%	97%
Nutritionist	51%	23%	35%	50%	64%	76%	85%	85%	88%
Physician	42%	15%	24%	41%	52%	69%	79%	85%	94%
Behavioral health professional	33%	6%	22%	26%	47%	49%	68%	80%	71%
Other environmental health scientist	27%	7%	17%	24%	32%	41%	65%	69%	70%
Information system specialist	24%	4%	9%	16%	24%	49%	69%	86%	88%
Epidemiologist	23%	4%	7%	11%	19%	50%	78%	91%	100%
Public Information specialist	19%	6%	7%	12%	20%	30%	50%	80%	88%

Source: Data from National Association of County and City Health Officials. *2008 National Profile of Local Health Departments.* Washington, DC: NACCHO; 2009.

- Public health programs and policies should incorporate a variety of approaches that anticipate and respect diverse values, beliefs, and cultures in the community.
- Public health programs and policies should be implemented in a manner that most enhances the physical and social environment.
- Public health institutions should protect the confidentiality of information that can bring harm to an individual or community if made public. Exceptions must be justified on the basis of the high likelihood of significant harm to the individual or others.
- Public health institutions should ensure the professional competence of their employees.
- Public health institutions and their employees should engage in collaborations and affiliations in ways that build the public's trust and the institution's effectiveness.

Information from national and state surveys indicates that the majority of public health workers lack formal education and training in public health. In 1980, HRSA determined that only 20% of the 250,000 professionals in the primary public health workforce had formal training in public health.[2] More than 2 decades later, there is little evidence that this situation has improved. While the proportion of those who have formal training varies by category of worker, the lack of formal training is striking in even some of the most critical categories. For example, a NACCHO survey in 1997 found that 78% of local health department leaders had no formal public health education or training.[12] A survey of Illinois local health jurisdictions in the year 2000 yielded similar results, with 79% of local health agency administrators lacking formal preparation in public health.[13]

Formal training for many public health workers focuses only on a specific aspect of public health practice, such as environmental health or community or school health nursing. Environmental health practitioners, nurses, administrators, and health educators account for the majority of public health workers with formal training in public health. Even among those with formal training in public health, public health workers with graduate degrees from schools of public health or other graduate public health programs represent only a small fraction of the total. In view of the number of master's-level graduates of schools of public health and other graduate-level public health degree programs—about 10,000 in 2008—this is not surprising.

Evidence of the lack of formal training within this workforce, however, does not necessarily lead to the conclusion that public health workers are unprepared.[14] Instead, public health workers enter the field having earned a wide variety of degrees and professional training credentials from academic programs and institutions unrelated to public health. Often overlooked, these institutions produce the bulk of the public health workforce and represent major assets for addressing unmet needs. On-the-job training and work experience contribute substantially to the overall competency and preparedness of the public health workforce. For example, public health workers are frequently involved in responses to earthquakes, floods, and other disasters and have increasingly acquired and demonstrated skills in assessing community health needs and devising community health improvement plans. These are skills that most public health workers acquired through real-world work experience rather than through their formal training.

TABLE 6–5 Estimated Size and Composition of Local Health Department (LHD) Workforce, United States, 2008

	Best Estimate	95% Confidence Interval	Percentage of All LHD Staff
Clerical staff	36,000	31,000–40,000	23.1%
Nurse	33,000	29,000–36,000	21.3%
Environmental health specialist (sanitarian)	12,000	10,000–13,000	7.5%
Manager/director	9,500	8,400–11,000	6.2%
Behavioral Health Professional	7,100	5,400–8,700	4.6%
Health educator	4,400	3,800–4,900	2.8%
Nutritionist	4,300	3,700–4,900	2.8%
Other Env Health scientist	3,200	2,400–3,900	2.0%
Physician	2,000	1,500–2,400	1.3%
Info system specialist	1,600	1,100–2,000	1.0%
Emergency preparedness coordinator	1,400	1,300–1,500	0.9%
Epidemiologist	1,200	900–1,500	0.8%
Public Information specialist	430	350–510	0.3%
All LHD staff	155,000	135,000–174,000	100%

Source: Data from National Association of County and City Health Officials. *2008 National Profile of Local Health Departments.* Washington, DC: NACCHO; 2009.

Continuing education and career development for public health workers has long been a cottage industry involving many different parties. Academic institutions certainly are contributors, but public health agencies at the state and local level, public health associations (national, state, and local), and other voluntary-sector health organizations participate as well. Many different entities offer credits for continuing education, including professional organizations, academic institutions, and hospitals, among others. Public health workers value continuing education credits as a means to satisfy requirements of their core disciplines in order to maintain some level of credentialing status (such as licensed physicians and nurses, certified health education specialists, and so on). A few states, such as New Jersey, enforce continuing education requirements for the public health disciplines licensed by that state. There is no formal system of public health-specific continuing education units (CEUs) and only fledgling efforts toward credentialing public health workers.

CHARACTERISTICS OF PUBLIC HEALTH OCCUPATIONS

This remaining sections of this chapter define and describe several key dimensions of public health occupations and organizations that provide the framework for examining specific positions and careers for public health workers. Information on the full spectrum of occupations in the public health workforce is available from a variety of sources, including federal health and labor agencies and national public health organizations.

Table 6–6 previews some public health titles, occupational categories, and careers. Standard occupation categories (SOCs) are explained later in this chapter.

There are many aspects of an occupation or career that are important to current and prospective public health workers. The framework used in this book includes

- Occupational classification: these are based on job titles and whether the duties of the job are primarily administrative, professional, technical, or supportive in nature. Many positions in public health practice have a variety of job titles associated with them. Similarly, the same job title can have a variety of regular duties and day-to-day responsibilities.
- Public health practice profile: The public health functions and essential public health services addressed by each occupational grouping are presented in a public health practice profile.
- Important and essential duties: These are the defining characteristics of any position describing what the worker does on a daily basis. Examples are derived from a sampling of job and position descriptions from a variety of sources.
- Minimum qualifications: Some positions require a specific academic degree or credential; many do not. Some require previous experience, while others do not. All require some particular minimum level of knowledge, skills, and abilities. Many also require specific physical capabilities. These characteristics will be identified for each public health occupation.
- Workplace considerations: This description will identify levels of government that employ significant numbers of workers in each occupational category as well as important nongovernmental work settings for public health workers. This section will also highlight considerations related to physical demands, work schedules, travel, and general working conditions.
- Salary estimates: Salary levels for public health workers are estimated based on information from current job postings and the May 2009 survey of employment and wages coordinated by the Labor Department's Bureau of Labor Statistics.
- Career prospects: Estimates as to current need and future demand for specific public health occupations and career paths are provided, based on the analyses performed by public health organizations and the Bureau of Labor Statistics' projections for various occupations.
- Additional information: Sources of additional information for each occupation or career are identified, including education and training opportunities.

The following sections briefly describe the type and source of information included for each of these characteristics.

Occupational Classifications

Throughout the economy, including the health sector, occupations are broadly classified as either white collar or blue collar depending on the degree of education and experience normally required. White collar occupations include five major occupational categories (professional, administrative, technical, clerical, and other), based on the subject matter of work, the level of difficulty or responsibility involved, and the educational requirements established for each occupation. Blue collar occupations are composed of the trades, crafts, and manual labor (unskilled, semiskilled, skilled), including foreman and supervisory positions entailing trade, craft, or laboring experience and knowledge as the paramount requirement.

The U.S. Office of Personnel Management tracks occupations in various industries using four general categories—professional, administrative, technical, and support.

- Professional occupations are those that require knowledge in a field of science or learning characteristically acquired through education or training equivalent to a bachelor's or higher degree with major study in or pertinent to the specialized field, as distinguished from general education. The work of a professional occupation requires the exercise of discretion, judgment, and personal responsibility for the application of an organized body of knowledge that is constantly studied to make new discoveries and interpretations, and to improve the data, materials, and methods. Professionals require specialized and theoretical knowledge. Well-known examples of professional job titles include physicians, registered nurses, dieticians, health educators, social workers, psychologists, lawyers, accountants, economists, system analysts, and personnel and labor relations workers. Professionals comprise the majority (56%) of public health workers (see Figure 6–2).
- Administrative occupations are those that involve the exercise of analytical ability, judgment, discretion, personal responsibility, and the application of a substantial body of knowledge of principles, concepts, and practices applicable to one or more fields of administration or management. Although these positions do not require specialized educational majors, they do involve the type of skills (analytical, research, writing, judgment) typi-

cally gained through a college-level general education, or through progressively responsible experience. Administrators set broad policies, oversee overall responsibility for the execution of these policies, direct individual departments or special phases of the agency's operations, or provide specialized consultation on a regional, district, or area basis. Common job titles for administrators include department heads, bureau chiefs, division chiefs, directors, deputy directors, and similar titles. Administrators and managers comprise 5% of all public health workers.

- Technical occupations are those that involve work that is not routine in nature and is typically associated with, and supportive of, a professional or administrative field. Such occupations involve extensive practical knowledge gained through on-the-job experience, or specific training less than that represented by college graduation. Work in these occupations may involve substantial elements of the work of the professional or administrative field but requires less than full competence in the field involved. Technical occupations require a combination of basic scientific or technical knowledge and manual skills. Titles include computer specialists, licensed practical nurses, inspectors, programmers, and a variety of technicians (environmental, laboratory, medical, nursing, dental, and so on). The technical occupations category also includes paraprofessionals who perform some of the duties of a professional or technician in a supportive role usually requiring less formal training and experience than that normally required for professional status. Included are outreach workers, research assistants, medical aides, child support workers, home health aides, emergency medical technicians, and so on. Workers in technical occupations account for 20% of all public health workers.
- Administrative support occupations are those that involve structured work in support of office, business, or fiscal operations; duties are performed according to established policies or techniques and require training, experience, or working knowledge related to the tasks to be performed. Clerical titles are often responsible for internal and external communication as well as recording and retrieval of data, information, and other paperwork required in an office. This category includes bookkeepers, messengers, clerk typists, stenographers, court transcribers, hearing reporters, statistical clerks, dispatchers, license distributors, payroll clerks, office machine and computer operators, telephone operators, legal assistants, and so on. In addition, workers in any of the blue-collar occupational categories are considered support workers within the public health workforce. About 19% of public health workers are in the administrative support category.

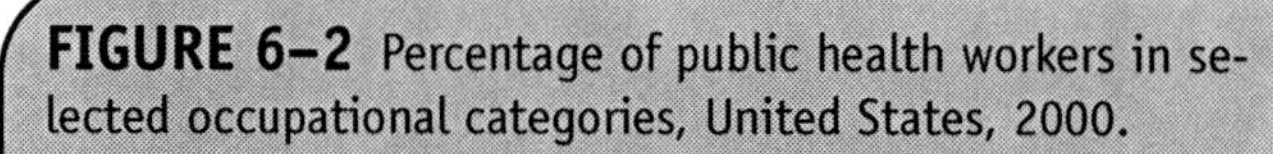
FIGURE 6–2 Percentage of public health workers in selected occupational categories, United States, 2000.

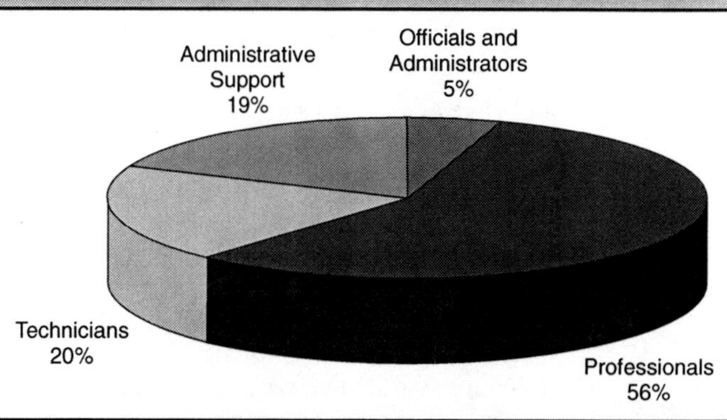

Source: Adapted from Health Resources and Services Administration, Bureau of Health Professions, National Center for Health Workforce Information and Analysis and Center for Health Policy, Columbia School of Nursing. *The Public Health Workforce Enumeration 2000.* Washington, DC: HRSA; 2000.

As indicated in Figure 6–2, 81% of public health workers fall into the professional, administrative, and technical categories. More than one half (56%) are classified as professionals, similar to the proportion of professionals among all 15 million health workers. Nursing and environmental health activities employ the largest number of public health workers when both professional and technical occupations are considered. Registered nurses (RNs) represent the largest professional category within the public health workforce.

The U.S. Department of Labor collects information on occupations throughout the economy, including the public sector. An official taxonomy for occupations allows the Department of Labor's Bureau of Labor Statistics (BLS) to track information on hundreds of standard occupational categories in terms of the number and location of jobs, salaries, and duties performed. BLS also develops projections for the number of future positions for these occupational categories based on economic and employment trends. Occupations generally can be found in a variety of industries, making it difficult to pinpoint trends

TABLE 6–6 Public Health Occupations and Careers

Career Category with Specific Public Health Titles Described	Bureau of Labor Statistics Standard Occupational Categories Relevant for Public Health
Public Health Administration • Health services manager • Public health agency director • Health officer	• Health services manager/administrator
Environmental and Occupational Health • Environmental engineer • Environmental health specialist (entry level) • Environmental health specialist (midlevel) • Environmental health specialist (senior level) • Occupational health and safety specialist	• Environmental engineer • Environmental engineering technician and technologist • Environmental scientist and specialist • Environmental science technician and technologist • Occupational health and safety specialist • Occupational health and safety technician
Public Health Nursing • Public health nurse (entry level) • Public health nurse (senior level) • Licensed practical/vocational nurse	• Registered nurse • Licensed practical/vocational nurse
Epidemiology and Disease Control • Disease investigator • Epidemiologist (entry level) • Epidemiologist (senior level)	• Epidemiologist • Statistician
Public Health Education and Information • Public health educator (entry level) • Public health educator (senior level) • Public information officer	• Health educator • Public relations/public information/health communications/media specialist
Other Public Health Professionals • Public health nutritionist/dietician • Public health social, behavioral, and mental health workers • Public health laboratory workers • Public health physicians • Public health veterinarians • Public health pharmacists • Public health dental workers • Administrative law judge/hearing officer • Dietician/nutritionist • Dietetic technician • Medical and public health social worker • Mental health and substance abuse social worker • Mental health counselor	• Substance abuse and behavioral disorder counselor • Microbiologist • Biochemist/biophysicist • Medical and clinical laboratory technologist • Medical and clinical laboratory technician • Public health physician • Public health veterinarian • Public health pharmacist • Public health dentist • Administrative law judge/hearing officer
Public Health Program Occupations • Public health program specialist/coordinator • Public health emergency preparedness and response coordinator • Public health policy analyst • Public health information specialists • Community outreach and other technical occupations	

and needs specific to the public health system. For example, registered nurses are the largest occupational category in the overall health workforce, with 2.6 million workers, but only a small percentage of all registered nurses (about 75,000) work in public health agencies. Many more work in hospitals and other health care organizations. This is also true for physicians, health services administrators, health educators, nutritionists, and many other occupations. Public health agencies, however, are the largest employers of several standard occupational categories, such as environmental health specialists and epidemiologists. For those occupational categories, BLS information is especially useful.

Standard occupational categories relevant for public health are identified in the second column of Table 6–6, with 28 specific categories listed.[15] These 28 occupational categories clearly do not cover all titles found in public health organizations. Nor do they capture the entire scope of work undertaken by public health workers.

Estimates of the number of current workers in each occupational category are synthesized from two sources. The Bureau of Labor Statistics conducts surveys of all standard occupational categories twice yearly, including information on the industries and levels of government that employ workers in each standard occupational category.[16] This source allows for estimates of the total number of workers in a particular standard occupational category who work for federal, state, and local agencies.

Projections for the number of positions for each occupational title in the year 2018 are also provided by the Bureau of Labor Statistics, allowing for estimates of job openings between now and 2018.

A second important source of estimates for public health workers in relevant standard occupational categories is the *Public Health Workforce Enumeration 2000* commissioned by the federal HRSA.[3] This enumeration collected information on workers of federal, state, and local public health agencies in the year 2000 based on existing data, reports, and surveys. As such, it was more of a qualitative and descriptive enumeration than a quantitative one. The year 2000 public health workforce enumeration identified a total of 450,000 public health workers, including 15,000 workers in voluntary sector organizations and 15,000 public health students. Occupational categories could not be established for 112,000 public health workers, making it difficult to project the actual number of workers in specific categories, such as public health nurses or epidemiologists.

To compare information with Bureau of Labor Statistics data, the year 2000 public health enumeration numbers were adjusted to assign an occupational category to all workers. Table 6–3 provides both the actual number of workers identified in specific occupational categories and the adjusted number after those in the unreported group are assigned to a category and title. Both sources provide insights useful for estimating the number of existing positions for each occupational category and title.

Public Health Practice Profile

Individual workers, as well as occupational categories, produce work important to achieving public health goals and objectives. Key public health goals and objectives address preventing disease and injury, promoting healthy behaviors, protecting against health risks and threats, responding to emergencies, and assuring the quality of health services.[4] This overall public health practice framework provides the basis for channeling contributions both by individuals and organizations toward common goals. The specific work tasks of different occupations and individuals generally fall into one or more of the 10 essential public health services. The essential public health services is characterized as the means to achieving public health ends, or how the work of public health is accomplished. It is useful to view these functions and essential public health services as an aggregate job description for the entire public health workforce, with the workload then divided among the many different professional and occupational categories composing the total public health workforce. An example of this format is provided in Table 6–7.

In this example, the public health occupational category is primarily involved in addressing three public health goals: preventing epidemics, preventing injuries, and promoting healthy behaviors. This public health occupational category works to address these goals largely through performing five essential public health services—monitoring health status, investigating health problems, educating people about health, evaluating effectiveness, and researching new solutions to health problems.

In this example, the assignment of specific public health purposes and essential public health services may appear somewhat arbitrary. In each case, however, judgments are made as to which purposes and essential services are most closely associated with each occupational category. Some occupational categories may appear to have a relatively limited focus (e.g., public health laboratory workers) in comparison with others (e.g., public health nurses) that may have very broad roles that could conceivably cover all purposes and services. For each occupational category and title, however, the number of purposes and essential services identified for each occupational category is limited to no more than one half the number possible (3 of 6 purposes, 5 of 10 essential public health services). Table 6–8 provides a composite profile that aggregates information from some public health occupations.

TABLE 6–7 Public Health Profile Example

(Example)
Public Health Practitioners
Make a Difference by:

Public Health Purposes

√ Preventing epidemics and the spread of disease
Protecting against environmental hazards
√ Preventing injuries
√ Promoting and encouraging healthy behaviors
Responding to disasters and assisting communities in recovery
Assuring the quality and accessibility of health services

Essential Public Health Services

√ Monitoring health status to identify community health problems
√ Diagnosing and investigating health problems and health hazards in the community
√ Informing, educating, and empowering people about health issues
Mobilizing community partnerships to identify and solve health problems
Developing policies and plans that support individual and community health efforts
Enforcing laws and regulations that protect health and ensure safety
Linking people with needed personal health services and assuring the provision of health care when otherwise unavailable
Assuring a competent public health and personal health care workforce
√ Evaluating effectiveness, accessibility, and quality of personal and population-based health services
√ Researching new insights and innovative solutions to health problems

Characterizing the work of an occupational category in this manner proves a functional view of the work performed. It also facilitates an understanding of how the work of one occupational category relates to the work of another category, and how it relates to the overall work performed across all public health occupational categories.

Important and Essential Duties

The most important aspect of any job or career is what workers do day in and day out. It is those basic and routine duties that best define positions in public health or any other field of endeavor. This list varies considerably from one position to another and often from one level of the same position to a higher level (e.g., from an entry level environmental health specialist to a midlevel environmental health specialist). Important and essential duties are based on information from a sampling of job and position descriptions from a variety of public health organizations.

Minimum Qualifications

Another key dimension of a position is a statement of the minimum qualifications necessary for that job. Often these minimum qualifications must be met in order for a worker to apply for a particular position. Minimum qualifications may emphasize experience or education or both. In any event, there is a battery of skills or competencies that are expected of those applying for and those working in public health positions. Additional qualifications, such as physical capabilities appropriate for specific jobs or job locations, are also presented. These qualifications are synthesized from a sampling of current position descriptions.

The range of public health occupations and careers extends from those requiring considerable education and training to those that require relatively little. For example, some state and local health officials may hold several degrees, such as a bachelor degree in science, a master's degree in public health, and a doctoral degree in medicine. At the same time, key staff performing investigations of communicable disease or environmental threats may have only an associate or bachelor's degree at the undergraduate level. It is not uncommon for some technical and clerical staff to have no more than a high school diploma with on-the-job training. As this book largely targets undergraduate and graduate-degree students, particular emphasis is on occupations and careers requiring at least an undergraduate degree.

TABLE 6–8 Composite Public Health Practice Profile for Public Health Occupations and Titles

	PH Adm	Env Hlth	PH Nurs	Epi	PH Ed	Nutr	Soc Beh MH	PH Lab	MD DVM Phar	Dent Wkrs	Adm Law Jdg	PH Prog Spec	ERC	PH Pol An	Hlth Info	Out Wkrs
Public Health Purposes																
Preventing epidemics and the spread of disease	√	√	√	√	√		√	√	√	√	√			√	√	√
Protecting against environmental hazards		√		√				√			√	√	√	√		
Preventing injuries		√		√	√							√	√			√
Promoting and encouraging healthy behaviors		√			√	√	√		√	√		√				√
Responding to disasters and assisting communities in recovery	√						√						√			
Assuring the quality and accessibility of health services	√		√			√	√	√	√	√	√			√	√	
Essential Public Health Services																
Monitoring health status to identify community health problems		√		√		√		√	√	√		√			√	
Diagnosing and investigating health problems and health hazards in the community		√	√	√				√	√			√	√			
Informing, educating, and empowering people about health issues		√			√	√	√			√				√	√	√
Mobilizing community partnerships to identify and solve health problems	√				√		√						√	√		√

(continued)

Workplace Considerations

Public health work takes place in many organizations and settings other than governmental public health agencies such as state health agencies or local public health departments. Many community and voluntary organizations collaborate with governmental public health agencies and employ staff whose work parallels that of workers in governmental public health agencies. This is true both for nongovernmental public health efforts here in the United States and those on the international level. Not much is known about public health workers and career opportunities in community and voluntary organizations. There is some information available for local, state, and federal public health agencies on measures such as numbers employed, occupational categories, work locations, salary, and specific duties.

Another important workplace consideration relates to special physical capabilities, travel requirements, and other unique aspects of specific jobs. For example, some positions may require the ability to lift and move items weighing up to 50 pounds. Other jobs may require the ability to walk great distances or to have normal vision or hearing. Others may require the ability to work outside in cold and inclement weather, or to work unusual hours.

Salary Estimates

Detailed and specific salary information is not widely available. Information will be provided based on limited sources, including BLS data and current job postings. This information should not be considered to be definitive or completely accurate. Variations in salary scales are wide from agency to agency depending on a variety of circumstances and conditions. Figure 6–3 indicates that the average salary of a full-time worker em-

TABLE 6–8 Composite Public Health Practice Profile for Public Health Occupations and Titles (*continued*)

	PH Adm	Env Hlth	PH Nurs	Epi	PH Ed	Nutr	Soc Beh MH	PH Lab	MD DVM Phar	Dent Wkrs	Adm Law Jdg	PH Prog Spec	ERC	PH Pol An	Hlth Info	Out Wkrs
Essential Public Health Services																
Developing policies and plans that support individual and community health efforts	√				√		√				√	√	√	√	√	
Enforcing laws and regulations that protect health and ensure safety	√	√						√		√	√					
Linking people with needed personal health services and assuring the provision of health care when otherwise unavailable			√			√	√		√	√			√		√	
Assuring a competent public health and personal health care workforce	√				√						√					
Evaluating effectiveness, accessibility, and quality of personal and population-based health services	√	√	√	√		√	√	√	√	√	√	√	√	√	√	
Researching new insights and innovative solutions to health problems			√	√		√		√	√		√				√	√

Notes: PH Adm—Public Health Administrator; Env Hlth—Environmental Health Practitioner; PH Nurs—Public Health Nurse; EPI—Epidemiologist; PH Ed—Public Health Educator; Nutr—Nutritionist; Soc Beh MH—Public Health Social, Behavioral, and Mental Health Workers; PH Lab—Public Health Laboratory Worker; MD DVM Phar—Public Health Physicians, Veterinarians, and Pharmacists; Dent Wkrs—Dental Health Workers; Adm Law Jdg—Administrative Law Judge; PH Prog Spec—Public Health Program Specialist; ERC—Emergency Response Coordinator; PH Pol An—Public Health Policy Analyst; Hlth Info—Health Information Specialist; and Out Wkrs—Outreach Workers.

ployed by a state or local health agency increased by nearly 45% to nearly $48,000 between 1998 and 2008. One trend contributing to this increase is a higher proportion of workers in professional and technical occupational titles in 2005 than a decade earlier.

Career Prospects

Current and future opportunities for public health careers, as do careers in all fields, depend on relationships among the population, the labor force, and the demand for public health programs and services.[17] The size and composition of the population strongly influences both the size of the workforce and the types of services needed by the population.

The U.S. population continues to increase, although at a slower rate than in recent decades. The average age of the population continues to increase as well, and the proportion of the population in the 55–64 year age category will increase more than 40% over the next 10 years. As this age group nears retirement, replacement of workers will create job opportunities and career advancement possibilities in addition to those created by the continued growth of the overall population.

Among the various sectors of the U.S. economy, the health sector is projected to grow faster and add more jobs than other sectors. About one in every four new jobs will be in the health sector. In the health sector, and in the overall economy, professional and related categories will exhibit the greatest growth and offer the greatest opportunities for new jobs and career advancement. In sum, the overall outlook for professional and technical occupations in public health is very bright for those now in or about to enter the job market.

The optimal number of public health workers is controversial and uncertain. There is widespread concern within the public health community that there will soon be a shortage of public health workers. Several key public

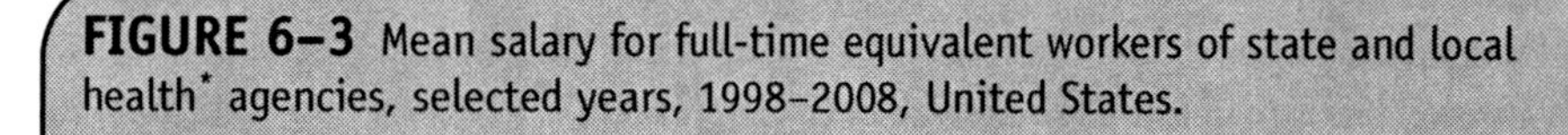

health occupational categories are currently in short supply, such as public health nurses and epidemiologists. The information provided in the career prospect section will identify specific occupational categories that have been identified (rightly or wrongly) as being in greatest need. Despite the uncertainties, the Bureau of Labor Statistics provides projections for the number of positions likely to be needed in 2018 and the number of job openings that will occur through new positions and retirements.

FIGURE 6–3 Mean salary for full-time equivalent workers of state and local health* agencies, selected years, 1998–2008, United States.

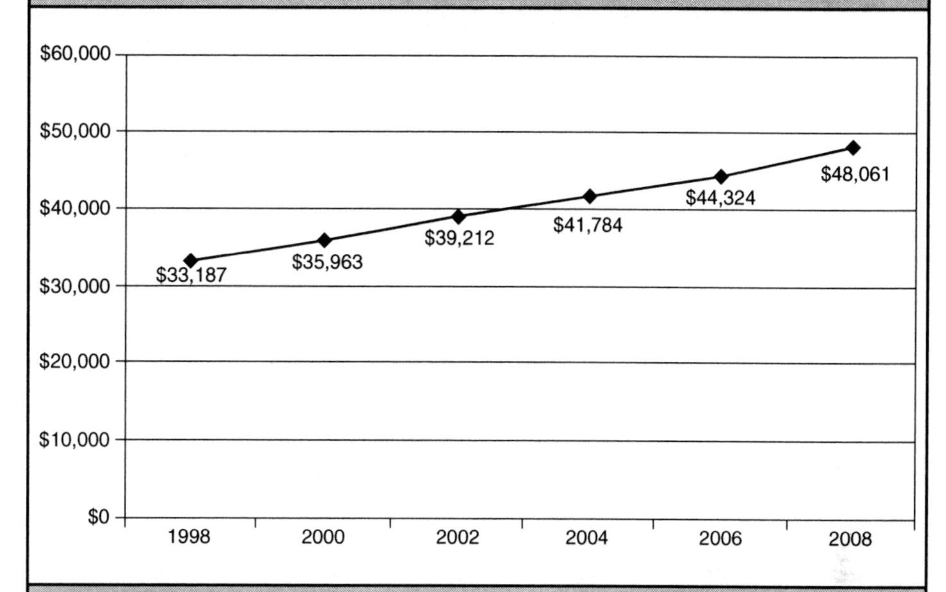

*Health: public health services, emergency medical services, mental health, alcohol and drug abuse, outpatient clinics, visiting nurses, food and sanitary inspections, animal control, other environmental health activities (e.g., pollution control), etc.
Source: Data from U.S. Bureau of the Census. Federal, state, and local governments, and public employment and payroll data. www.census.gov/govs/www/apes. Accessed June 15, 2010.

Careers in public health, like those in many fields, are not always straightforward. Individual workers can begin in one career pathway and then move into another. For example, administrators of public health agencies could come up through the ranks of program and agency management or from one of the public health professional categories, such as environmental health, nursing, or health education. This section will identify some of these paths and career ladders for public health workers.

Additional Information

Most public health occupational categories and careers have excellent sources for more detailed information. Career development opportunities through education, training, and credentialing are also provided for each public health workforce category.

PUBLIC HEALTH WORKFORCE GROWTH PROSPECTS

Will the public health workforce increase or decrease in size over the next 10 years? There should be little debate over this question, but there is. One reason for controversy derives from the lack of accurate information on the size of the public health workforce between 1980 and 2000. Another relates to the many complex forces within public health and the broader economy that influence the number of public health workers needed.

In hindsight, it is clear that the frequently cited figure that the workforce numbered 500,000 in 1980 lacked precision in terms of what was included and how it was generated. This is unfortunate, as the 500,000 figure from 1980 is frequently cited as documentation that the public health workforce must be shrinking because only 450,000 public health workers were enumerated in 2000. As previously discussed, the HRSA 1980 estimate actually indicated that only 250,000 of the 500,000 public health workers were in the primary public health workforce consisting of federal, state, and local public health agency workers and selected others who devoted most of their work efforts on public health activities.[2] Within this 250,000 figure, there were faculty and researchers at academic institutions; occupational health physicians and nurses working for various private companies; health educators teaching in schools; and administrators working in hospitals, nursing homes, and other medical care settings. The actual number of public health professionals working for federal, state, and local public health agencies in 1980, after adjusting for these inclusions, was closer to 140,000. The total for the comparable categories from the *Public Health Workforce Enumeration 2000* was 260,000, a figure that indicates the public health workforce is growing rather than shrinking. Data from the employment census of governmental agencies support this conclusion, showing there has been a steady increase in full-time equivalent (FTE) workers of governmental health agencies over the past decade (see Table 6–1 and Figure 6–1).

These findings indicate that the public health workforce has been increasing since 1980, throughout the 1990s, and into the early years of the current decade. This is consistent with the documented expansion of the health sector within the overall economy, which continues to grow at a more rapid rate than the rest of the economy. If public health activities continue to maintain their small share of total health spending, funding for public health activities and public health workers will grow commensurately. It is conceivable that public health activities could even increase their share of overall health spending, fostering even more rapid growth of employment opportunities.

There are concerns, however, that the growth of the public health workforce may be slowing or even reversing. It is somewhat surprising that the infusion of bioterrorism preparedness funding after 2001 didn't result in even greater numbers of state and local public health workers than are reflected in Table 6–1. It appears that state and local governments initially shifted some workers onto federal bioterrorism grant payrolls, thereby saving state and local resources or possibly shifting resources from public health to other priorities such as education. The severe national economic downturn in 2009 forced many states and localities to suspend hiring and even lay off workers. Bureau of Labor Statistics data documents a decline between 2008 and 2009 in government employment for virtually all public health occupations, including emergency management specialists.[16] The long-term impact of this recession on the national public health workforce will be clearer after 2011, although surveys conducted by ASTHO and NACCHO in 2009 and 2010 suggest that state and local health departments suffered significant staff reductions.

This example illustrates how federal funding to states and localities for bioterrorism preparedness serves as a temptation to replace or supplant state and local support for public health with federal money. The funding of epidemiologists further illustrates this phenomenon. In 2004, federal bioterrorism funds paid the salaries of 460 epidemiologists; among 390 epidemiologists working on bioterrorism and emergency response activities, 62% were funded by the federal government. Infectious disease epidemiologists did not increase between 2001 and 2004, but in 2004 nearly 20% were paid through federal bioterrorism funds.[18] This scenario may also be true for several other public health occupational categories, such as laboratory workers and emergency response coordinators. It underscores the important role of the underlying financial health of state and local governments in determining the size of the public health workforce.

Two additional modern forces affect public health workforce size. These are the expansion of information technology and the resulting increase in worker productivity. Public health practice, by its very nature, is information dependent and information driven. Enhanced information technology tools and increased individual worker productivity mean fewer workers are needed to support the work of administrators, professionals, and technical staff. This trend would tend to increase the proportion of professionals within the public health workforce; however, these trends also mean fewer professionals are needed to perform the same volume of work. The net effect is therefore difficult to predict in terms of the number and types of workers needed.

The impact of these trends will be affected by events and forces within the overall economy, the health system, and the public sector in general. Public health workers and public health agencies are key components of the public health system, but it is important to consider the larger context in which they operate. This larger environment is in constant flux, undergoing changes that impact the public health system and its components. For example, information and communication technologies advance continuously. These developments enable public health agencies and workers to carry out their duties in a more efficient and effective manner. The work of public health is especially information dependent. The speed at which information is accessed and communicated significantly affects how well public health achieves its mission and objectives. Advances in information and communications technology improve public health practice and public health outcomes. There is every reason to believe that these advances will continue at least at levels achieved in recent decades. The net effect is to make public health workers more effective and productive. The challenge is to assure that public health workers have access to the education and training resources that assure this happens.

Trends within the health sector will also continue to affect public health workers. Health is highly valued both as a personal and societal goal. The economic value placed on health exceeds $2.5 trillion annually, or about $8,000 per person in the United States. There is no indication that health will assume a lower priority within the American social value system. In recent years, for example, expenditures for health purposes have grown faster than the rate for the overall economy. In effect, health is becoming an even greater priority. Between the two general strategies to achieve health—preventive and therapeutic approaches—the balance may be slowly shifting toward more prevention. There is still a notable imbalance, with a 20 to 1 ratio; however, this shift is likely to continue. Taken together with an increased priority on health itself, public health activities, including those carried out by public health agencies and workers, should continue to increase in size, importance, and value to society.

The value placed on public health activities can be measured in economic terms, such as funding levels for programs, services, and the workers who implement public health programs and services. To sustain or even enhance public health funding, national leadership is necessary. Federal health agencies such as the Centers for Disease Control and Prevention (CDC) and HRSA within the Department of Health and Human Services (DHHS) are especially important in the area of public health workforce development. In addition to national leadership, state and local governments must remain committed to and invested in public health objectives. However, states and local governments face difficult economic circumstances and tough choices across the United States and are looking to cut back services that are either low priority or that have other funding sources. If state and local governments supplant their own funding with the new federal funds, the overall effort will be less than it should be.

Beyond funding, administrative and bureaucratic obstacles challenge public health workforce development efforts in the public sector. State and local agencies are often the source of some of the most significant recruitment and retention problems facing the public health workforce. These include slow hiring by governmental agencies, civil service systems, hiring freezes, budget crises affecting state and local government, and the lack of career ladders, competitive salary structures, and other forms of recognition that value workers for their skill and performance.

Despite the uncertainties inherent in these influences, past trends and current forces suggest that professional and administrative jobs and careers in public health are likely to grow over the next decade. Unfortunately, it will be difficult to measure the progress that has been made without deployment of a standard taxonomy for public health occupations and more comprehensive enumeration strategies and tools that provide better information on the key dimensions of the public health workforce, including its size and distribution in official agencies and private and voluntary organizations.

In addition to the size of the public health workforce, its distribution and composition are important to current and future public health workers. Key questions include: (1) Where will public health job opportunities be most abundant? and (2) Which occupational categories are likely to grow most rapidly and be in greatest demand?

Job opportunities generally track with population density and demographic shifts. Within the health sector, job opportunities cluster around metropolitan areas. Public health positions also follow this pattern. There are more positions, and therefore more opportunities, in metropolitan areas than there are in rural areas. General demographic trends indicate a continuing shift of population from the Northeast and Midwest regions of the United States to the South, Southwest, and West Coast. It is likely that health sector jobs and public health positions will also follow this pattern.

The ratio of positions to population, however, can be higher in rural areas (and states that have higher proportions of their population living in nonmetropolitan areas). This occurs because there is a basic core staffing that must be present regardless of the size of the population and because rural and remote communities often lack other public health resources and assets. For example, local public health agencies in small as well as large communities will have an agency administrator, director of nursing, and environmental director. Public health agencies serving larger communities may have more total workers, but the ratio of workers to population is often lower due to the effect of core (or overhead) staffing. In addition, nongovernmental resources are often lacking in rural communities. Governmental agencies may constitute a larger proportion of a rural community's overall resources than for urban or suburban communities. A higher public health worker to population ratio in rural areas raises issues of efficiency in terms of scarce resources, including public health professionals, and can be used as an argument for consolidation of several small local public health agencies into one large agency.

Table 6–8 provides a snapshot describing the distribution and composition of the public health workforce from a different perspective by aggregating public health practice profiles. This composite profile illustrates the breadth of roles in addressing public health's broad purposes and essential services as well as the contribution of the various public health occupational categories and titles.

This composite highlights the importance of preventing the spread of disease and assuring the quality of health services as public health purposes. The majority of public health occupations place significant emphasis on these purposes. Only a few public health occupations and titles focus on emergency response as a primary duty. Virtually all, however, have roles in responding to public health emergencies as a secondary-level responsibility.

Among the 10 essential public health services, nearly all public health occupations and titles are actively involved in evaluating the effectiveness, accessibility, and quality of personal and population-based health services. Eight other essential public health services are widely distributed across the

TABLE 6–9 Percentage of Local Health Departments (LHDs) Employing Selected professional Occupations, 1990 and 2005

	1989	2005
Physicians—All LHDs	62%	43%
<50,000	51%	27%
50,000–499,999	75%	62%
500,000+	99%	91%
Epidemiologists—all LHDs	11%	25%
<50,000	3%	7%
50,000-499,999	8%	41%
500,000+	87%	94%
Health educators—all LHDs	37%	55%
<50,000	22%	37%
50,000–499,999	54%	78%
500,000+	95%	94%
Public information specialists—all LHDs	6%	18%
<50,000	2%	5%
50,000–499,999	5%	29%
500,000+	52%	78%

Source: Data from National Association of County and City Health Officials. *2005 National Profile of Local Health Departments*. Washington, DC: NACCHO; 2006.

various occupational categories and titles. Only a few public health occupations focus extensively on assuring a competent workforce.

Some health sector occupations will grow more rapidly than others, even while the health sector grows more rapidly than the rest of the economy. Among the many public health occupations, several appear to be growing rapidly and several others appear to be in danger of their supply not keeping pace with anticipated demand.

It is not surprising that public health nurses and environmental health practitioners are repeatedly identified as the positions in greatest demand. Indeed, these occupational categories are the largest in the public health workforce, and it is only natural that these categories undergo greater turnover than others. For registered nurses, there is substantial evidence of a current national shortage. For environmental health practitioners, this is not so clear.

The demand for many public health professional occupations is growing steadily. Between 1990 and 2005, an increasing number of LHDs are employing epidemiologists, health educators, and public health information officers (Table 6–9).

The aftermath of terrorist events of 2001, including the series of anthrax spore attacks through the postal system, spotlighted the need for two professional positions in particular. The first, emergency response coordinators, is new to the list of public health occupations; the second, epidemiologists, is one of the oldest public health professional occupations. State and local public health agencies are rapidly hiring emergency response coordinators. These people come to these new positions with a wide range of academic and experiential qualifications. Epidemiologists, on the other hand, have more restrictive qualifications in terms of academic preparation such as master's and doctoral degrees. Concerns over the past few decades that epidemiologists were in short supply and great demand are now heightened as agencies seek to quickly hire these specialists. The number of epidemiologists coming out of graduate programs does not appear to be keeping pace with the need, despite an increase in interest as measured by the number of applications for epidemiology training programs.

Prior to 2001, health educators and community health planners were steadily growing professional categories in the public health workforce. Expansion of health education and promotion services, and an increase in community health planning and community health improvement activities account for this trend. It is not clear whether this trend will continue in view of the current emphasis on bioterrorism and public health emergency preparedness.

PUBLIC HEALTH PRACTITIONER COMPETENCIES

Beyond workforce size, distribution, and composition are issues related to the core competencies and skills that will be most important in public health practice and how these skills are best acquired. Establishing and promoting competencies for public health workers is tricky business. For one thing, public health workers come from a variety of professional backgrounds, many of which have their own core competencies. For example, public health nursing has a set of core competencies, and health educators use a sophisticated competency framework for purposes of certification. The same can be said for public health physicians, administrators, epidemiologists, and several other public health professional occupations. Identifying a common core for these various professional categories generally leads to a framework with very general and nonspecific competencies that are difficult to relate to a specific situation or problem. The Council on Linkages between Academia and Public Health Practice spent 2 decades grappling with this problem before arriving at the set of core competencies for public health professionals summarized in Table 6–10 for entry-level workers.

The national public health organizations endorsed and adopted these core competencies, which track to the essential public health services framework, as the basis for assessing and enhancing the skills of public health workers. Core public health practice competencies serve as a useful benchmark for competency frameworks developed to serve state or local public health systems or to guide the development of more focused skills, such as in public health law, informatics, genomics, and emergency preparedness.

There are several important and practical uses for competency frameworks. Core competencies can serve as models whenever an agency's job descriptions are developed, updated, or revised. As competency-oriented job descriptions become more widely used, core competencies can guide orientation and training activities for new employees. Core competencies are also useful in employee self-assessment activities as well as in personnel evaluation activities when supervisors review the past performance of employees and set performance expectations for the next cycle. The use of competencies within personnel and human resources systems is growing slowly within the public sector, although widespread implementation could take decades.

The identification of core competencies for public health practice and for emergency preparedness and response demonstrate the support for competency-based training among practice organizations. A companion effort to identify a panel of core competencies for graduates of master's of public health (MPH) programs in schools of public health was compiled in 2006 under the auspices of the Association of Schools of Public Health (ASPH). This panel of competencies addresses discipline-specific competencies for behavioral sciences, health administration, epidemiology, biostatistics, environmental health, and public health biology as well as crosscutting competencies in the areas of communication, informatics, cultural proficiency, ecologic determinants of health, leadership, policy development, professionalism, program development and evaluation, and systems thinking.

Despite this progress, formidable challenges lie ahead.[19,20] These include the establishment of mechanisms to support workforce planning and training in all states and local jurisdictions, and refinement and validation of public health practice competencies associated with each of the various disciplines that compose the workforce. Enhanced competencies are necessary to improve basic, advanced, and continuing education curricula for public health workers. Also needed are strategies to certify competencies among practitioners. In addition, large-scale assessments of current levels of workforce preparedness as measured by core competencies are lacking. For education and training of the public health workforce to be taken seriously, both academic and practice interests must view public health workforce development as an important priority.

Education and training opportunities for public health workers are widely available today and likely to expand even further over the next decade. The first school of public health was established in 1916 at the Johns Hopkins School of Hygiene and Public Health with the support of the Rockefeller Foundation. In 1969, there were only 12 schools of public health, but that number grew to 43 by mid-2010, with a dozen new schools in the pipeline. The number of accredited programs offering the MPH and equivalent degrees exceded 80 in 2010. Many unaccredited programs also exist.

Before 1970, students in public health training were primarily physicians or members of other disciplines with professional degrees. In recent decades, however, more than two thirds of the students enter public health training in order to obtain their primary postgraduate degrees. Public health training evolved from a second degree for medical professionals to a primary health discipline. Schools of public health that initially emphasized the study of hygiene and sanitation have expanded their curricula to address five core disciplines—biostatistics, epidemiology, health services administration, health education/behavioral science, and environmental science.

The number of individuals earning graduate degrees in public health tripled between 1975 and 2010, from 3,000 to more than 10,000.[7] Surprisingly, this increase has not had a significant impact on the number and proportion of professionals trained in public health in the primary public health workforce. In the 1970s, about one half of MPH graduates took jobs with governmental public health agencies, the primary public health workforce. Currently, only about one in five MPH graduates take jobs with governmental public health agencies.

Despite this impressive growth of public health schools and programs, most public health workers continue to receive their professional preparation elsewhere. This is not surprising in view of the number of training programs for key occupational categories in the public health workforce. There are more

TABLE 6–10 Core Competencies for Tier 1 (Entry-Level) Public Health Workers

Analytic/Assessment Skills

- Identifies the health status of populations and their related determinants of health and illness
- Describes the characteristics of a population-based health problem
- Uses variables that measure public health conditions
- Uses methods and instruments for collecting valid and reliable quantitative and qualitative data
- Identifies sources of public health data and information
- Recognizes the integrity and comparability of data
- Identifies gaps in data sources
- Adheres to ethical principles in the collection, maintenance, use, and dissemination of data and information
- Describes the public health applications of quantitative and qualitative data
- Collects quantitative and qualitative community data
- Uses information technology to collect, store, and retrieve data
- Describes how data are used to address scientific, political, ethical, and social public health issues

Policy Development/Program Planning Skills

- Gathers information relevant to specific public health policy issues
- Describes how policy options can influence public health programs
- Explains the expected outcomes of policy options
- Gathers information that will inform policy decisions
- Describes the public health laws and regulations governing public health programs
- Participates in program planning processes
- Incorporates policies and procedures into program plans and structures
- Identifies mechanisms to monitor and evaluate programs for their effectiveness and quality
- Demonstrates the use of public health informatics practices and procedures
- Applies strategies for continuous quality improvement

Communication Skills

- Identifies the health literacy of populations served
- Communicates in writing and orally, in person, and through electronic means, with linguistic and cultural proficiency
- Solicits community-based input from individuals and organizations
- Conveys public health information using a variety of approaches
- Participates in the development of demographic, statistical, programmatic, and scientific presentations
- Applies communication and group dynamic strategies in interactions with individuals and groups

Cultural Competency Skills

- Incorporates strategies for interacting with persons from diverse backgrounds
- Recognizes the role of cultural, social, and behavioral factors in the accessibility, availability, acceptability and delivery of public health services
- Responds to diverse needs that are the result of cultural differences
- Describes the dynamic forces that contribute to cultural diversity
- Describes the need for a diverse public health workforce
- Participates in the assessment of the cultural competence of the public health organization

Community Dimension of Practice Skills

- Recognizes community linkages and relationships among multiple factors (or determinants) affecting health
- Demonstrates the capacity to work in community-based participatory research efforts
- Identifies stakeholders
- Collaborates with community partners to promote the health of the population
- Maintains partnerships with key stakeholders
- Uses group processes to advance community involvement
- Describes the role of governmental and nongovernmental organizations in the delivery of community health services
- Identifies community assets and resources
- Gathers input from the community to inform the development of public health policy and programs
- Informs the public about policies, programs, and resources

(continued)

TABLE 6–10 Core Competencies for Tier 1 (Entry-Level) Public Health Workers *(continued)*

Public Health Sciences Skills
- Describes the scientific foundation of the field of public health
- Identifies prominent events in the history of the public health profession
- Relates public health science skills to the core public health functions and ten essential services of public health
- Identifies the basic public health sciences (including, but not limited to biostatistics, epidemiology, environmental health sciences, health services administration, and social and behavioral health sciences)
- Describes the scientific evidence related to a public health issue, concern, or, intervention
- Retrieves scientific evidence from a variety of text and electronic sources
- Discusses the limitations of research findings
- Describes the laws, regulations, policies, and procedures for the ethical conduct of research
- Partners with other public health professionals in building the scientific base of public health

Financial Planning and Management Skills
- Describes the local, state, and federal public health and healthcare systems
- Describes the organizational structures, functions, and authorities of local, state, and federal public health agencies
- Adheres to the organization's policies and procedures
- Participates in the development of a programmatic budget
- Operates programs within current and forecasted budget constraints
- Identifies strategies for determining budget priorities based on federal, state, and local financial contributions
- Reports program performance
- Translates evaluation report information into program performance improvement action steps
- Contributes to the preparation of proposals for funding from external sources
- Applies basic human relations skills to internal collaborations, motivation of colleagues, and resolution of conflicts
- Demonstrates public health informatics skills to improve program and business operations
- Participates in the development of contracts and other agreements for the provision of services
- Describes how cost-effectiveness, cost-benefit, and cost-utility analyses affect programmatic prioritization and decision making

Leadership and Systems Thinking Skills
- Incorporates ethical standards of practice as the basis of all interactions with organizations, communities, and individuals
- Describes how public health operates within a larger system
- Participates with stakeholders in identifying key public health values and a shared public health vision as guiding principles for community action
- Identifies internal and external problems that may affect the delivery of essential public health services
- Uses individual, team, and organizational learning opportunities for personal and professional development
- Participates in mentoring and peer review or coaching opportunities
- Participates in the measuring, reporting, and continuous improvement of organizational performance
- Describes the impact of changes in the public health system and that of the larger social, political, economic environment on organizational practices

Note: Tier 1 core competencies apply to public health professionals who carry out the day-to-day tasks of public health organizations and are not in management positions. Responsibilities of these public health professionals may include basic data collection and analysis, fieldwork, program planning, outreach activities, programmatic support, and other organizational tasks. In general, an individual at the Tier 1 level may be educated at the baccalaureate level or educated at a higher level with limited experience as a public health professional.

Source: From Council on Linkages between Academia and Public Health Practice; 2010.

than 1,500 basic RN training programs at the bachelor, associate, or diploma level; well in excess of 1,000 LPN training programs; more than 150 programs in health administration; and several hundred programs offering training in environmental health sciences.

In summary, educational resources contribute to a national network of nearly 150 accredited schools and other graduate training programs in public health, and as many as 500 other graduate-level education programs in areas related to public health, such as health administration, public health nursing, and environmental engineering.

Training activities that focus on public health workers rather than students are also extensive. HRSA has long been the primary federal health agency supporting development of the various health professions, although the public health workforce has never been a priority for that agency. Because many public health workers come from other health disciplines, however, HRSA support for training other health professionals also benefits the public health workforce. Throughout the 1990s, HRSA training activities for public health focused increasingly on strengthening links between schools of public health (SPH) and public health agencies. Early in the 1990s, HRSA initiated support for the Council on Linkages between Academia and Public Health Practice, which has grown to include representation from many prominent public health academic and practice organizations. Since 1999, HRSA has funded Public Health Training Centers, which are multistate training collaborations involving SPHs and health agencies, with 14 such centers (with approximately $5 million in annual funding) operating in late 2010. Beginning in 2002, HRSA also funded states and several large cities to support hospital bioterrorism planning and provided funds for curriculum development and training for health care professionals and for community-wide planning related to bioterrorism and other public health emergencies.

During the 1990s, the CDC became increasingly engaged in supporting capacity development and improving state-based public health systems through the establishment of national and regional leadership development projects in the early 1990s. CDC also provided direct financial assistance to state public health systems for emergency preparedness later in that decade. CDC encouraged states and large cities to utilize this funding to improve the capacity of their public health infrastructures in order to respond to a wide range of both emergency and routine threats, including bioterrorism preparedness. CDC increasingly emphasized and supported public health workforce development as the cornerstone of infrastructure improvement. Between 2000 and 2010, through its cooperative agreement with the ASPH, CDC awarded substantial grants (approximately $1 million per center per year) to more than two dozen academic Centers for Public Health Preparedness.

Since 1998, funding for public health workforce development through SPHs has increased dramatically, from under $1 million (primarily from HRSA) in 1997 to more than $30 million (mainly from CDC) in 2005. Approximately another $70–$80 million for public health training is available in the bioterrorism grants awarded to states and several large cities, an estimated 10% of those grants. A total of more than $100 million is being programmed specifically for public health workforce development in 2010 in addition to resources that prepare other health professionals to participate in responses to public health emergencies.[14]

The extent of organized workforce development activities within state and local health departments and other public health organizations is unknown. Nonetheless, virtually all public health organizations provide some form of orientation, training, and support of continuing education for their workers. Costs for these activities are often buried in agency budgets as human resources, administrative support, and employee travel expenditures encompassing both direct and indirect, or opportunity costs for time spent away from performing official duties. Aggregating these costs would likely represent a significant pool of resources.

Efforts to forge links between academic and training partners and public health practice agencies at all levels of government are advancing, although unevenly from state to state. Comprehensive approaches that serve the entire public health workforce with an extensive menu of options for workers at varying stages of career development are lacking. More limited approaches that increase the number of workers who can acquire formal public health training through degree programs or that provide advanced skills to specific categories of workers within the public health workforce are useful but not sufficient. These efforts serve a relatively small portion of the overall public health workforce. More comprehensive and systems-based approaches are needed.

PUBLIC HEALTH WORKFORCE DEVELOPMENT

Although education and training are key components of public health workforce strategies, they are not by themselves sufficient. Comprehensive public health workforce development efforts assess and promote competencies in addition to enhancing them (Figure 6–4). Efforts to promote the acquisition of public health competencies focus on several fronts but necessarily emphasize the workplace and the organizations that employ workers. Critical skills and core competencies are promoted in the workplace through job descriptions and performance appraisals that are organized around those skills and competencies. Managers and supervisors work with their employees to manage the professional development of workers and build skills that are necessary for career advancement. These administrative and personnel policies and practice create a culture that values competent performance and the acquisition of new skills.

A complementary approach to promote competencies relies on external bodies to validate and recognize skill levels through credentialing programs. There are many different forms of credentials for various categories of public health workers. For example, nutritionists may earn the RD (registered dietician) credential, health educators may become CHES (Certified Health Education Specialists), physicians may achieve board certification in preventive medicine and public health, and many different credentials are available to environmental health practitioners. With discipline-specific credentials available to so many different public health worker occupational categories, it should come as no surprise that there are now efforts to develop credentials specific to public health.

FIGURE 6–4 Components of a public health workforce preparedness management system.

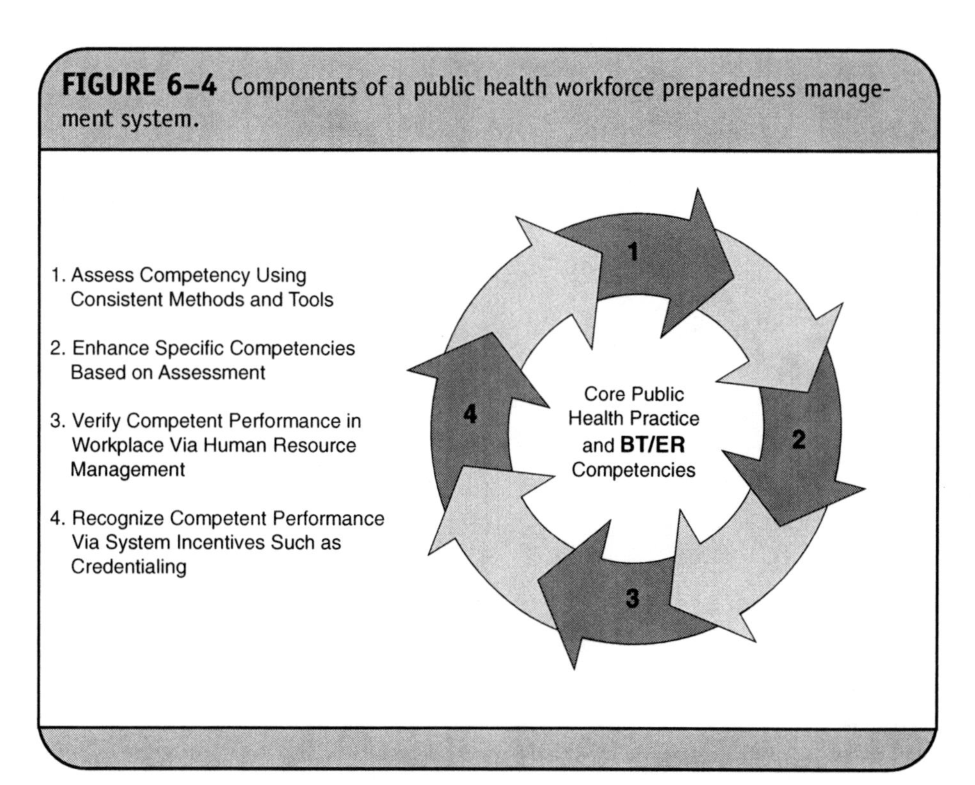

The intent of any credential is to distinguish someone who is eligible for some status from others who are not. Identifying individuals who have demonstrated practice-relevant competencies at a specified level (from front-line workers to senior professionals, specialists, and leaders) provides an incentive for individuals to enhance their skills. Health professions have taken various approaches to credentialing that include licensing (for physicians and nurses), certification (for health education specialists), and registration (for dieticians and sanitarians). These examples suggest that credentialing is already widely used for public health workers; examples include board-certified preventive medicine physicians, certified community health nurses and health education specialists, and certified, registered environmental health practitioners. There is still a need for credentials for those who would not fit into these specialty-specific credentials, such as public health physicians not certified in preventive medicine, or health educators who are not certified health education specialists. Because many, indeed most, workers will not be able to meet the specific requirements for specialty credentialing, such as the 3-year residency for physicians or completion of a health education degree at the undergraduate or graduate level for certified health educators, a midlevel public health-specific credential could be attractive to many public health disciplines. Fledgling competency-based credentialing programs for public health managers and for public health emergency response coordinators exist in one state using an independent certification board.[21] In 2008, the newly established National Board of Public Health Examiners initiated a credential (CPH or Certified in Public Health) for graduates of MPH degree programs based on a national test. These and other models focus more on public health practice competencies rather than on a worker's core discipline, making them fertile ground for turf battles with professional organizations. Considerable input from these professional organizations and from professionals in practice will be needed, however, for any framework to be valued and widely used. A three-prong credentialing strategy emerged from the National Public Health Workforce Development Conference in early 2003 calling for recognition of public health competency at a basic or Public Health 101 level and at a leadership level as well as expansion of existing credentialing activities for public health disciplines to cover those not now included.[22]

For workers to value credentials and the competencies upon which they are based, employers and health agencies must find value in them as well and base decisions about hiring, promotion, salaries, and the like on an individual worker's demonstration of those competencies. Improving workers' ability to perform their functions competently relies on both worker training and work management strategies[14]; these relationships are illustrated in Figure 6–5. As performance standards for public health organizations and public health systems gain headway through initiatives such as the National Public Health Performance Standards

FIGURE 6–5 The structure of a public health work-doing system.

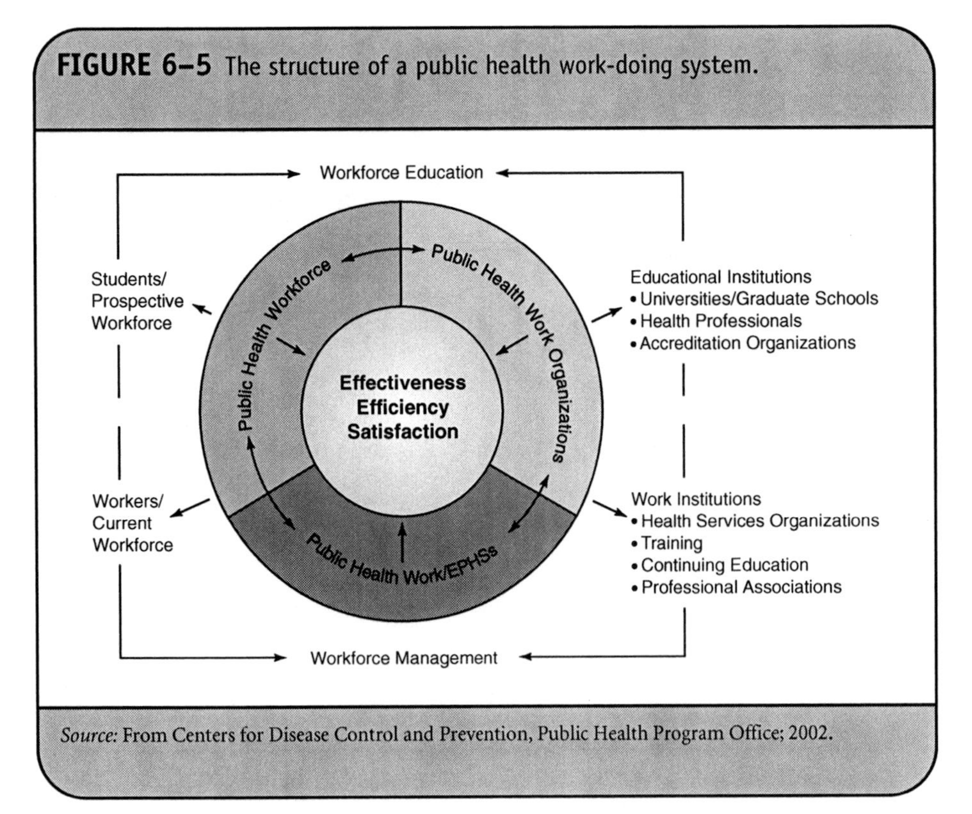

Source: From Centers for Disease Control and Prevention, Public Health Program Office; 2002.

Program and the National Association of County and City Health Officials' (NACCHO's) Mobilizing for Action through Planning and Partnerships (MAPP) process, competency-based performance standards for workers will increasingly be viewed as key ingredients of organizational and system performance.

An innovative NACCHO program, Public Health Ready, contributed significantly, promoting public health workforce preparedness. Public Health Ready recognizes public health agencies that meet standards for worker competency, agency preparedness plans, and regular exercises of those plans.[23] Workers can demonstrate preparedness competencies during those drills and simulations, furthering the ability of the agency to verify and document the preparedness levels of the organization and its staff. As this approach expands, it could serve to focus public health workforce development efforts through its emphasis on the work, workers, and work organizations that constitute the governmental public health enterprise.

Although several forms of incentives are slowly advancing, one key element of a system of incentives remains lacking—there is no common currency in the form of a public health continuing-education unit (CEU) that assures quality and consistency of training activities nationally. Neither CDC, nor any of the national public health organizations, has sought to serve in this capacity. A common currency that has credibility in the practice sector and is linked with organized workforce development strategies and funding from recent bioterrorism preparedness legislation would provide a considerable incentive for competency-based approaches to public health workforce development. Nonetheless, the obstacles and inertia that have accrued over several decades remain formidable challenges for the public health system.

As demonstrated in Figure 6–5, comprehensive workforce development strategies must focus not only on the worker, but on the organizations in which the work of public health is performed.

CONCLUSION

Recent decades have witnessed an increase in the number of public health workers employed by both governmental and nongovernmental agencies, caused by expanded public health priorities and partnerships. This expansion of the workforce, however, leaves many questions unanswered as to the number, distribution, training, and preparedness of the public health workforce, making these issues of public concern.[19,20] Some of these concerns have persisted since the late 1800s, as suggested by an editorial appearing in the *Journal of the American Medical Association* more than 110 years ago:

> It is unfortunate that in the absence of epidemics or pestilence, too little attention is paid to the protection of the public health, and as a necessary consequence, to the selection of those whose duties require them to guard the public health.[24(p189)]

Other concerns are of more recent vintage. The economic recession of 2009 displaced millions of workers in both the public and private sectors of the economy. State and local governments were especially hard hit, with the budget crises facing many states threatening future employment opportunities for public health workers. Sources point to the aging of the public health workforce, current shortages of public health nurses and epidemiologists, and the imminent retirement of many public health professionals. On the other hand, national health reform legislation enacted in 2010 included several provisions for stabilizing and strengthening the public health workforce through scholarship and loan repayment programs to push more public health professionals through the pipeline and into positions in state and local agencies.

Responses to these developments, however, reflect a view that public health workforce development strategies must produce more public health workers. Although strategies that focus on the pipeline are necessary and useful, they will never be sufficient to assure an effective public health workforce over the long term. Strategies that focus on the workforce itself are also needed. The public health workforce is growing and will continue to grow for years to come. Many public health occupational categories will see a steady increase; others will grow even more rapidly. As a population-based enterprise, public health jobs should mirror demographic changes in terms of both location of job opportunities and the diversity and cultural proficiency of workers. Core public health practice competencies will increasingly influence education and training programs and find their way into the human resource activities and personnel systems of governmental public health agencies. Worker recognition initiatives based on relevant competencies, such as credentialing and certification programs, will also grow in order to address the need for both heightened accountability and expanded career pathways. The recent influx of resources to support public health workforce development will continue only if measurable progress and impact can be demonstrated. Without those resources, however, the progress of public health workforce development efforts could stall. In the end, the most important asset of the public health system remains its workforce.

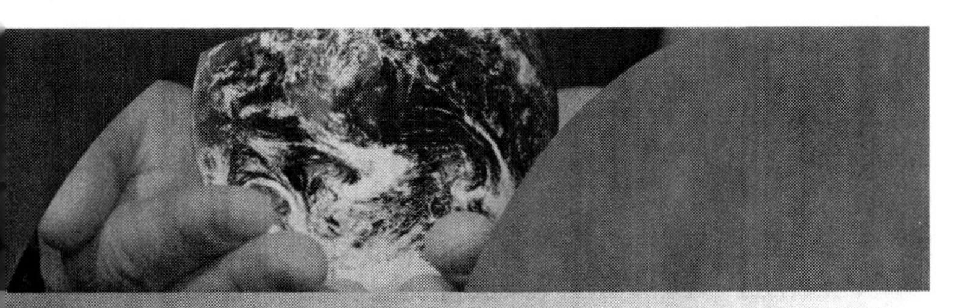

Discussion Questions

1. Choose a recent (within the last 3 years) outbreak or other public health emergency situation that has drawn significant media attention. Describe how specific occupational categories in the public health infrastructure contributed to either the emergency situation or its solution. The *MMWR Morbidity and Mortality Weekly Report* contents for recent weeks would be a good place to look for recent outbreaks; various print and electronic media may also be useful sources of information.
2. What distinguishes a public health professional from a professional working for a public health organization?
3. Are public health professionals viewed as change agents in their communities today? Why or why not? Do you hold the same opinion for public health organizations? Why or why not?
4. What factors determine the optimum size of the public health workforce in your community?
5. How have the needs for different public health occupations changed over the past century? How will the need for various public health occupations change over the next 2 decades?

REFERENCES

1. Institute of Medicine, National Academy of Sciences. *The Future of Public Health*. Washington, DC: National Academy Press; 1988.
2. Health Resources and Services Administration, U.S. Department of Health and Human Services. *Public Health Personnel in the United States, 1980: Second Report to Congress*. Washington, DC: U.S. Public Health Service; 1982.
3. Health Resources Services Administration, U.S. Department of Health and Human Services. *Public Health Enumeration 2000*. Washington, DC: Government Printing Office; December 2000.
4. Public Health Functions Steering Committee. I. Washington, DC: U.S. Public Health Service; 1995.
5. Kennedy VC, Moore FI. A systems approach to public health workforce development. *J Public Health Manage Pract*. 2001;7:17–22.
6. U.S. Bureau of the Census. *Federal, State, and Local Governments, Public Employment and Payroll Data*. www.census.gov/govs/apes/. Accessed September 27, 2010.
7. Centers for Disease Control and Prevention, National Center for *Health Statistics. Health United States, 2009*. Hyattsville, MD: National Center for Health Statistics; 2009.
8. National Association of County and City Health Officials. *2005 National Profile of Local Health Departments*. Washington, DC: National Association of County and City Health Officials; 2006.
9. National Association of County and City Health Officials. *2008 National Profile of Local Health Departments*. Washington, DC: National Association of County and City Health Officials; 2009.
10. Gerzoff RB, Baker EL. The use of scaling techniques to analyze U.S. local health department staffing structures, 1992–1993. *Proceedings of the Section on Government Statistics and Section on Social Statistics of the American Statistical Association*. 1998:209–213.
11. Thomas JC, Sage M, Dillenberg J, Guillory VJ. A Code or ethics for public health. *Am J Public Health*. 2002;92:1057–1059.
12. Gerzoff RB, Richards TB. The education of local health department top executives. *J Public Health Manage Pract*. 1997;3:50–56.
13. Turnock BJ, Hutchison KD. *The Local Public Health Workforce: Size, Distribution, Composition, and Influence on Core Function Performance, Illinois 1998–1999*. Chicago IL; Illinois Center for Health Workforce Studies; 2000.
14. Turnock BJ. Roadmap for Public Health Workforce Preparedness. *J Public Health Manage Pract*. 2003;9:471–480.
15. Bureau of Labor Statistics, U.S. Department of Labor. *Standard occupational classification*. www.bls.gov/soc/. Accessed May 15, 2010.
16. Bureau of Labor Statistics, U.S. Department of Labor. *May 2008 and May 2009 national, state, and metropolitan occupational employment and wage estimates*. www.bls.gov/oes/current/oes_nat.htm. Accessed June 17, 2010.
17. Bureau of Labor Statistics, U.S. Department of Labor. *Occupational outlook handbook*. www.bls.gov/oco/. Accessed May 15, 2010.
18. Council of State and Territorial Epidemiologists. *2004 National Assessment of Epidemiologic Capacity: Findings and Recommendations*. Washington, DC: Council of State and Territorial Epidemiologists; 2004. http://www.ste.org/Assessment/ECA/pdffiles/ECAfinal05.pdf. Accessed September 27, 2010.
19. Tilson H, Gebbie KM. The public health workforce. *Ann Rev Public Health*. 2004;25:341–356.
20. Gebbie KM, Turnock BJ. The public health workforce, 2006: new challenges. *Health Aff (Millwood)*. 2006;25:923–933.
21. Turnock BJ. Competency-based credentialing of public health administrators in Illinois. *J Public Health Manage Pract*. 2001;7:74–82.
22. Cioffi JP, Lichtveld MY, Thielen L, Miner K. Credentialing the public health workforce: an idea whose time has come. *J Public Health Manage Pract*. 2003;6:451–458.
23. National Association of County and City Health Officials. *Project Public Health Ready*. http://www.naccho.org/topics/emergency/pphr.cfm. Accessed September 27, 2010.
24. American Medical Association. Editorial. *JAMA*. 1893;20:189.

CHAPTER 7

Non-communicable Diseases

Learning Objectives

By the end of this chapter the reader will be able to:

- Describe the most important non-communicable diseases
- Discuss the importance of these diseases to global health
- Discuss the burden of non-communicable diseases worldwide
- Outline the costs and consequences of non-communicable diseases, tobacco use, and excessive drinking of alcohol
- Review measures that can be taken to address the burden of non-communicable diseases in cost-effective ways
- Describe some successful cases of dealing with non-communicable diseases

VIGNETTES

Roberto was 45 years old and lived in Bogota, Colombia. He had been overweight for most of his adult life. He enjoyed eating and had a government desk job. Because he lived in the heart of the city, he got little exercise. He had read about increasing rates of diabetes but thought this was largely a disease of people in rich countries. Last year, Roberto started feeling thirsty all the time, had dry mouth, and felt weak after any exertion. He went to his doctor and was diagnosed as having adult onset diabetes.

Shanti was 35 years old and lived in Sri Lanka. She had grown up in a village, had worked hard on her family's small farm, and had been healthy for all of her adult life. She had two children and had not had any problems during either pregnancy. During a recent visit to the local health center, however, the doctor discovered that Shanti had high blood pressure. The doctor talked with Shanti about changing her diet and also prescribed medication for her. The medicine she needed is not expensive, but, unfortunately, Shanti has to take this medicine for the remainder of her life.

Alexei was 47 years old and lived in Moscow, Russia. Alexei had been smoking one pack of cigarettes a day since he was 16 years old. He heard on television and on the radio about the bad effects that cigarettes have on health. Urged by his children to stop smoking, he tried unsuccessfully on several occasions to quit. Over the last few months, Alexei developed a continuous cough and was often short of breath. Alexei had lung cancer.

Lai Ying lived in Guandong Province, China, and was a factory worker. Until recently she had been a happy and healthy young woman. More recently, however, Lai Ying had felt very unhappy. She did not feel like getting out of bed in the morning, did not want to go to work, and had no energy when she was at work. She thought from time to time of death and considered suicide. Lai Ying's family noticed that she was not eating properly and that she was "not herself." However, they thought she was having a difficult time at work or with a boyfriend and that she would soon be fine. After some months of this behavior, Lai Ying committed suicide by taking an overdose of sleeping pills.

THE IMPORTANCE OF NON-COMMUNICABLE DISEASES

Non-communicable diseases are of considerable and growing importance worldwide. In fact, the burden of non-communicable diseases is now greater than the burden of communicable diseases in low- and middle-income countries, as well as in high-income countries. This is a relatively recent fact which contradicts the notion that low-income countries are so overwhelmed with the burden of communicable disease that they do not face a significant burden of non-communicable disease. Among the most important of the non-communicable health conditions that low- and middle-income countries face are cardiovascular disease, diabetes, cancers, and mental disorders.[1]

The risk factors for non-communicable diseases relate in significant ways to lifestyle, much of which is within people's control. We will discuss, for example, the importance of diet, physical activity, tobacco use, and alcohol abuse to the onset of certain non-communicable diseases. By engaging in appropriate health behaviors, it is possible for people to considerably reduce the risk of getting heart disease, some cancers, or diabetes.

Some non-communicable diseases can be prevented at relatively low cost, but these diseases are often very expensive to treat. It is possible, for example, to significantly reduce the chances of getting lung cancer by making a modest investment in smoking cessation therapy and by quitting smoking. By contrast, the cost of treating lung cancer through drugs and surgery is considerably more.

This chapter will focus on non-communicable diseases. It will pay particular attention to cardiovascular disease, cancer, diabetes, and mental disorders because of their important and growing contribution to the global burden of disease, including in low- and middle-income countries. Because of the importance of tobacco and alcohol as risk factors for non-communicable diseases, the chapter will also contain specific sections on these topics.

The chapter will first introduce you to definitions of selected health conditions. It will then examine the burden of non-communicable diseases and the risk factors for those diseases. Following that, it will comment on some of the most important costs and consequences of these diseases. It will then review what steps can be taken to address the burden of non-communicable diseases effectively and efficiently, and will discuss several examples of successful efforts to prevent and deal with non-communicable diseases. The chapter will conclude with comments on some of the future challenges that must be addressed if the burden of non-communicable diseases is to be reduced.

TABLE 7-1 Key Terms and Definitions

Blood Glucose—Blood sugar, the main source of energy for the body.
Cancer—One of a large variety of diseases characterized by uncontrolled growth of cells.
Cardiovascular Disease—A disease of the heart or blood vessels.
Cholesterol—A fat-like substance that is made by the body and is found naturally in animal-based fods such as meat, fish, poultry, and eggs.
Diabetes—An illness caused by poor control by the body of blood sugar.
Hypertension—High blood pressure, with a reading of 140/90 or greater.
Ischemic Heart Disease—A disturbance of the heart function due to inadequate supply of oxygen to the heart muscle.
Stroke—Sudden loss of function of the brain due to clotting or hemorrhaging.

Source: The Author. Modified from: Global Cardiovascular Infobase Glossary. Available at: http://www.cvdinfobase.ca/cvdbook/En/Glossary.htm. Accessed 14, 2007; National Institutes of Health. Obesity, Physical Activity, and Weight-control Glossary. Available at: http://win.niddk.nih.gov/publications/glossary/AthruL.htm. Accessed April 14, 2007.

KEY DEFINITIONS

Communicable diseases are illnesses caused by an infectious agent that spread from a person or an animal to another person or animal. **Non-communicable diseases** are, in many respects, the opposite of communicable diseases. First, they can not be spread from person to person by an infectious agent, even if they might be associated with one. Second, they tend to last a long time. Third, they can be very disabling, can seriously impair the ability of people to engage in day to day activities, and they often lead to death if they are not treated appropriately.

The terms "chronic disease" and "degenerative disease" are often used interchangeably with non-communicable disease. In this book, however, we shall consistently use the term "non-communicable disease." The most recent studies of the burden of disease include the following under non-communicable diseases: malignant neoplasms (cancers); diabetes; endocrine disorders; neuropsychiatric disorders, such as mental disorders, epilepsy, and Alzheimer's disease; and sense organ disorders, such as hearing loss, glaucoma, or cataracts.

You are already familiar with most of the terms used in this chapter. However, a few key terms with which you may be less familiar are defined in Table 7-1.

THE BURDEN OF NON-COMMUNICABLE DISEASES

Cardiovascular Disease

Cardiovascular disease (CVD) caused 16.4 million deaths in 2001 and is now the leading cause of death in the world.[1]

CVD is the cause of about 30% of all deaths worldwide, and it is predicted that by 2020, more than half of all deaths worldwide will be associated with CVD.[1] As noted earlier, it is now the leading cause of death in low- and middle-income countries, as well as in richer countries. CVD is associated with about 30% of all deaths in high-income countries and about 28% of deaths in low- and middle-income countries.[1]

CVD is the largest cause of death in all regions, except in Sub-Saharan Africa. CVD is the cause of about 58% of all deaths in Europe and Central Asia and about 30% of all deaths in East Asia and the Pacific, but only about 10% of the total deaths in Sub-Saharan Africa.[1] CVD rates are higher in Eastern Europe than in Western Europe, although the rates of CVD are falling in some Eastern European countries. The highest rates of CVD are in the former Soviet Union, where they are contributing to declines in life expectancy.[1] The rate of prevalence of CVD tends to be higher in urban than in rural areas.

About 80% of the burden of CVD worldwide is due to three conditions: ischemic heart disease (IHD), stroke, and congestive heart failure.[1] In most regions, ischemic heart disease is the most important contributor to death due to all cardiovascular diseases. In the Middle East and North Africa, for example, three people die from IHD for every one who dies from stroke. Stroke, however, is the dominant contributor to deaths in both Sub-Saharan Africa and in China.[2] In India, CVD appears in people at younger ages more than in high-income countries. Whereas in high-income countries only about 22% of CVD deaths are in people under 70 years of age, in India, about 50% of the CVD deaths occur in people under 70.[3]

To help get a better understanding of the importance of CVD to the burden of disease, Table 7-2 shows the burden of deaths and DALYs worldwide and by regions that are associated with CVD, compared to some of the other leading causes of death and DALYs lost, including diabetes, cancer, TB, HIV, and malaria.

Diabetes

There are several types of **diabetes**. The two most common are called type I and type II diabetes. Type I diabetes is "a life-long condition in which the pancreas stops making insulin. Without insulin, the body is not able to use glucose (blood sugar) for energy. To treat the disease, a person must inject

TABLE 7-2 Death and DALYs from Leading Causes, by Region, 2001 as Percentage of Total Deaths and DALYs

Region	CVD	Diabetes	Cancer	TB	HIV	Malaria
East Asia & Pacific						
Deaths	31%	2%	16%	4%	1%	<1%
DALYs	15%	1%	9%	3%	<1%	<1%
Europe & Central Asia						
Deaths	58%	1%	15%	1%	<1%	0%
DALYs	33%	1%	10%	1%	1%	<1%
Latin America & the Caribbean						
Deaths	28%	5%	15%	1%	3%	<1%
DALYs	11%	3%	7%	1%	2%	<1%
Middle East & No. Africa						
Deaths	35%	2%	9%	1%	<1%	1%
DALYs	14%	1%	4%	1%	<1%	1%
South Asia						
Deaths	25%	1%	7%	4%	2%	<1%
DALYs	13%	1%	3%	3%	2%	1%
Sub-Saharan Africa						
Deaths	10%	1%	4%	3%	19%	10%
DALYs	4%	<1%	2%	2%	16%	10%

Source: Data with permission from The World Bank. Lopez AD, Mathers CD, Murray CJL. The burden of disease and mortality by condition: data, methods, and results for 2001. In: Lopez AD, Mathers CD, Ezzati M, Jamison DT, Murray CJL, eds. *Global Burden of Disease and Risk Factors.* New York: Oxford University Press; 2006:126–233.

insulin, follow a diet plan, exercise daily, and test blood sugar several times a day."[4] Type I diabetes usually begins before the age of 30. This type of diabetes was previously known as 'insulin-dependent diabetes mellitus' or 'juvenile diabetes.'[4] 'Type II diabetes was previously known as 'noninsulin-dependent diabetes mellitus' or 'adult-onset diabetes.' Type II diabetes is the most common form of diabetes mellitus, present in about 90–95% of all diabetics. People with type II diabetes produce insulin; however, they either do not make enough insulin or their bodies do not use the insulin they do make."[4] As will be examined further later, type I diabetes is genetic; type II is related to "lifestyle" issues, particularly obesity.

It is estimated that about 5.1% of adults aged 20 to 79 worldwide had diabetes in 2003.[5] The prevalence rate of diabetes among this group was generally higher in high-income countries than in low- and middle-income countries. It ranged from a low of 2.4% in Sub-Saharan Africa to a high of 7.6% in Europe and Central Asia.[5] Almost 200 million people worldwide suffered from diabetes in 2003.[5]

Diabetes has a number of important and costly complications. Among the most common are eye problems that can cause blindness, kidney problems, circulatory problems that can result in amputation of the lower extremities, stroke, and coronary heart disease. About two thirds of the people with diabetes have some disability, compared to less than one third of the people without diabetes.[6] For this reason, the DALYs lost from diabetes are far greater than would be suggested just by the prevalence of the disease. In fact, it is estimated that almost 20 million DALYs were lost to diabetes worldwide in 2001, which is similar, for example, to the DALYs lost for measles; a little less than is lost due to maternal conditions; and about 50% less than are lost due to nutritional deficiencies. The prevalence of diabetes worldwide is increasing at a rapid rate, mostly associated with the rapid increase in the amount of obesity in the world.[7] Some students of global health now refer to diabetes as being an "epidemic." Table 7-3 shows the number of people with diabetes in 2000 and the number of people projected to have diabetes in 2030.

Type I diabetes appears to have an important genetic component. Studies have been done on other factors that might be linked with type I diabetes, but they are not conclusive. The risk factors for type II diabetes may also include a genetic component. However, they do include low birth weight and having been bottle-fed. The best studies of the risk factors associated with diabetes include obesity and weight gain, as well as physical inactivity.[8] In high-income countries, less-educated and lower-income individuals have higher rates of diabetes than better-educated and wealthier people.[9]

Cancer

There are many different types of cancers. Among the most important in terms of the burden of disease worldwide are cancers of the lung, colon, breast, prostate, liver, stomach, and cervix. There are many risk factors for cancer and they vary by type of cancer. Some cancers are associated with tobacco use, such as lung and esophageal cancers. Other cancers are associated with infectious agents. Liver cancer, for example, is associated with the hepatitis B virus, cervical cancer is associ-

TABLE 7-3 Number of People with Diabetes, 2000, and Projected Number with Diabetes in 2030

Region	2000 Number of People with Diabetes	2030 Number of People with Diabetes	Percentage of Change in Number of People with Diabetes	Percentage of Change in Total Population
Established Market Economies	44,268	68,156	54	9
Former Socialist Economies	11,665	13,969	20	–14
India	31,705	79,441	151	40
China	20,757	42,321	104	16
Sub-Saharan Africa	7,146	18,645	161	97
Latin America & the Caribbean	13,307	32,959	148	40
Middle Eastern Crescent	20,051	52,794	163	67
World	171,228	366,212	114	37

Source: © 2004 American Diabetes Association for *Diabetes Care.* Vol. 27. 2004;1047–1053. Reprinted with permission from the American Diabetes Association.

ated with the human papillomavirus, and stomach cancer is associated with the bacteria *Helicobacter pylori.* Liver cancer is associated with schistosomiasis, a parasitic worm that is also called *bilharzia,* which infects more than 200 million people worldwide.[10] There are also numerous environmental and occupational carcinogens, such as asbestos, which was the cause of lung cancer in many roofing workers in the United States, for example.

In 2001, it was estimated that about seven million people worldwide died of cancer, with about five million of those in low- and middle-income countries.[11] At the same time, there were about 10 million new cases of cancer worldwide. The number of deaths caused by different types of cancers varies by region, as shown in Table 7-4, which indicates the first, second, and third leading causes of cancer deaths in each region.

It is clear from the table that lung and breast cancers are two of the five most common types of cancers in both developed and developing countries.

Generally, the higher the income of a country, the more likely it is that the leading forms of cancer deaths will be associated with tobacco use, environmental factors, diet, and lifestyle, whereas there will be a higher preponderance of cancers linked with infectious agents in low-income countries. In high-income countries, for example, lung cancer is the predominant cause of cancer deaths and colon and breast cancer are the next most common causes of cancer deaths. East Asia and the Pacific is the only region in which stomach cancers, often linked with infection with *Helicobacter pylori,* are the most common cause of cancer deaths. As you can also see, the leading cause of cancer deaths in Sub-Saharan Africa is liver cancer, linked in many cases to infection with the hepatitis B virus. In South Asia, the leading cause of cancer deaths are oral cancers, often associated with the use of betel, a nut that is chewed by many people in the region.[12]

Mental Disorders

As noted earlier, one of the major categories of non-communicable diseases is neuropsychiatric disorders. This includes a number of neurological disorders, such as epilepsy. It also includes alcohol and drug abuse. Mental disorders are also included in this category. Together, neuropsychiatric disorders are very important to the burden of disease, causing about 10% of all DALYs lost in low- and middle-income countries in 2001.[13] Covering a wide range of neuropsychiatric disorders, however, is beyond the scope of this book. This part of the book, therefore, will only cover selected mental disorders.

Mental disorders have generally been given less attention in global health than they deserve when considering their contribution to the overall burden of disease. One reason for this is the extent to which health providers and global health

TABLE 7-4 Leading Causes of Cancer Deaths by Region, Number of Deaths in Thousands, 2001

Region	Cancer Type	Deaths	Cancer Type	Deaths	Cancer Type	Deaths
East Asia & Pacific	Stomach	442	Trachea, Bronchus & Lungs	387	Liver	373
Europe & Central Asia	Trachea, Bronchus & Lungs	165	Other Malignant Neoplasms	82	Stomach	101
Latin America & the Caribbean	Other Malignant Neoplasms	82	Stomach	57	Trachea, Bronchus & Lungs	55
Middle East & No. Africa	Other Malignant Neoplasms	26	Trachea, Bronchus & Lungs	20	Stomach	18
South Asia	Mouth & Oropharynx	140	Trachea, Bronchus & Lungs	129	Other Malignant Neoplasms	99
Sub-Saharan Africa	Other Malignant Neoplasms	55	Liver	46	Prostate	40
High Income Countries	Trachea, Bronchus & Lungs	456	Other Malignant Neoplasms	257	Colon & Rectal	257

Source: Data with permission from The World Bank. Lopez AD, Mathers CD, Murray CJL. The Burden of Disease and Mortality by Condition: Data, Methods, and Results for 2001. In: Lopez AD, Mathers CD, Ezzati M, Jamison DT, Murray CJL, eds. *Global Burden of Disease and Risk Factors.* New York: Oxford University Press; 2006:126-233.

actors have historically underestimated the burden of mental disorders. Recent work on the global burden of disease, however, indicates that four of the most common mental disorders contribute about 5% of the total DALYs lost in low- and middle-income countries, about equal to the burden of HIV/AIDS, diseases of vision and hearing, or ischemic heart disease.[14] Depression alone is estimated to be associated with 3.4% of the DALYs lost, which would make it the fourth most important burden[15] of any health condition globally.[16] One reason for this large burden is the large number of people who suffer mental disorders. Another, however, is that mental disorders start at relatively young ages, they go on for a long time, they are often not "cured," and they, therefore, produce large amounts of disability. There is also some mortality, largely from suicide, that is associated with mental disorders.

Four mental disorders contribute the largest share to the burden of mental disorders. These are unipolar depressive disorders, which will be referred to here as depression, schizophrenia, panic disorder, and bipolar affective disorder. These conditions are defined briefly in Table 7-5.

There is only limited data on the burden of mental disorders from low- and middle-income countries. Nonetheless, when assessing the burden of these four disorders per million people, it is clear that South Asia has the highest rate of depression among all regions. The rate of depression is fairly consistent across better-off regions, somewhat lower in East Asia and the Pacific, and only about half as high in Sub-Saharan Africa as in Europe and Central Asia.[15] The rates of schizophrenia range from about 1600 DALYs per one million people in Europe and Central Asia to about 2100 DALYs per one million people in East Asia and the Pacific.[15] Bipolar disorder ranges from 1400 DALYs per million people in Europe and Central Asia to 1830 DALYs per million people in the Middle East and North Africa.[15] The range for panic disorders is very narrow, with all regions clustering in the range of 700 to 800 DALYs per million people.[15]

There appear to be both genetic and non-genetic risk factors for mental disorders. It is clear that women suffer from depression more than men, as noted earlier. Early childhood abuse, violence, and poverty may be important environmental risk factors for depression. However, there is still very little definitive evidence on the risk factors for schizophrenia, depression, bipolar disorder, or panic disorders.

TABLE 7-5 Key Mental Health Terms and Definitions

Bipolar Disorder—A serious mood disorder characterized by swings of mania and depression

Depression—A mental state characterized by feelings of sadness, loneliness, despair, low self-esteem, and self-reproach

Panic Disorders—An anxiety disorder characterized by attacks of acute intense anxiety

Schizophrenia—A mental illness, the main symptoms of which are hallucinations, delusions, and changes in outlook and personality

Source: Modified from Ohio Psychological Association Psychological Glossary. Available at: http://www.ohpsych.org/Public/glossary.htm. Accessed April 14, 2007; The Royal College of Psychiatrists. Diagnoses or conditions. Available at: http://www.rcpsych.ac.uk/mentalhealthinformation/definitions/diagnosesorconditions.aspx. Accessed April 14, 2007.

Tobacco Use

Tobacco is such an important risk factor for cardiovascular disease and diabetes that it bears specific mention of its own. It is estimated that about five million deaths annually are associated with the use of tobacco, of which about half are in low-income countries.[17] It is also estimated that 1 in 5 males over 30 and 1 in 20 females over 30 who die worldwide, die of tobacco-related deaths.[18] Ultimately, one half to two thirds of those who smoke will die of causes related to tobacco.[17] In addition, half of all tobacco-related deaths occur among people aged 35 to 69.[17] The most common tobacco-related deaths are from CVD; diseases of the respiratory system, such as emphysema; and from cancers.

Most tobacco is used through smoking either cigarettes or *bidis*, which are hand-rolled cigarettes used largely in South Asia. It is estimated that about 1.1 billion people smoke worldwide.[19] The rate of prevalence of smoking for all adults varies from 18% in Sub-Saharan Africa to 35% in Europe and Central Asia. In all regions of the world, men smoke more than women do. This is most pronounced in low-income countries, in which a relatively small share of women smoke. Prevalence for men varies from 29% in Sub-Saharan Africa to 63% in East Asia and the Pacific. The rates for women vary from 5% in East Asia and the Pacific and the Middle East and North Africa to 24% in Latin America and the Caribbean.[17]

The extent to which people take up smoking varies not only by sex, but also by socioeconomic status and level of educational attainment. The higher the socioeconomic status and the higher the level of education, the less likely a person is to smoke. Most people who smoke start when they are teens. In addition, it is important to note that tobacco is physically addictive and once one starts to smoke, it is difficult to stop.[20]

In some countries, the use of tobacco has been declining, such as Canada, Poland, Thailand, the United Kingdom, and the United States. However, usage is increasing among men in developing countries and among women in all regions. Unless steps are taken to stop the spread of tobacco use, we are likely to see continued growth in CVD and cancers related to smoking, many of which are avoidable.

Abuse of Alcohol

Although we may be familiar with the idea that "a glass of red wine a day is protective against heart disease," on balance alcohol is a major public health problem. About 4% of the global burden of disease, in fact, is attributable to alcohol, which is about the same amount as that related to tobacco and hypertension and somewhat more than is attributed to depression.[21]

High risk drinking is defined as drinking 20 grams or more per day of pure alcohol for a woman and 40 grams a day for a man.[22] This is equal to about one quarter of a bottle of wine for a woman and one half a bottle of wine for a man. High-risk drinking may also be defined to include the total amount that is consumed, the frequency with which it is consumed, and the extent to which one engages in binge drinking.

High-risk drinking has a negative effect on people's health in a number of ways. Among other things, it increases the risks for hypertension, liver damage, pancreatic damage, hormonal problems, and heart disease.[21] In addition, alcohol intoxication is associated with accidents, injuries, accidental death, and a variety of social problems, including the first sexual encounters of teens, unprotected sex, and intimate partner violence. It is also possible to become dependent on alcohol, with a number of negative psychological and physical consequences. Moreover, fetal alcohol syndrome is associated with low birth weight babies who are at risk of developmental disabilities.

The prevalence of high risk drinking varies by region. Men in Europe and Central Asia have the highest rates of high risk drinking: 21.4% between ages 45 to 59. People in the Middle East and North Africa have the lowest rates, which are reported to be very low. South Asia also has a very low prevalence of high risk drinking.[23] The prevalence rate of high risk drinking also varies by age, with fewer people engaging in high risk drinking after age 60 than at younger ages. In each region, high-risk drinking is higher among men than in women, except in South Asia.[23]

There is very little evidence about the determinants of high risk drinking, especially in low-income settings. Studies done in high-income countries suggest that lower socioeconomic status and lower educational attainment are risk factors for drinking to the level of intoxication.[24]

THE COSTS AND CONSEQUENCES OF NON-COMMUNICABLE DISEASES, TOBACCO USE, AND ALCOHOL ABUSE

The economic costs of non-communicable diseases are substantial and are growing, given the increasing burden of cardiovascular disease and diabetes. These costs include the direct costs of treating non-communicable diseases, which by their nature require many years of treatment. They also include indirect costs that result from lost productivity. These are also very substantial, given that non-communicable diseases often start at relatively younger ages, often cause substantial disability, and then persist for many years.

In addition, many actors in the global health arena previously carried out their work as if rich countries faced the burden and costs of non-communicable diseases and poor countries faced only the burden and costs of communicable diseases. However, in light of the increasing amount of non-communicable disease and injury and accidents in developing countries, it is clear that most low-income countries do not have the luxury of facing *either* communicable *or* non-communicable disease. Rather, even low-income countries now *simultaneously* face the burden and costs of communicable diseases, non-communicable diseases, and injuries. Some additional comments follow on the costs and consequences of non-communicable diseases.

Cardiovascular Disease

Only a small number of studies have been done on the direct and indirect costs of CVD in low- and middle-income countries. A study conducted in South Africa suggested that the direct costs of treating cardiovascular disease were about 25% of all healthcare expenditures, which was equal to between 2–3% of GDP in that country.[25] The indirect costs of cardiovascular disease on the economy are likely to be substantial, given the relatively low age at which such diseases affect people in many countries. South Africa is a middle-income country, with a section of the economy that is very advanced. We should, therefore, expect that the costs of cardiovascular disease in most low-income countries will be a lower share of GDP than it is in South Africa. However, we should also expect that the costs of addressing cardiovascular disease in low- and middle-income countries will increase as the burden of such diseases continues to grow in those countries.

Diabetes

It is estimated that the direct costs of treating diabetes vary between 2.5% and 15.0% of health expenditures in different countries, depending on the prevalence of disease and the extent and costs of treatment available.[5] Given the level of development of different regions, it is likely that the Latin America and the Caribbean region has the highest expenditure on diabetes per capita and Sub-Saharan Africa the lowest such expenditures.[5] The indirect costs of diabetes in low- and middle-income countries are probably substantial because many people in those countries are living with diabetes without proper treatment and therefore suffer from disability and loss of productivity. The direct and indirect costs of diabetes will continue to grow for some time in all regions as the number of people with diabetes increases, as noted earlier.

Mental Disorders

There are relatively few reliable data on the direct and indirect costs of mental disorders. In addition, the studies that have been done largely refer to developed countries. Nonetheless, they are indicative of the large and usually unappreciated costs of mental illness in all countries. A study done in the United States estimated that the direct and indirect costs of mental illness were equal to about 2.5% of GNP, and a similar study done in Europe estimated that the costs of mental illness there was between 3–4% of GNP.[26] Studies done in Canada, the United Kingdom, and the United States showed that about half of the total costs of mental illness were direct costs and about half were indirect costs. These indirect costs are so substantial for mental illness that one study done in the United States estimated that almost 60% of the productivity losses that come from illness, accidents, or injuries are linked with mental illness.[26] Studies done in the United States and the United Kingdom showed, in addition, that workers suffering from depression lost 40 to 45 days of work in a year as a result of their illness.[26]

Tobacco Use

Calculating the costs of smoking to an economy can be very complicated.[27] The simplest way to do so is to calculate gross costs, which includes all the costs that are associated with smoking-related diseases. Studies on the costs of smoking have largely focused on the costs of smoking in the developed world. These studies suggested that the gross costs of smoking to various economies in high-income countries range from 0.1–1.1% of GDP and that the costs to low- and middle-income countries might be just as high.[27] The prevalence rates of smoking are increasing among women everywhere and among men in low-income countries. We should expect, therefore, that the economic costs of smoking in those countries will increase for some time to come. In fact, it is estimated that 70 million people died of smoking-related causes between 1950 and 2000 but that, if present trends in tobacco use continue, an additional 150 million people will die of smoking-related causes between 2000 and 2025. Of course, the economic costs of this will be enormous. In addition, it is important to note that the economic burden of smoking in the future is likely to have a disproportionate impact on relatively poorer people, in relatively poorer countries, because they smoke at higher rates than do better-off people.[28]

Alcohol Abuse

For the economic costs of alcohol abuse, as for many other issues, there are relatively few data for low- and middle-income countries. Excessive alcohol use, as discussed earlier, is linked with health problems of the drinker. In addition, it is linked with violence and injuries caused by the drinker, such as when driving while intoxicated. When calculating the economic costs of excessive alcohol drinking, therefore, one has to take account of the costs of health care of the user and on others whose injuries or health condition were caused by the user. The indirect costs of excessive alcohol drinking will include the productivity losses not only of the drinker, but also of people hurt by the drinker because of excessive drinking. The limited studies that have been done on the costs of alcohol abuse can only be considered indicative because they did not follow any standard methodology. However, they all reveal substantial costs of alcohol abuse, as a share of GDP:

Canada—1.1%
France—1.4%
Italy—5.6%
New Zealand—4.0%
South Africa—2.0%[29]

ADDRESSING THE BURDEN OF NON-COMMUNICABLE DISEASES

There are also relatively few data available about cost-effective investments to address the burden of non-communicable diseases, including tobacco and alcohol-related illness, in the developing world. However, there is an increasing amount of information about efforts to address these issues in developed countries. Although the circumstances in these high-income countries may be quite different from those in low- and middle-income countries, the efforts undertaken to date may provide some useful lessons for low- and middle-income countries as they seek to prevent the burden of non-communicable diseases from growing. In considering how to address non-communicable diseases, it is important to note that some interventions can be made at the level of the population, whereas others are based on personal contact with an individual. Since smoking tobacco and excessive alcohol drinking are such important risk factors for cancer, cardiovascular disease, and diabetes, the following section starts with a discussion about measures that can be taken to reduce smoking and excessive alcohol consumption.[30]

Tobacco Use

Experiences in the developed world suggest a number of steps can be taken to reduce the use of tobacco. Almost all countries tax cigarettes; however, low- and middle-income countries tend to tax cigarettes at lower rates than do higher income countries. Public demand for cigarettes is sensitive to price, and the poorer the country, the more price increases will affect demand. Studies conducted in low- and middle-income countries indicate that a 10% increase in cigarette taxes can lead to an 8% reduction in the demand for cigarettes. Under these circumstances, taxing cigarettes would be an effective policy for reducing cigarette consumption.[31]

For countries where there is weak government enforcement of laws, it will be more difficult to enforce restrictions on smoking; however, an increasing number of countries are undertaking these measures. Studies suggest that countries that can enforce legal restrictions can reduce the number of cigarettes smoked between 5–25% and can reduce smoking uptake by about 25%.[31] The effectiveness of these actions is likely to be enhanced in settings in which there are also strong social norms against smoking.

There is also evidence from high-income countries that consumption of cigarettes can be reduced by about 6% through a total ban on cigarette advertising, which is another step that low- and middle-income countries might consider.[31] Countries should also provide the public with information about the negative effects of smoking tobacco. There is evidence from high-income countries that such efforts led to short run reduction in cigarette consumption of between 4–9% and long-run declines of 15–30%.[31]

High-income settings that have had the biggest impact on reducing tobacco consumption have undertaken comprehensive tobacco control programs that generally included efforts to prevent young people from starting smoking, encourage all smokers to quit smoking, reduce exposure to passive smoking, and eliminate disparities in smoking among different population groups by helping those most at risk to reduce tobacco consumption.[32] It remains critically important to stop people from taking up smoking. However, in order to reduce tobacco-related deaths in the near future, it is essential to reduce consumption among those already smoking. Preventing young people from taking up smoking will only have an impact on tobacco-related deaths in the more distant future.

Abuse of Alcohol

Despite the high burden of disease and economic costs that are related to excessive drinking of alcoholic beverages, very few countries have embarked on coherent efforts to reduce alcohol consumption. Those that have done so generally focused their attention on policy and legislative actions, such as taxation, laws on drunk driving, and restricting alcohol sales to selected places, times, and age limits. Controlled advertising and tightened law enforcement, such as through more widespread breath testing of drivers, have also been imposed. Another successful part of their program was to encourage counseling by healthcare providers through "brief interventions with individual high risk drivers."[33]

Just as is the case for cigarette taxation, increased taxation on alcohol will likely lead to a decrease in the purchase and consumption of alcohol. Whereas in the case of tobacco, increased taxation can lead to the smuggling of untaxed cigarettes, in the case of alcohol, increased taxation can lead to a rise in the consumption of illicit alcohol. This is an issue that countries must take into account in considering raising taxes on alcohol.

In selected high-income countries, studies suggest that reducing the number of hours when alcohol can be sold can lead to a 1.5–3% decrease in high risk drinking and to a 1.5–4% decrease in alcohol-related traffic deaths.[34] Government authorities have to assess the extent to which such measures could be implemented effectively, especially in low- and middle-income countries with weak governance, as well as the extent to which such measures might also drive people to seek illicit alcohol.

Bans on alcohol advertising can be put into effect, as discussed for tobacco; however, it appears that such bans have had relatively little effect on the consumption of alcohol.[35] In health care settings in a number of countries, efforts have been made to engage high-risk drinkers in brief but specific education and counseling about the risks of excessive drinking. Even when taking relapses into account, it appears that such counseling is effective in reducing excessive consumption by 14–18%, compared to no treatment at all.[35] Although this approach might be effective in middle-income countries, it is unlikely to be effective in many low-income countries, given the scarcity of effective health services, the lack of health providers, and the already excessive demands on their weak health systems.

High Blood Pressure, High Cholesterol, and Obesity

The majority of risk associated with cardiovascular disease relates to a combination of high blood pressure, high cholesterol, high body mass index, low intake of fruits and vegetables, physical inactivity, and tobacco and alcohol use. The single most important risk factor for type II diabetes is obesity. The following section comments on measures that can be taken to improve diet and to reduce obesity.

To reduce the burden of CVD and diabetes, healthy eating and maintaining a healthy weight is key. Generally, this requires eating more fruits and vegetables and decreasing the intake of salt and foods that are high in saturated fat and trans fats. It also entails limiting the intake of sugar and replacing refined grains with whole grains. People who are overweight generally need to consume fewer calories each day and need to become more active physically.[53]

The lack of regular physical activity, in fact, is associated, among other things, with CVD, stroke, type II diabetes, and colon and breast cancer. Urbanization, motorization, and television watching all reduce physical activity. Countries can use public policies to try to limit the role of automobiles, promote walking and biking, and design communities in ways that encourage healthy lifestyles. In Singapore and London, for example, taxes are levied on cars that enter the center of the city to reduce the use of vehicles and their attendant traffic and pollution. Many cities promote the use of bicycles and have bicycle lanes, as one can see in a number of European cities such as Amsterdam. Some communities in the United States, for example, have no sidewalks, little public transport, and services that are very spread out, all of which provide an incentive for people to use automobiles to get from place to place, rather than to walk or bicycle.[53]

One way to promote healthier diets is through population-based "health education." Large-scale education efforts of this type, often through the mass media, have had mixed results because it is difficult on a large scale to successfully promote the reduction of obesity.[36] Generally, mass programs are more effective when they are combined with direct communication with individuals.

Few efforts to undertake population-based education measures have been studied. However, a study on a project to reduce salt intake among men in one part of China found a reduction in both hypertension and obesity after 5 years. In another effort, the government of Mauritius encouraged the population to switch from cooking with palm oil, which is high in saturated fat, to soybean oil, which has less saturated fat. Over a 5-year period, the intake of saturated fat decreased and the total cholesterol levels of the population fell.[37] Regulations and legislation on labeling food products and the reduction of unhealthy ingredients in commercial food products can also contribute to reducing obesity.

Studies suggest that if large scale health education efforts are to succeed in changing what people eat, then it is important that such programs:

- have a realistic time frame that takes account of the time it takes to change deeply ingrained behaviors;
- be carried out by a respected organization and headed by a competent manager, with clear responsibility;
- encourage different organizations and agencies to work together to maximize the reach of the program and ensure that messages get disseminated in appropriate ways; and
- involve the food industry and enhance food labeling.[38]

Some countries, such as Brazil and Mexico, simultaneously face substantial burdens of underweight and overweight children and women. It may be politically and socially difficult for countries that face such a double burden to get the support they need to address problems of overweight, as many people believe that obesity is a problem that only affects wealthier people. There are few examples to date of best practices for addressing the two problems simultaneously.

Even as countries undertake the steps noted, they will still need to treat those who already have CVD, or who have some of the key risk factors for CVD, including hypertension. Most low- and some middle-income countries do not have the level of health system or the financial resources needed to carry out sophisticated medical procedures. In such settings, however, an important reduction in risks and in the burden of disease can be realized through preventive interventions such as getting people to take an aspirin a day and to get people with high cholesterol and hypertension to take inexpensive medicines to lower blood pressure and cholesterol.

Further Addressing Diabetes

There is no evidence that type I diabetes can be prevented; however, avoiding being overweight is the single most important way to avoid type II diabetes. Although large scale efforts to reduce obesity have generally not been very successful, a pilot project that used intensive personal counseling to promote weight loss through healthier eating and more physical activity was successfully carried out in China, Finland, Sweden, and the United States. The average weight loss after almost 3 years of participation in this study was about 10 pounds more than in the control group. In addition, the study group had a 58% lower rate of type II diabetes than the control group.[9]

Treatment for people with diabetes is needed in all countries. Treating people with type I diabetes with insulin is a cost-effective investment, although difficult to afford or manage in the poorest countries, especially for people living outside of the main cities. For all diabetics, it is cost-effective to control hypertension because the combination of the two diseases can produce major vascular complications. Diabetics are also subject to foot problems from circulation difficulties associated with their diabetes, and appropriate foot care is another cost-effective investment. The cost of not doing this can be ulcers and eventual amputation of the foot.[9] Those countries with greater resources and a health system that can deliver additional interventions can also consider other cost-effective measures for treating diabetes, including vaccination against influenza and pneumococcal infections, diagnosis and treatment of retinal problems associated with diabetes, and treating hypertension with ACE inhibitors to prevent kidney problems from getting worse.[9]

Cancer

Tobacco control is overwhelmingly the first priority for preventing cancer, as noted earlier. Countries can also try to reduce the burden of cancer by addressing infectious agents that are associated with cancers, such as hepatitis B, which is vaccine-preventable; *H. pylori*, which is treatable with antibiotics; and schistosomiasis, which is also treatable with drugs.[39] An increasing number of countries are adding the hepatitis B vaccine to their national immunization programs. This is especially important in countries where a relatively large share of the population carries hepatitis B. Many countries have schistosomiasis control programs, and some of the most successful efforts against schistosomiasis have been undertaken in Egypt and China. *H. pylori* is important in settings like Japan, China, or Colombia where there is a significant amount of stomach cancer linked with this bacteria. In these settings, it might be cost-effective to carry out a screening and treatment program for *H. pylori*.

Mental Disorders

Unfortunately, there are few public health measures that can prevent mental disorders. For the mental disorders that have been discussed, treatment through medication, combined with psychosocial support, is the best way to try to address these illnesses. Providing such treatment and psychosocial support, however, will be difficult in many low- and middle-income countries, given their weak health systems, a historic lack of attention to mental disorders, and a lack of staff at every level to address mental health in effective and efficient ways.

Given the important burden of disease associated with mental disorders, the World Health Organization recommends that countries take a number of steps to address mental health issues. These include:

- Having a mental health policy
- Ensuring there is a unit of government responsible for mental health
- Budgeting for mental health programs—including program development, training, drug procurement, and program monitoring
- Training primary healthcare workers in mental health
- Integrating mental health into the primary healthcare program[39]

In addition, a number of public health measures can be taken to address some of the factors that are associated with mental disorders. Reducing abuse of women and children can reduce the burden of mental illness among the abused. Curtailing bullying of students in schools can also be important. Improving parenting skills is helpful to the healthy development of children. Appropriate care and counseling for children and adults affected by war, conflict, and other complex emergencies can also reduce the risks of mental illness.

To the extent possible, treatments should be made available for the different mental disorders discussed in this chapter. Of the different treatments available, the most cost-effective include those for:

Schizophrenia—combining an older antipsychotic drug with psychosocial treatment
Bipolar disorder—providing an older mood stabilizing drug, plus psychosocial treatment
Depression—providing a newer antidepressant drug
Panic disorder—providing a newer antidepressant drug[40]

It is estimated that including the above in primary healthcare packages could cost between about $3 in Sub-Saharan Africa and $9 per capita in Latin America.[40] This represents a significant share of the current level of public health expenditure in the poorest countries of Sub-Saharan Africa and would be difficult to finance from their own resources. Other developing countries with more resources may be better able to provide needed treatments with their own funds.

Unfortunately, there is often an inadequate understanding of the importance of mental health, a lack of funds, a shortage of people who understand mental health issues, and stigma around mental disorders. As a result, there has been little progress in most low-income countries in addressing mental disorders.[41]

CASE STUDIES

Most efforts to try to reduce the burden of non-communicable diseases, alcohol abuse, and tobacco use have taken place in high-income countries. However, middle- and low-income countries are beginning to gather evidence about what works most effectively in preventing non-communicable diseases. The following section examines efforts to reduce tobacco use in Poland. It will be followed by a review of the cataract blindness control program in India. The last case study is about a program to integrate mental health into primary health care in Uganda.

The Challenge of Curbing Tobacco Use in Poland

Background

More than three quarters of the world's 1.2 billion smokers live in low- and middle-income countries, where smoking is on the rise.[42] In the late 1970s, Poland had the highest rate of smoking in the world, with the average Pole smoking 3500 cigarettes a year and nearly three quarters of Polish men smoking daily. The impact on the nation's health was staggering. In 1990, the probability of a 15-year-old boy in Poland reaching his 60th birthday was lower than in most countries, including China and India.[43] Lung cancer rates were among the highest in the world. But because tobacco production, run by the state, provided a significant source of revenue, the government did not fully disclose to the population the negative consequences of smoking. The fall of communism further exacerbated smoking because tobacco, the first industry to be privatized, was taken over by powerful multinational corporations who flooded the market with international brands, spent vast sums on advertising, and kept prices so low that cigarettes cost less than a loaf of bread.

The Intervention

As the tobacco epidemic escalated, Poland's scientific community laid the foundation of the anti-tobacco movement. Research in the 1980s by the Marie Sklodowska-Curie Memorial Cancer Centre and Institute of Oncology contributed to the first Polish report on smoking, highlighting the link between tobacco and the country's alarming rise in cancer. A series of international workshops and scientific conferences in Poland further strengthened these findings. Civil society was experiencing a renewal at the time, with the formation of anti-tobacco groups such as the Polish Anti-Tobacco Society that began to interact with international bodies, such as WHO and the International Union Against Cancer. In addition, the Health Promotion Foundation was established to lead public efforts on health issues and anti-tobacco education efforts.

With the fall of the Berlin Wall, the media became free to cover health topics and played an important role in disseminating information, raising awareness about the dangers of smoking, and shaping public opinion. When tobacco control legislation was introduced in 1991, a heated public debate ensued between health advocates and the powerful tobacco lobby, increasingly viewed by the public as a contest between David and Goliath. In 1995, groundbreaking legislation was finally passed, requiring sweeping measures such as large health warnings on cigarette packs and bans on smoking in enclosed workspaces and health centers, on electronic media advertising, and on tobacco sales to minors. A 30% increase in taxes levied on cigarettes was subsequently passed in 1999 and 2000, and advertising was completely banned. In parallel, the Health Promotion Foundation also launched extensive health education and consumer awareness efforts. These included an annual "Great Polish Smoke-Out" competition to encourage smokers to quit, with incentives like winning a week-long stay in Rome and a chance to meet the Polish-born Pope John Paul II. In a decade of smoke-outs, nearly 2.5 million smokers have quit smoking. Since the first smoke-out in 1991, more than 2.5 million poles have permanently snuffed out their cigarettes because of the campaign.

The Impact

Cigarette consumption dropped 10% between 1990 and 1998, and the number of smokers declined from 14 million in the 1980s to under 10 million by the end of the 1990s. The reduction in smoking led to 10,000 fewer deaths each year, a 30% decline in lung cancer among men aged 20 to 44, a nearly 7% decline in CVD, and a reduction in infant mortality and low birth weight.[44] Life expectancy in the 1990s increased by 4 years.

Lessons Learned

Poland's experience shows that once smoking is seen for what it is—the leading cause of preventable deaths among adults worldwide—then governments do act. Working in concert with civil society and using state-of-the-art communication strategies, the Polish government succeeded in countering the powerful economic influence of the tobacco industry and inducing major shifts in smoking, an addictive behavior that was also then an ingrained social norm. Poland's sweeping legislative measures came to serve as a model for other countries. The experience of South Africa provides an interesting parallel: once the African National Congress came to power in 1994, the antismoking movement gained a powerful ally in Nelson Mandela and his first health minister, ultimately leading to the passage of strict tobacco control legislation and dramatic price control measures that increased the real value of cigarette taxes by 215%. As a result, cigarette consumption fell by more than 30%, from 1.9 billion packs in 1991 to 1.3 billion packs in 2002. As a South African researcher noted, "You need the right combination of science, evidence, and politics to succeed. If you have one without the other, you don't see action."[45] For a more detailed discussion of these Polish efforts see *Case Studies in Global Health: Millions Saved.*

Cataract Blindness Control in India

This chapter has focused on a limited number of the leading causes of deaths and DALYs lost due to non-communicable diseases. This chapter, however, does not cover vision disorders, despite the large number of DALYs lost to them in low- and middle-income countries. As you would expect, there are few people who die of diseases related to vision disorders. However, the burden of disability of these diseases, especially in low- and middle-income countries in which they are not generally treated in a timely manner, is great. In fact, about 45 million people worldwide are blind and another 135 million people are visually impaired.[46] The total number of DALYs lost from cataracts alone in low- and middle-income countries is almost the same as those lost to nutritional deficiencies, is slightly more than those lost to maternal conditions, and is about 15% fewer than the amount lost to TB. It is also just under the number of DALYs lost to road traffic injuries.[47]

Background

About one quarter of the total number of people in the world who are blind live in India and the case study that follows deals with controlling cataract blindness there.[48] The blindness control program in India has been one of the most extensive such programs in low-income countries for many years. In addition, over the last decade, this program has emerged, in many respects, as a public health "success story." Those wishing to examine this case in greater detail can read further about it in *Case Studies in Global Health: Millions Saved.*

History

Cataracts are the leading cause of blindness in India. About 80% of all of the people in India who are blind are blind due to cataracts. In addition, there are another 10 million people in India who are visually impaired due to untreated cataracts.

In the simplest terms, a cataract is a clouding of the lens of the eye. It blurs the image on the retina, producing a visual effect that is like looking through a window that is frosted or fogged with steam. Cataracts form when protein clumps in the lens of the eye. This is associated with age, excessive exposure to sunlight, diabetes, undernutrition, and other risk factors. Cataracts can affect one or both eyes.

Cataracts are treatable through surgery. One form of surgery requires a large incision in the eye and the removal of the lens and lens capsule. This form of surgery (ICCE) is relatively easy to perform and relatively inexpensive; however, it requires that the patient wear thick eyeglasses after surgery, and it has a high rate of complications. Nonetheless, it has been the form of surgery traditionally done in low-income settings. The other form of surgery is more technically sophisticated (ECCE); however, it has a lower rate of complications when done by trained surgeons. In addition, recent research in India showed that those having ECCE surgery were 2.8 times more likely to have a good outcome than those having ICCE surgery.[49]

Intervention

India's response to the problem of blindness has been impressive in breadth and duration. India's first intervention in 1963 aimed specifically at controlling trachoma, a highly contagious eye infection. By the end of the decade, the government expanded its approach to include all visual impairment. In 1975, the Central Council of Health declared that "one of the basic human rights is the right to see. In 1976, India formed the National Program for the Control of Blindness (NPCB) to expand access to surgical treatment of vision disorders and to increase ophthalmologic services.

India's first international collaboration in eye care was with DANIDA, the Danish International Development Assistance Agency. Until 1989, DANIDA assisted India in funding the improvement and expansion of its cataract blindness control program through the provision of equipment, mobile units, training, and enhancements of monitoring and evaluation. The program focused then on mass ECCE surgeries in camps that were mostly set up in areas with limited health infrastructure. This demonstrated the ability of the government to lead mass screening and treatment camps, even in rural areas. It also generated enormous demand for cataract surgeries, even among the poor and rural. However, the limited amount of time a camp was stationed in a particular location, as well as the nature of field work, meant that post-surgical follow-up was difficult to implement. Consequently, although the efforts succeeded in reaching many people, only about 75% of those who got surgery returned to an acceptable level of vision.[50]

In 1994, building on its experience with DANIDA, the Government of India began to collaborate with the World Bank to finance a 7-year Cataract Blindness Control Project. The project focused on seven Indian states that had the highest prevalence of blindness and, in simple terms, it meant to assist India in moving its cataract blindness control program from a focus on quantity to a focus on quality and outcomes. The aims of the program were to improve surgical outcomes by shifting from ICCE to ECCE, strengthen India's capacity to provide high quality surgery done by competently trained staff, and increase the coverage of the program to areas which had previously been underserved. Much greater attention was paid than before to monitoring the outcomes of surgery.

The program also focused on trying to achieve its aims through enhancing collaboration between the public and the private sectors. Some surgeries were done in public facilities. The government financed other surgeries that were conducted by the private and NGO sectors. In addition, NGOs such as Sight Savers International, Lions Clubs International, and Christoffel Blinden Mission also financially supported eye hospitals, training institutes, and the development of school vision-screening programs and outreach. The Aravind Eye Hospital in Madurai, India, was a world famous leader in eye care and became increasingly involved in training and other assistance to the NPCB.

Impact

Over 15 million cataract operations were performed in connection with the Cataract Blindness Control Project. In addition, ECCE surgeries increased as a share of the total surgeries from between 15–65% across different states in 1998–1999 to between 44–91% in 2001–2002.[50] Moreover, by 2001, 92% of surgeries occurred in fixed facilities where better outcomes can be expected. Most importantly, surgical outcomes have improved, with the introduction of improved procedures, well-equipped surgical procedures, and trained personnel. The ability to see at an acceptable level after surgery grew from 75% in 1994 to 82% from 1999 to 2002. The number and quality of surgeries was associated with a decrease in the prevalence of cataract blindness by 26%.

Cost Effectiveness

The World Bank-assisted intervention cost $136 million, with close to 90% coming from the Bank and the remainder from the government of India. When done correctly and in areas of high prevalence, cataract surgery is among the most highly cost-effective interventions.[51] ECCE surgery is estimated to cost about $60 per DALY averted in the South and East Asia regions. Through the combination of serving those most in need and their educational and awareness raising campaigns, NGOs operating under the project used their financial resources very effectively.

Lessons Learned

The efforts in India demonstrate the benefits of collaboration among different public and private sectors and international institutions. The government of India and its political commitment to the problem in the 1960s was a requirement for success, as it offered a "big push" to combating cataract blindness. In addition, even though the government's early efforts were not always at the level of quality desired, they provided a baseline for further studies of how the program could be improved and expanded in a higher quality manner. Finally, the involvement of the NGOs helped to bring innovative approaches to the project and continually encouraged the government to improve and maintain quality services.

Integrating Mental Health into Primary Care in Uganda

Mental disorders are neglected in most developing countries. They are difficult to diagnose and treat, they carry considerable stigma, and low-income countries often lack the skilled personnel and financial resources needed to address mental health issues. Uganda is one of the few low-income countries that has made an effort to tackle the important burden of mental disorders and the case study that follows describes this effort and some of the outcomes associated with Uganda's move to integrate mental health concerns into its primary healthcare program.

Background

In 1986, Uganda came out of a 5-year civil conflict that had been preceded by 8 years of government led by General Idi Amin, which were characterized by misrule and violence. Although the civil conflict was for the most part over in the southern parts of the country, the conflict continued in the north, with abduction of children and terrorizing of the communities carried out by the Lord's Resistance Army. At about the same time, Uganda was increasingly being impacted by the emerging HIV/AIDS epidemic.

According to the 1995 Uganda Burden of Disease study, over 75% of life years lost from premature deaths was the result of preventable communicable disorders.[47] However, it was also recognized that there was a simultaneous surge in the occurrence of non-communicable disorders, such as hypertension, diabetes, cancer, and mental disorders. It was also becoming clearer that HIV/AIDS and the prolonged armed conflict created an increased need for attention to be paid to mental health.

In order to address the increasing burden of mental disorders, the Ministry of Health decided to promote the integration of mental health into primary health care. This involved developing standards and guidelines for the management of eight priority mental disorders for the community, district, and national referral levels of care. This was part of Uganda's efforts to address health care in an effective and efficient manner through the establishment of a minimum healthcare package.

The Intervention

The process of integrating mental health into primary health care was to be implemented through training all healthcare workers to recognize and manage common mental disorders, as well as establishing and strengthening a referral and supportive supervision system. The initiative was outlined in the Uganda Health Sector Strategic Plan 1999 to 2004.[52]

Central level activities included the creation of a Mental Health Coordinating Committee whose main responsibilities were the development of standards and guidelines for the management of common mental disorders, developing materials for the training of health workers, and developing and participating in the referral and supervision system. Central level activities also included participation in the creation of a Core Team on Psychosocial Disorders, a group of representatives of two government sectors; the Ministry of Health and the Ministry of Gender, Labor, and Social Development, which was responsible for child protection; five NGOs working in the field of psychosocial disorders; and UNICEF.

The Core Team carried out an assessment of the psychosocial situation of the conflict-affected population in eight districts of northern Uganda, disseminated the results to the district leaders, and facilitated the affected districts in the development of psychosocial components to be included in District Development Plans. The Core Team developed indicators, as well as a monitoring and evaluation plan, that they then implemented. The Core Team was instrumental in the coordinated safe return and reintegration of abducted children into their communities.

As a result of having mental health in the Health Sector Policy and the Health Sector Strategic Plan, a budget line for mental health was created. Although the allocation to mental health from the Government of Uganda was only 0.7% of the total health budget, having mental health as a budget item made it easier for other funding agencies to support mental health efforts in Uganda.

The African Development Bank (AfDB) provided a loan to the Government for support in the integration of mental health into primary health care. This AfDB assisted project is to provide $17.73 million to mental health efforts in Uganda over a 5-year period. Activities include rehabilitation of Butabika National Referral Psychiatric Hospital, down-sizing it from a 900-bed to a 450-bed hospital, as well as the construction of 6 regional mental health units. The project includes provision of essential mental health medications and support to the training of healthcare workers at all levels of the care system, from training primary healthcare nurses in the recognition and management of common mental disorders, to the training of specialized personnel, such as psychiatrists, psychologists, and psychiatric social workers.[52]

Lessons Learned

It is often thought that mental health is not a priority in low-income countries, or that feasible mental health interventions are not available. This case study, however, demonstrates that mental disorders are of importance in low-income countries, especially those affected by disasters, complex emergencies, and HIV/AIDS. It also demonstrates that countries, even with few resources, can take measures to considerably improve mental health services.

This case study also suggests that it is possible to design and implement a strategy for dealing with mental disorders that builds on an existing healthcare system. As a result of the investments made, resources for mental health are better allocated in Uganda than before, and funds for mental health have moved from the large psychiatric institution to the regional levels, where services are more accessible to the populations that require them.

Nonetheless, there remain great challenges in trying to provide appropriate mental health services in Uganda. These include the need to strengthen information and public education so the population is aware of what constitutes mental disorders, as well as where help can be sought. A further challenge is likely to be sustainability of the established services. The AfDB project provides the infrastructure and the start-up costs; however, the Government of Uganda will have to ensure that recurrent costs for staff, maintenance of equipment and infrastructure, referral and supervision, and other inputs such as drugs are provided for in the long-term.

FUTURE CHALLENGES

The world must face a number of challenges if it is to reduce the burden of non-communicable diseases in low- and middle-income countries. First, the number of people with new cases of non-communicable diseases will grow in low- and middle-income countries as a result of lifestyle changes and the aging of the population. In addition, because non-communicable diseases are chronic, the number of people with these diseases will also rise. The increasing number of people who will be at risk of and living with chronic diseases in low- and middle-income countries will pose a huge challenge to the health of these countries, to their health systems, and to their national finances.

Related to this, a number of low-income countries will have to deal with the challenge of addressing increasing amounts of non-communicable disease simultaneously with having to address substantial burdens of communicable diseases. This will severely tax the managerial, technical, and financial capacity of many developing countries. It will also require greater attention by low-income countries to non-communicable diseases and to improved surveillance of these diseases, as well.

In addition, it will be important to spread as rapidly as possible to low-and middle-income countries the lessons that the high-income countries have already learned about how to address non-communicable diseases in cost-effective ways. This body of evidence, especially for low-cost interventions that have a high payback, needs to be disseminated in low- and middle-income countries as rapidly as possible. Ongoing mechanisms need to be established to ensure, as well, that cost-effective diagnostics and drugs continuously get disseminated as early as possible to low- and middle-income countries.

Having said this, however, it will also be important that low- and middle-income countries take the measures that are known to prevent non-communicable diseases as soon as they can. They should not wait to build the political consensus that they need to undertake a comprehensive approach to reducing tobacco smoking, for example. Nor do they need to wait to do the same for excessive alcohol consumption. Even in the face of undernutrition, a number of countries will need to promote healthier diets and more physical activity for people who are overweight. Some of the low-cost but effective treatments for cardiovascular disease, such as aspirin, can also be promoted.

MAIN MESSAGES

Non-communicable diseases now constitute the largest burden of disease worldwide. In all regions of the world, except Sub-Saharan Africa, the burden of these diseases is greater than the burden of communicable diseases. Cardiovascular disease is the single largest cause of death worldwide. Diabetes, some forms of cancer, and mental disorders are also major causes of disability and death from non-communicable diseases. In fact, about 14% of the DALYs lost in 2001 were attributable to CVD, about 7% to cancer, 1.3% to diabetes, and about 5% to the four mental disorders discussed earlier.

The leading risk factors for cardiovascular disease are hypertension, obesity, high cholesterol, and tobacco use. A lack of physical activity contributes to CVD and obesity, and the main risk factor for diabetes is obesity. Some cancers are associated with an infectious agent, such as hepatitis B, *h.pylori*, or the human papilloma virus. Other cancers are linked with tobacco use. Little is known about the non-genetic risk factors that are associated with mental disorders.

The costs of non-communicable diseases and the use of tobacco and alcohol abuse are substantial. They have a considerable impact on people in their productive years of life. In addition, mental disorders and diabetes are associated with very large amounts of disability. The costs of trying to prevent the burden of non-communicable diseases include efforts to promote "healthier lifestyles," including a healthy diet and maintaining an appropriate weight and increasing physical activity, while trying to reduce obesity, cigarette consumption, and excessive drinking. The costs of treating non-communicable diseases can be high both because of the high cost of some medical treatments for specific episodes of illness, as well as the need to treat some diseases and conditions for many years. Mental disorders, for example, frequently start early in life and often continue throughout a life. Nonetheless, aspirin and some medicines used for hypertension, for example, are highly cost-effective at dealing with CVD, even in low- and middle-income settings.

The single most important step that countries can take to reduce the burden of non-communicable diseases is to reduce the consumption of tobacco. There is good evidence from high-income and some lower-income countries that taxing cigarettes more heavily, banning smoking from public places, and trying to educate the population about the impact of tobacco on health can all contribute to reducing tobacco consumption.

Reducing the burden of non-communicable diseases will also require that obesity be reduced through healthier diets, fewer calories, increased intake of fruits and green leafy vegetables, and more physical activity. Other measures to reduce obesity can be complemented with food labeling legislation and legislation to encourage the use of healthier ingredients in food products.

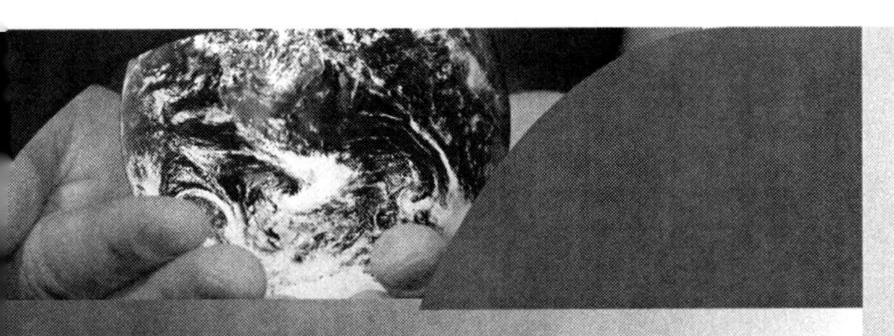

Discussion Questions

1. How important are non-communicable diseases to the global burden of disease?
2. Why are non-communicable diseases less important to that burden in Sub-Saharan Africa?
3. What are the leading risk factors for cardiovascular disease?
4. What are the most important cancers that affect low-income countries?
5. What are the most important risk factors for cancers?
6. What factors are causing the "epidemic" of diabetes that is occurring worldwide?
7. Why are mental disorders so important to the burden of disease if so few people die of them?
8. What measures have proven effective in reducing the use of tobacco?
9. What lessons of Uganda's approach to mental health concerns are important for other resource-poor countries?
10. What measures have been effective in reducing the abuse of alcohol?

REFERENCES

1. Lopez AD, Mathers CD, Murray CJL. The burden of disease and mortality by condition: data, methods, and results for 2001. In: Lopez AD, Mathers CD, Ezzati M, Jamison DT, Murray CJL, eds. *Global Burden of Disease and Risk Factors.* New York: Oxford University Press; 2006:45–240.
2. Gaziano TA., Srinath Reddy K, Paccaud F, Horton S, Chaturvedi V. Cardiovascular disease. In: Jamison DT, Breman JG, Measham AR, et al., eds. *Disease Control Priorities in Developing Countries.* 2nd ed. New York: Oxford University Press; 2006:649–650.
3. Gaziano TA., Srinath Reddy K, Paccaud F, Horton S, Chaturvedi V. Cardiovascular disease. In: Jamison DT, Breman JG, Measham AR, et al., eds. *Disease Control Priorities in Developing Countries.* 2nd ed. New York: Oxford University Press; 2006:650.
4. National Institutes of Health. Obesity, Physical Activity, and Weight-control Glossary. Available at: Available at: http://win.niddk.nih.gov/publications/glossary/MthruZ.htm. Accessed April 15, 2006.
5. International Diabetes Association. *Diabetes Atlas.* 2nd ed. Brussels: International Diabetes Federation; 2003.
6. Ryerson B, Tierney EF, Thompson TJ, et al. Excess physical limitations among adults with diabetes in the U.S. population, 1997–1999. *Diabetes Care.* 2003;26(1):206–210.
7. Mathers C, Stein C, Fat CMF, et al. *Global Burden of Disease 2000: Version 2 Methods and Results.* Geneva: World Health Organization; 2000.
8. Haffner SM. Epidemiology of type 2 diabetes: risk factors. *Diabetes Care.* 1998;21 Suppl 3:C3–6.
9. Venkat Narayan K, Zhang P, Kanaya AM, et al. Diabetes: the pandemic and potential solutions. In: Jamison DT, Breman JG, Measham AR, et al., eds. *Disease Control Priorities in Developing Countries.* 2nd ed. New York: Oxford University Press; 2006:645–662.
10. Centers for Disease Control and Prevention. Fact Sheet—Schistosomiasis. Available at: http://www.cdc.gov/ncidod/dpd/parasites/schistosomiasis/default.htm. Accessed April 20, 2006.
11. Jamison DT, Breman JG, Measham AR, et al., eds. *Priorities in Health.* Washington, DC: TheWorld Bank; 2006.
12. Lopez AD, Mathers CD, Murray CJL. The burden of disease and mortality by condition: data, methods, and results for 2001. In: Lopez AD, Mathers CD, Ezzati M, Jamison DT, Murray CJL, eds. *Global Burden of Disease and Risk Factors.* New York: Oxford University Press; 2006:158.
13. Lopez AD, Mathers CD, Murray CJL. The burden of disease and mortality by condition: data, methods, and results for 2001. In: Lopez AD, Mathers CD, Ezzati M, Jamison DT, Murray CJL, eds. *Global Burden of Disease and Risk Factors.* New York: Oxford University Press; 2006:128.
14. Lopez AD, Mathers CD, Murray CJL. The burden of disease and mortality by condition: data, methods, and results for 2001. In: Lopez AD, Mathers CD, Ezzati M, Jamison DT, Murray CJL, eds. *Global Burden of Disease and Risk Factors.* New York: Oxford University Press; 2006:230.
15. Hyman S, Chisholm D, Kessler R, Patel V, Whiteford H. Mental disorders. In: Jamison DT, Breman JG, Measham AR, et al., eds. *Disease Control Priorities in Developing Countries.* 2nd ed. New York: Oxford University Press; 2006:605–625.
16. Lopez AD, Mathers CD, Murray CJL. The burden of disease and mortality by condition: data, methods, and results for 2001. In: Lopez AD, Mathers CD, Ezzati M, Jamison DT, Murray CJL, eds. *Global Burden of Disease and Risk Factors.* New York: Oxford University Press; 2006:228–233.
17. Jha P, Chaloupka FJ, Moore J, et al. Tobacco addiction. In: Jamison DT, Breman JG, Measham AR, et al., eds. *Disease Control Priorities in Developing Countries.* 2nd ed. New York: Oxford University Press; 2006:870.
18. Jha P, Chaloupka FJ, Moore J, et al. Tobacco addiction. In: Jamison DT, Breman JG, Measham AR, et al., eds. *Disease Control Priorities in Developing Countries.* 2nd ed. New York: Oxford University Press; 2006:869.
19. Jamison DT, Breman JG, Measham AR, et al., eds. *Priorities in Health.* Washington, DC: The World Bank; 2006.
20. Jamison DT, Breman JG, Measham AR, et al., eds. *Priorities in Health.* Washington, DC: The World Bank; 2006.
21. Rehm J, Chisholm D, Room R, Lopez AD. Alcohol. In: Jamison DT, Breman JG, Measham AR, et al., eds. *Disease Control Priorities in Developing Countries.* 2nd ed. New York: Oxford University Press; 2006:887.
22. Rehm J, Chisholm D, Room R, Lopez AD. Alcohol. In: Jamison DT, Breman JG, Measham AR, et al., eds. *Disease Control Priorities in Developing Countries.* 2nd ed. New York: Oxford University Press; 2006:888.
23. Rehm J, Chisholm D, Room R, Lopez AD. Alcohol. In: Jamison DT, Breman JG, Measham AR, et al., eds. *Disease Control Priorities in Developing Countries.* 2nd ed. New York: Oxford University Press; 2006:889.
24. Rehm J, Chisholm D, Room R, Lopez AD. Alcohol. In: Jamison DT, Breman JG, Measham AR, et al., eds. *Disease Control Priorities in Developing Countries.* 2nd ed. New York: Oxford University Press; 2006:890.
25. Rodgers A, Lawes CM, Gaziano TA, Vos T. The growing burden of risk from high blood pressure, cholesterol, and bodyweight. In: Jamison DT, Breman JG, Measham AR, et al., eds. *Disease Control Priorities in Developing Countries.* 2nd ed. New York: Oxford University Press; 2006:854.
26. World Health Organization. *Investing in Mental Health.* Geneva: World Health Organization; 2003.
27. Lightwoood J, Collins D, Lapsley H, Novotny TE. Estimating the costs of tobacco use. In: Jha P, Chaloupka FJ, eds. *Tobacco Control in Developing Countries.* London: Oxford University Press; 2000:107–153.
28. Chaloupka FJ, Tauras JA, Grossman M. The economics of addiction. In: Jha P, Chaloupka FJ, eds. *Tobacco Control in Developing Countries:* London: Oxford University Press; 2000:107–153.
29. World Health Organization. *Global Status Report on Alcohol 2004.* Geneva: World Health Organization; 2004.
30. Jha P, Chaloupka FJ, Moore J, et al. Tobacco addiction. In: Jamison DT, Breman JG, Measham AR, et al., eds. *Disease Control Priorities in Developing Countries.* 2nd ed. New York: Oxford University Press; 2006:869–885.
31. Jha P, Chaloupka FJ, Moore J, et al. Tobacco addiction. In: Jamison DT, Breman JG, Measham AR, et al., eds. *Disease Control Priorities in Developing Countries.* 2nd ed. New York: Oxford University Press; 2006:876.
32. Jha P, Chaloupka FJ, Moore J, et al. Tobacco addiction. In: Jamison DT, Breman JG, Measham AR, et al., eds. *Disease Control Priorities in Developing Countries.* 2nd ed. New York: Oxford University Press; 2006:881.
33. Jha P, Chaloupka FJ, Moore J, et al. Tobacco addiction. In: Jamison DT, Breman JG, Measham AR, et al., eds. *Disease Control Priorities in Developing Countries.* 2nd ed. New York: Oxford University Press; 2006:893.
34. Rehm J, Chisholm D, Room R, Lopez AD. Alcohol. In: Jamison DT, Breman JG, Measham AR, et al., eds. *Disease Control Priorities in Developing Countries.* 2nd ed. New York: Oxford University Press; 2006:887–906.
35. Rehm J, Chisholm D, Room R, Lopez AD. Alcohol. In: Jamison DT, Breman JG, Measham AR, et al., eds. *Disease Control Priorities in Developing Countries.* 2nd ed. New York: Oxford University Press; 2006:894.
36. Rodgers A, Lawes CM, Gaziano TA, Vos T. The growing burden of risk from high blood pressure, cholesterol, and bodyweight. In: Jamison DT, Breman JG, Measham AR, et al., eds. *Disease Control Priorities in Developing Countries.* 2nd ed. New York: Oxford University Press; 2006:863.
37. Rodgers A, Lawes CM, Gaziano TA, Vos T. The growing burden of risk from high blood pressure, cholesterol, and bodyweight. In: Jamison DT, Breman JG, Measham AR, et al., eds. *Disease Control Priorities in Developing Countries.* 2nd ed. New York: Oxford University Press; 2006:856.
38. Rodgers A, Lawes CM, Gaziano TA, Vos T. The growing burden of risk from high blood pressure, cholesterol, and bodyweight. In: Jamison DT, Breman JG, Measham AR, et al., eds. *Disease Control Priorities in Developing Countries.* 2nd ed. New York: Oxford University Press; 2006:855–856.
39. World Health Organization. *Policies and Managerial Guidelines.* Geneva: National Cancer Control Programme; 2002.
40. Hyman S, Chisholm D, Kessler R, Patel V, Whiteford H. Mental disorders. In: Jamison DT, Breman JG, Measham AR, et al., eds. *Disease Control Priorities in Developing Countries.* 2nd ed. New York: Oxford University Press; 2006:621–622.
41. Hyman S, Chisholm D, Kessler R, Patel V, Whiteford H. Mental disorders. In: Jamison DT, Breman JG, Measham AR, et al., eds. *Disease Control*

Priorities in Developing Countries. 2nd ed. New York: Oxford University Press; 2006:620.

42. Jha P, Chaloupka FJ. The economics of global tobacco control. *BMJ.* 2000;321(7257):358–361.

43. Witold Z. *Evolution of Health in Poland Since 1988.* Warsaw: Marie Sklodowska-Curie Memorial Cancer Center and Institute of Oncology, Department of Epidemiology and Cancer Prevention; 1998.

44. Zatonski W. Democracy and health: tobacco control in Poland. In: de Beyer J, Brigden LW, eds. *Tobacco Control Policy, Strategies, Successes and Setbacks.* Washington, DC: The World Bank and International Development Research Center; 2003:97–119.

45. Malan M, Leaver R. Political Change in South Africa: New Tobacco Control and Public Health Policies. In: deBeyer J, Waverly Brigden LW, eds. *Tobacco Control Policy: Strategy, Success, and Setbacks.* Washington, DC: The World Bank and International Development Research Center; 2003.

46. World Health Organization. *Global Initiative for the Prevention of Avoidable Blindness.* Geneva: World Health Organization; 1997. WHO/PBL/97.61.

47. Lopez AD, Mathers CD, Murray CJL. The burden of disease and mortality by condition: data, methods, and results for 2001. In: Lopez AD, Mathers CD, Ezzati M, Jamison DT, Murray CJL, eds. *Global Burden of Disease and Risk Factors.* New York: Oxford University Press and The World Bank; 2006:180–185.

48. Thomas R, Paul P, Rao GN, Muliyil J, Matahai A. Present status of eye care in India. *Surv Ophthalmol* 2005;50(1):85–101.

49. Bachani D, Gupta GK, Murthy G, Jose R. Visual outcomes after cataract surgery and cataract surgical coverage in India. *Int Ophthamol.* 1999;23(1):49–56.

50. The World Bank. *Cataract Blindness Control Project Implementation Completion Report.* Washington, DC: The World Bank; 2002.

51. Javitt J, Venkataswamy G, Sommer A. The economic and social aspect of restoring sight. In: Henkind P, ed. *ACTA: 24th International Congress of Ophthalmology.* New York: JP Lippincott; 1983:1308–1312.

52. Government of Uganda. *Uganda Health Sector Strategic Plan 1999–2004*: Uganda: Government of Uganda; 1999.

53. Willett WC, Koplan JP, Nugent R, Dusenbury C, Puska P, Gaziano TA. Prevention of Chronic Disease by Means of Diet and Lifestyle Changes. In: Jamison DT, Breman JG, Measham AR, et al., eds. *Disease Control Priorities in Developing Countries.* 2nd ed. New York: Oxford University Press; 2006:833-850.

CHAPTER 8

Communicable Diseases

Learning Objectives

By the end of this chapter the reader will be able to:

- Discuss the determinants of selected communicable diseases
- Understand key concepts concerning the prevention and transmission of those diseases
- Review the costs and consequences of communicable diseases of importance
- Outline some of the most important examples of successful interventions against communicable diseases
- Understand key challenges to the future prevention and control of these diseases

VIGNETTES

Henrietta was a 35-year-old Kenyan mother of four who lived in Mombassa. Over the last 4 months, Henrietta was barely able to digest her food, had frequent bouts of diarrhea, and had been losing weight. She worried about having HIV. Henrietta went to a local clinic where she was tested and found to be HIV-positive. She had been infected by her husband, who was a truck driver.

Maria was 33 years old and lived in the mountains of Peru. For some time, she had not been feeling well. She often had a fever, was coughing a lot, and had night sweats. Maria had TB earlier and worried that this might be TB again. Maria was correct. In fact, this time she had drug-resistant TB, which would be difficult and expensive to cure. When Maria was sick the first time, she took most of her drugs. However, because she felt much better after the first 2 months of drugs, she did not take the rest of them.

Wole was 4 years old and lived in southwestern Nigeria. He had flu-like symptoms, a fever, and a headache. His mother suspected he might have malaria but decided she would see if he got better before taking him to the doctor. In another few days, however, Wole was much sicker and weaker. He was also dizzy and, shortly thereafter, lapsed into a coma. His mother then rushed him to the local health center but he died within a few hours. Unfortunately, Wole had the most virulent form of malaria.

Sanjay was 18 months old and lived in Lucknow, India. His mother was a day laborer and his father was a rickshaw driver. They lived in a hut in a large slum with little access to water and no sanitation. Sanjay was below the normal height and weight for his age and looked only 12 months old. Over the past year, Sanjay had four bouts of severe diarrhea.

THE IMPORTANCE OF COMMUNICABLE DISEASES

Communicable diseases are immensely important to the global burden of disease and account for about 40% of the disease burden in low- and middle-income countries.[1] Annually, HIV/AIDS kills about 3 million people, diarrhea kills 1.8 million, tuberculosis kills 1.6 million, and malaria kills 1.2 million.[1] Parasitic infections also account for an enormous burden of disease and disability.

Communicable diseases are the most important burden of disease in Sub-Saharan Africa. They are also especially important in South Asia. These diseases disproportionately affect the poor. Better-off people have the knowledge and income to protect themselves from diseases spread by unsafe water. They do not live in the crowded circumstances that can spread TB, and they also protect themselves as much as possible against malaria. In additon, they immunize their children against vaccine-preventable diseases at rates that are much higher than poor people do.

Communicable diseases are also of enormous economic consequence. These diseases constrain the physical and mental development of infants and young children and reduce their future economic prospects. The impacts on adult productivity of HIV, TB, and malaria are also exceptionally large. In addition, the direct and indirect costs of treatment for the infected person are often a substantial share of their income, causing them to borrow money or sell their already limited assets, and forcing them to sink into poverty. High rates of communicable diseases are also impediments to the investment needed to spur economic growth.

Much of the burden of communicable diseases is unnecessary because many of these diseases can easily be prevented or treated. Vaccines are an extremely cost-effective way to prevent a number of communicable diseases in children. The safe use of water can reduce the burden of diarrhea and certain parasitic diseases. There are inexpensive, safe, and effective treatments for TB, malaria, and some parasitic infections. Unfortunately, these technologies are not sufficiently used in low- and middle-income countries, especially by the poor.

Given their importance and their impact on the poor, the communicable diseases are of immense relevance to the MDGs, as noted in Table 8-1.

This chapter will introduce the reader to some of the major communicable diseases and the burden of morbidity, disability, and mortality associated with them in low- and middle-income countries. It will also outline how selected communicable diseases can be controlled and will elaborate on some success stories in addressing them effectively. The chapter will conclude by reviewing some of the remaining challenges the world faces in the control of these diseases. This chapter will focus on HIV/AIDS, TB, malaria, and a set of parasitic and bacterial infections often referred to as "neglected diseases." Finally, it will offer some brief comments on avian influenza as an example of new and emerging infectious diseases.

This chapter is only introductory. Communicable diseases are a very important topic about which an exceptional amount of material has been written. Those interested in gaining a deeper understanding of these diseases are encouraged to read some of the materials cited in this chapter.

KEY TERMS, DEFINITIONS, AND CONCEPTS

As you begin to explore communicable diseases in greater detail, there are a number of terms and concepts with which one should be familiar. These are defined in Table 8-2. It is also important to recall that a **communicable disease** is a disease that is transmitted from an animal to another animal, an animal to a human, a human to another human, or a human to an animal. Transmission can be direct, such as through respiratory means, or indirect through a vector, such as a mosquito as in the case of malaria. Most people use the term "communicable disease" in a manner that is synonymous with "infectious disease." However, others prefer to speak separately about diseases caused by infectious agents, such as TB, and those caused by parasites, such as hookworm. This chapter will consistently use the term "communicable disease" to refer to infectious and parasitic diseases.

As we examine the basic concepts concerning communicable diseases, it is also important to know how such diseases can be spread. This is shown in the following list, which includes examples of diseases spread in each manner:

- Food-borne—Salmonella, *E. coli*, *Entamoeba histolitica*
- Waterborne—cholera, rotavirus
- Sexual or blood-borne—hepatitis, HIV
- Vector-borne—malaria, onchocerciasis
- Inhalation—tuberculosis, influenza, meningitis
- Non-traumatic contact—anthrax
- Traumatic contact—rabies

In addition, it is critical to understand the ways in which communicable diseases can be controlled. These are noted below, also with examples of relevant diseases:

- Vaccination—smallpox, polio, measles, pediatric tuberculosis, diphtheria, pertussis, tetanus, hepatitis B, yellow fever, meningitis, influenza
- Mass chemotherapy—onchocerciasis, hookworm, lymphatic filariasis
- Vector control—malaria, dengue, yellow fever, onchocerciasis, west nile virus
- Improved water, sanitation, hygiene—diarrheal diseases
- Improved care seeking, disease recognition—maternal health, neonatal health, diarrheal disease, respiratory disease
- Case management (treatment) and improved care giving—diarrheal disease, acute respiratory illness
- Case surveillance, reporting, and containment—avian influenza, meningitis, cholera
- Behavioral change—HIV, sexually transmitted infections

A final concept of exceptional importance when discussing communicable diseases is the concept of **drug resistance**. When considering the concerns of this book, this generally refers to the extent to which infectious and parasitic agents develop an ability to resist drug treatment. These agents naturally evolve over time to resist the treatments against them. Penicillin, for example, was previously used as the drug of choice against a variety of bacterial infections. Some of these bacteria over time, however, became resistant to the penicillin and this drug can no longer be used effectively against them. It is critical when considering public health approaches to major burdens of disease to understand that the improper use of drugs hastens the pace at which drug resistance develops. This has contributed to the development of TB strains that are resistant to the drugs normally used to treat TB. Similarly, some strains of malaria are no longer susceptible to treatment with chloroquine. A fundamental goal of interventions in public health is to avoid the development of drug resistance as much as possible. As indicated in the opening vignette about Maria, drug resistant strains of disease are difficult to treat, expensive to treat, and sometimes even impossible to treat.

TABLE 8-1 Communicable Diseases and the MDGs

Goal 1: Eradicate Extreme Hunger and Poverty
Communicable diseases are associated with high rates of morbidity and mortality. Communicable diseases can be part of a cycle of disease and malnutrition. In addition, communicable diseases reduce one's ability to work, thereby decreasing productivity and family income. In addition, illness causes people to spend an important share of their income on health care.

Goal 2: Achieve Universal Primary Education
Enrollment, attendance, and performance of children in schools is closely linked with health status. Communicable diseases are the leading cause of illness among the poor in Sub-Saharan Africa and South Asia.

Goal 4: Reduce Child Mortality
The three leading causes of death among children in the developing world are respiratory infections, diarrheal diseases, and malaria.

Goal 5: Improve Maternal Health
Malaria can cause anemia and mortality in pregnant women and is a major cause of poor maternal outcomes.

Goal 6: Combat HIV/AIDS, Malaria, and Other Diseases
Reducing the burden of communicable diseases is at the core of meeting this development goal.

Goal 8: Develop a Global Partnership for Development
The most important communicable diseases are being addressed through public-private partnerships or through product-development partnerships, such as Roll Back Malaria; Stop TB; The Global Fund to Fight Against AIDS, TB, and Malaria; The Global Polio Eradication Program; The Global Alliance for TB Drug Development; The Malaria Vaccine Initiative; and The International Partnership on Microbicides.

Source: Author commentary on the Millennium Development Goals. Available at: http://www.un.org/millenniumgoals/goals. Accessed July 11, 2006.

THE BURDEN OF COMMUNICABLE DISEASES

Communicable diseases account for about 36% of total deaths and about 40% of total DALYs lost annually in low- and middle-income countries.[1] Table 8-3 summarizes the major causes of deaths from communicable diseases for the world and in low- and middle-income countries.

The relative importance of communicable diseases, compared to non-communicable diseases and injuries, varies considerably by region. Figure 8-1 indicates the share of the total deaths by region that is represented by communicable diseases. Figure 8-1 further highlights the fact that South Asia and Sub-Saharan Africa have the highest burden of deaths from communicable diseases, relative to other causes of death. Communicable diseases are the largest cause of death only in Sub-Saharan Africa.

The relative importance to the burden of disease of specific communicable diseases also varies by region. HIV/AIDS is of exceptional importance in Sub-Saharan Africa, as is malaria. The "neglected" diseases are also much more important in Sub-Saharan Africa than in any other region.

TABLE 8-2 Communicable Disease Definitions

- **Case**—An individual with a particular disease.
- **Case Fatality Rate**—The proportion of persons with a particular condition (cases) who die from that condition.
- **Control (Disease Control)**—Reducing the incidence and prevalence of a disease to an acceptable level.
- **Eradication (of Disease)**—Termination of all cases of a disease and its transmission and the complete elimination of the disease-causing agent.
- **Palliative Care**—End of life care.
- **Parasite**—An organism that lives in or on another organism and takes its nourishment from that organism.

Source: The Author and Centers for Disease Control and Prevention: Reproductive Health Glossary. Available at: http://www.cdc.gov/reproductivehealth/EpiGlossary/glossary.htm. Accessed April 15, 2007.

TABLE 8-3 Leading Causes of Death from Selected Communicable Diseases, 2001, by Number of Deaths in Thousands

Condition	World	Low- and Middle-Income
Lower Respiratory Conditions	3753	3408
HIV/AIDS	2574	2552
Diarrheal Diseases	1783	1777
Tuberculosis	1606	1590
Malaria	1208	1207
Measles	763	762

Source: Data with permission from The World Bank. Lopez AD, Mathers CD, Ezzati M, Jamison DT, Murray CJL. Measuring the global burden of disease and risk factors 1990–2001. In: Lopez AD, Mathers CD, Ezzati M, Jamison DT, Murray CJL, eds. *Global Burden of Disease and Risk Factors.* New York: Oxford University Press; 2006:8.

FIGURE 8-1 Deaths from Selected Infectious and Parasitic Diseases, as Percent of Total Deaths, by Region 2001 (Includes Infectious and Parasitic Infections and Lower Respiratory Infections)

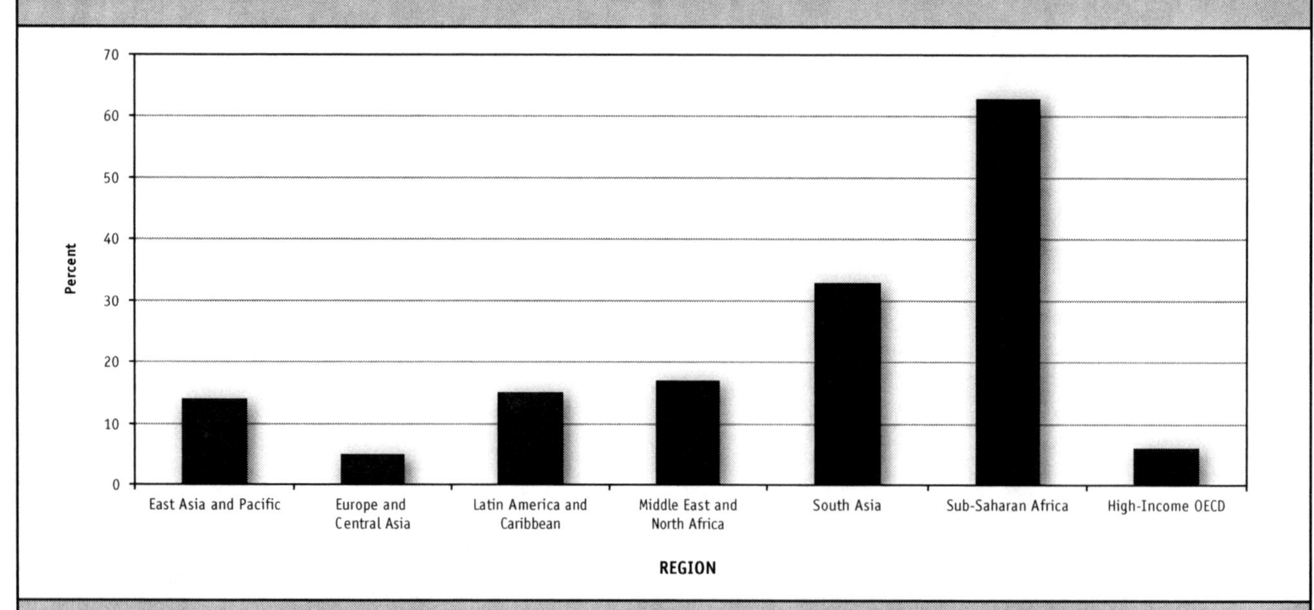

Source: Data with permission from The World Bank. Lopez AD, Mathers CD, Murray CJL. The burden of disease and mortality by condition: data, methods, and results for 2001. In: Lopez AD, Mathers CD, Ezzati M, Jamison DT, Murray CJL, eds. *Global Burden of Disease and Risk Factors.* New York: Oxford University Press; 2006:126–179.

The burden of specific communicable diseases varies by age group. Diarrheal disease, malaria, lower respiratory infections, and measles are most important for young children. HIV/AIDS and TB are most important for people who are 15 to 59 years old, although there is also a substantial TB burden for people older than that. In Table 8-4, one can see the leading causes of deaths from communicable diseases in low- and middle-income countries, by broad age group.

There are relatively small differences in the distribution of deaths from communicable diseases between males and females in low- and middle-income countries. However, it is consistently the case that TB affects males more than females. It is also true that the HIV/AIDS epidemic is being increasingly feminized and that HIV/AIDS is now a more important cause of death for women than for men. These can be seen in Table 8-5.

The section that follows offers additional comments on the burden of disease from specific communicable diseases.

HIV/AIDS

Human Immunodeficiency Virus (HIV) and Acquired Immune Deficiency Syndrome (AIDS) can justifiably be considered the plague of the 21st century. Rarely has a single pathogen had a greater impact on the human condition than HIV. No cure exists for it. Although effective drugs are available to keep HIV/AIDS under control, drug regimens require careful adherence and have significant side effects.

Some of the basic facts about HIV/AIDS are presented in Table 8-6. HIV is a virus that can be spread through:

- unprotected sex
- mother-to-child-transmission, during birth or through breastfeeding

TABLE 8-4 Leading Causes of Death in Low- and Middle-Income Countries by Broad Age Group, 2001, as Percent of Total Deaths

Aged 0–14		Aged 15–59	
Cause	**Percent of Total Deaths**	**Cause**	**Percent of Total Deaths**
Perinatal conditions	20.7	HIV/AIDS	14.1
Lower respiratory infections	17.0	Ischemic heart disease	8.1
Diarrheal diseases	13.4	Tuberculosis	7.1
Malaria	9.2	Road traffic accidents	5.0
Measles	6.2	Cerebrovascular disease	4.9
HIV/AIDS	3.7	Self-inflicted injuries	4.0
Congenital anomalies	3.7	Violence	3.1
Whooping cough	2.5	Lower respiratory infections	2.3
Tetanus	1.9	Cirrhosis of the liver	2.2
Road traffic accidents	1.5	Chronic obstructive pulmonary disease	2.2

Source: Data with permission from The World Bank. Lopez AD, Mathers CD, Murray CJL. The burden of disease and mortality by condition: data, methods, and results for 2001. In: Lopez AD, Mathers CD, Ezzati M, Jamison DT, Murray CJL, eds. *Global Burden of Disease and Risk Factors.* New York: Oxford University Press; 2006:70–71.

TABLE 8-5 Leading Causes of Death by Sex, Low- and Middle-Income Countries, 2001, as Percent of Total Deaths

Males		Females	
Cause	**Percent of Total Deaths**	**Cause**	**Percent of Total Deaths**
Ischemic heart disease	11.8	Ischemic heart disease	11.8
Cerebrovascular disease	8.5	Cerebrovascular disease	10.7
Lower respiratory infections	6.7	Lower respiratory infections	7.4
Perinatal conditions	5.4	HIV/AIDS	5.2
HIV/AIDS	5.4	Chronic obstructive pulmonary disease	5.1
Chronic obstructive pulmonary disease	4.7	Perinatal conditions	4.9
Tuberculosis	4.1	Diarrheal diseases	3.7
Diarrheal diseases	3.6	Malaria	2.8
Road traffic accidents	3.1	Tuberculosis	2.4
Malaria	2.3	Diabetes Mellitus	1.8

Source: Data with permission from The World Bank. Lopez AD, Mathers CD, Murray CJL. The burden of disease and mortality by condition: data, methods, and results for 2001. In: Lopez AD, Mathers CD, Ezzati M, Jamison DT, Murray CJL, eds. *Global Burden of Disease and Risk Factors.* New York: Oxford University Press; 2006:70.

- blood, including by transfusion and needle sharing
- transplantation of infected tissue or organs

The main risk factors for HIV are unprotected sex with an HIV-positive person; being born to and breastfed by an HIV-positive woman; exposure to the blood of an infected person through, for example, transfusion, the sharing of needles with an infected person, or a needlestick injury. Being an uncircumcised male also increases risk. Females are also at greater biological and social risk than males of being infected with HIV. Having a sexually transmitted disease also increases the risk of HIV infection.

The efficiency with which the virus is transmitted varies. The virus is spread most efficiently from exposure to infected blood products and through the sharing of infected needles. There is a 90% probability of being infected from a transfusion of blood from an HIV-positive person.[2] The efficiency of transmission is also relatively high from sharing needles with an HIV-infected person. Sexual transmission depends on the type of sexual act and whether the HIV-positive person is male or female. Male-to-female transmission is higher than female-to-male transmission. The risk of unprotected receptive anal intercourse is about 30 times greater than it is for receptive or insertive vaginal intercourse.[2]

HIV attacks the human immune system. The time from becoming infected until one is diagnosed with AIDS can vary from as little as 1 year to as many as about 15 years. However, without treatment for HIV, about half of those infected will be diagnosed with AIDS in 10 years. Infectiousness is high during the initial period of infection and also increases as the immune system weakens and in the presence of other sexually transmitted infections.[3]

As the immune system of an HIV-positive person deteriorates, that person will suffer from a variety of what are called opportunistic infections, because they take advantage of the person's compromised immunity. As their HIV disease reaches a fairly advanced state, for example, HIV-positive people who are not on antiretroviral therapy may fall ill with TB, herpes infections, a variety of cancers, and an array of significant communicable diseases such as toxoplasmosis and cryptococcal meningitis.[4]

The main routes of transmission of HIV vary by location. In the first phases of the epidemic in high-income countries and in Brail, HIV was largely spread through unprotected sex among men who have sex with men. In Sub-Saharan Africa, the disease has been spread overwhelmingly through unprotected sex between men and women, especially among those engaging in "high-risk behaviors," such as sex workers and their clients and men engaging in sex with multiple female partners. In China, the epidemic was centered originally in a group of people who received transfusions from blood that had been infected with the blood of HIV-positive people. From there, it spread largely through sex between men and women but also through injecting drug use. In Russia and much of the former Soviet Union, the epidemic is being driven by injecting drug users who are HIV-positive and who share needles. The epidemic is spreading from them largely through unprotected sex.

HIV/AIDS epidemics are categorized as either a "concentrated epidemic," in which less than 1% of the population of adults is HIV positive, or a "generalized epidemic," in which more than 5% of the adult population is infected. When HIV first appears in a population, it is generally concentrated in certain groups, such as sex workers, truckers, men who have sex with men, or injecting drug users. If the virus is controlled in these groups, then the spread to the general population can be limited. A generalized epidemic means that HIV/AIDS has spread to the general population, transmission is widespread, and prevalence is high. South Africa and Zimbabwe, for example, have generalized epidemics. India and Vietnam have concentrated epidemics.

It is estimated that about 40 million people worldwide are now infected with the HIV virus, and in the year 2005 about 2.3 million people died of HIV. It is also estimated that about 4.3 million people were newly infected with HIV in

TABLE 8-6 HIV/AIDS—Basic Facts

Number of AIDS cases to date—69 million
Number of AIDS deaths to date—20 million
Number of people living with HIV/AIDS—39.5 million
Number of new HIV infections in 2006—4.3 million
Prevalence among adults—0.1% in East Asia to 5.9% in Sub-Saharan Africa
Prevalence—Two thirds of those living with HIV are in Sub-Saharan Africa
Distribution of infection by sex—21.8 million men; 17.7 million women
Children under 15 with HIV—2.3 million
Number of HIV-positive people on treatment with antiretroviral therapy—1.6 million

Source: Data from UNAIDS. AIDS Epidemic Update 2006. Available at: http://data.unaids.org/pub/EpiReport/2006/02-Global_Summary_2006_EpiUpdate_eng.pdf. Accessed November 21, 2006. UNAIDS. Global Facts and Figures. Available at: http://data.unaids.org/pub/EpiReport/2006/20061121_EPI_FS_GlobalFacts_en.pdf. Accessed November 21, 2006.

2005.[5] The prevalence of HIV varies considerably by region and by country. The prevalence rate of HIV by country is shown in Figure 8-2.

The highest rates of prevalence of HIV/AIDS are in Central and Southern Africa. Relatively high rates of HIV/AIDS are also found in several other African countries and in parts of the Caribbean. With about 25 million infections, Sub-Saharan Africa has about 62.5% of the total number of infections in the world and about 75% of the AIDS-related deaths.[5] There is also considerable concern that the HIV/AIDS epidemics in China and India could become generalized. In addition, there is enormous worry about HIV/AIDS in Russia and other parts of the former Soviet Union. This stems largely from concerns over social disruptions linked with increasing poverty, commercial sex, and injecting drug use, all of which fuel the spread of HIV.

New HIV infections occur predominantly in people aged 15 to 24.[5] They also occur among infants due to maternal-to-child transmission. In the high-income countries, efforts have been made to address maternal-to-child transmission and there are almost no such cases any longer. In the highest prevalence countries, however, infants continue to be infected through maternal-to-child transmission, although efforts have begun to reduce it through drug therapy.

Tuberculosis

Some of the basic facts concerning TB are noted in Table 8-7.

Almost one third of the world, or about two billion people, are infected with tuberculosis. One person is infected with TB every second. This leads to about 30 million new infections annually and about 9 million people in the world with active tuberculosis.[6]

Tuberculosis is caused by the bacteria *Mycobacterium tuberculosis*, and it is spread through aerosol droplets. People breathe in the TB bacteria from other infected people. Tuberculosis can affect all organs of the body, but 80% of cases infect the lungs.

Not everyone infected with TB becomes sick with it. Rather, the TB remains latent in the bodies of about 90% of those infected and they do not have active TB disease. People

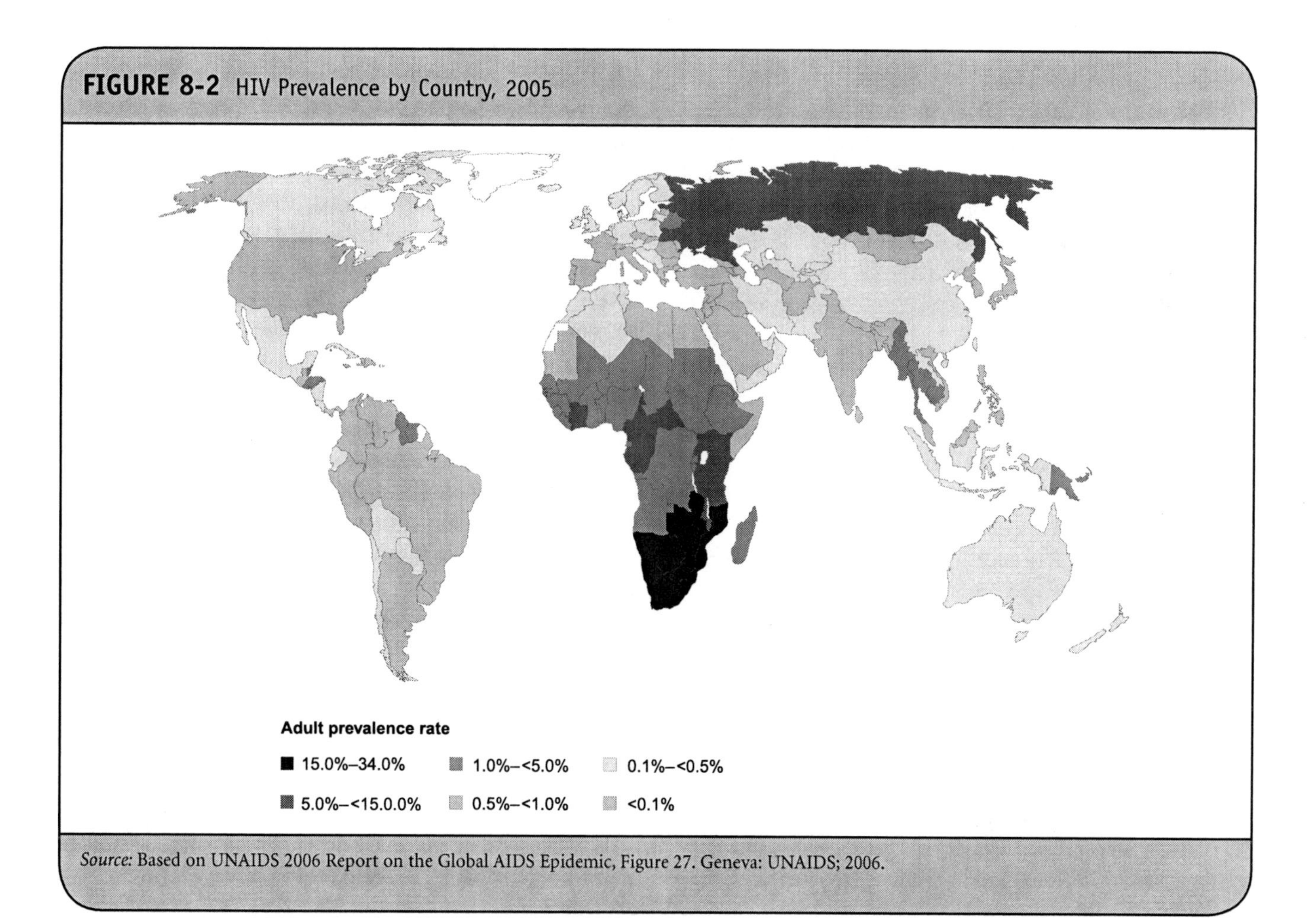

FIGURE 8-2 HIV Prevalence by Country, 2005

Source: Based on UNAIDS 2006 Report on the Global AIDS Epidemic, Figure 27. Geneva: UNAIDS; 2006.

TABLE 8-7 TB—Basic Facts

Number of people infected worldwide—2 billion
Number of new TB cases each year—9 million
Growth in incidence—1% per year
Number of TB deaths each year—2 million, equal to 5000 per day
Number of new multi-drug resistant TB cases each year—450,000
Global distribution of prevalence—29% of cases in Sub-Saharan Africa; half of all new cases in Bangladesh, China, India, Indonesia, Pakistan, and the Philippines
Global TB targets—70% detection of smear positive cases and 85% cure of those cases
Recommended approach to treatment—DOTS (Directly Observed Therapy, Short Course)

Source: Data from: WHO. 2006 Tuberculosis Facts. Available at: http://www.who.int/tb/publications/2006/tb_factsheet_2006_1_en.pdf. Accessed November 15, 2006.

with latent TB do not spread TB to others.

The nature of latent TB is extremely important, especially in an age of HIV, because latent TB can become active when people's immune systems become weak. This could occur because of immune suppressing drugs or because of illness such as some cancers, diabetes, or HIV. Thus, the large pool of people in the world with latent TB infection presents a very significant risk of developing active TB infection if they become infected with HIV.

An untreated person with active pulmonary TB can infect 10 to 15 people annually. If left untreated, about one third of those with active TB will die, one third will self-cure, and one third will remain infectious to others. Pulmonary TB can be spread from person to person, but people with TB in other organs generally do not spread TB. Active TB is characterized by a persistent cough for more than 3 weeks, decreased appetite, general weakness, and profuse night sweats.

In terms of the extent to which people can spread pulmonary TB, there are two forms of TB disease. One is called smear positive and the other is called smear negative. The recommended means for diagnosing TB in low- and middle-income settings is through a microscopic examination of smears of sputum from a person suspected of having TB. Smear positive TB cases are those in which the presence of TB bacteria is confirmed by microscopic examination. They are the most contagious, and in resource-poor settings, they receive priority for treatment.[6]

The TB-HIV interface is a very important public health issue in terms of TB transmission and morbidity and mortality for both TB and HIV. The *lifetime* risk of developing active TB for a person who is *not* infected with HIV is 10%. If a person is HIV-positive, however, the *annual* risk of developing active TB is 10%; thus, after 8 years, the HIV-positive individual has an 80% chance of developing active TB. HIV/AIDS is also associated with a higher proportion of TB that is not pulmonary, compared to TB in people who are not HIV-positive. In addition, TB in HIV-positive people is often very difficult to diagnose.

Tuberculosis kills between two and three million people each year, equal to one person every 10 seconds, and is responsible for 30–40% of the mortality from HIV/AIDS. Most of the infections, cases, and deaths are in adults. Africa has the highest estimated incidence with 356 new cases per 100,000 population, but the most populous countries of Asia, such as Bangladesh, China, India, Indonesia, Pakistan, and the Philippines annually comprise half of the total number of new cases in the world.[6]

TB is the fifth most important cause of death worldwide, with 1.6 million deaths annually. Seventy-five% of the TB infections and deaths occur in the most productive age group—those who are 15 to 54 years old.[6] There are about 8.8 million new cases of TB each year and about half are sputum-smear-positive. TB accounts for 36 million DALYs annually, which is 2.3% of the world's total. Men are more frequently infected than women with TB, possibly because of reporting, but also because of exposure and, perhaps, susceptibility. Nonetheless, TB is also a leading killer of women, with about 550,000 female deaths attributed to TB annually.[7,8]

The number of cases of TB is declining in most high-income countries and new cases there are often among immigrants from low-income countries. However, in much of the developing world the number of cases is increasing, largely fueled by HIV/AIDS. Cases had also been growing in Russia and the former Soviet Union, also driven by HIV/AIDS, the social dislocation noted earlier, and breakdowns in the health system.

The main risk factors for TB are exposure to a person infected with TB, living in crowded circumstances, undernutrition, HIV, inadequate health care, and other conditions that weaken the immune system. TB is overwhelmingly a disease of the poor because it is they who have the most exposure to these risk factors.

There has been an increase in TB infections that are resistant to one or more TB drugs. These forms of TB are called drug-resistant TB, multidrug-resistant TB (MDR TB), and extensively drug-resistant TB (XDR TB). An underlying cause for the development of resistant forms of TB is the failure to complete TB treatment, as was the case for Maria in one of the opening vignettes. However, it is also possible to be infected with drug-resistant TB directly from another person. Drug-resistant strains are found in many countries and are difficult and expensive to treat. Drug resistance is especially important in countries in which TB programs are weak or have fallen into disarray, as in many of the very poor countries, Russia, and in countries with high rates of HIV. In 2006, a number of cases of XDR TB were found in South Africa among HIV patients, and 52 of 53 patients died within 25 days, despite being on HIV treatment. This caused considerable alarm in the public health community.[9] A global effort is now underway to determine the extent of XDR TB.

Malaria

Malaria is caused by parasites in the genus *Plasmodium* and there are four species of malaria parasites that infect humans. They are *Plasmodium falciparum*, *Plasmodium vivax*, *Plasmodium ovale*, and *Plasmodium malariae*. These parasite species exist in different proportions in different regions of the world. *Plasmodium falciparum*, for example, dominates in Africa, *Plasmodium vivax* occurs in temperate zones, and *Plasmodium ovale* is found in South Asia and tropical Africa. The disease is spread by the bite of the female *Anopheles* mosquito. Essentially, the mosquito carries the parasite from an infected person to an uninfected person.

Malaria infects 300 to 500 million people annually, kills 1.2 million people each year, and causes over 40 million DALYs lost annually, which is equal to 2.9% of the global total.[10] Malaria is the ninth leading cause of death in low- and middle-income countries and the fourth leading cause of death in children aged 0 to 14 in those countries. Sub-Saharan African children account for 82% of the malaria deaths worldwide. About 11% of the childhood deaths worldwide are attributed to malaria.[10]

The most important risk factor for malaria is being bitten by mosquitoes that carry malaria. This risk varies with the feeding habits of various species of mosquitoes, the climate, and the time of year. Some people have a degree of immunity to malaria from having grown up in malarial zones and the risks of contracting malaria increase if one does not have such immunity.

Pregnant women are at high risk of giving birth to low birthweight children, and they and their fetuses are at high risk of anemia and death because of malaria. It is estimated that 45 million pregnancies occur annually in malaria endemic areas of Africa and 23 million occur in high malaria transmission areas. 3 to 15% of African mothers suffer severe anemia, accounting for 10,000 malaria-related anemia deaths per year. Globally, malaria causes about 30% of low birth weight in newborns and between 75,000 and 200,000 infant deaths per year.[11]

Diarrheal Disease

Diarrhea is caused by certain bacteria, viruses, and/or parasites that are transmitted by contaminated water or food through the fecal-oral route, such as *Shigella sp.*, *Salmonella sp.*, *Cholera vibrio*, rotavirus, and *Escherichia coli*. Diarrheal disease agents can be spread by dirty utensils, dirty hands, or flies. Diarrhea causes severe dehydration and a loss of body water and can kill infants and young children very quickly. Poor recognition of the extent of illness, failed home care, and lack of knowledge about simple therapies increase the severity of diarrhea. Diarrheal diseases can be prevented by access to safe drinking water, improved sanitation, and the carrying out of more hygienic personal behaviors, such as hand washing.

Diarrheal diseases most significantly impact the poor, especially children in developing countries.[12] Poor housing, crowding, lack of safe water and sanitation, cohabitation with domestic animals, lack of refrigeration for food storage, and poor personal and community hygiene all contribute to the transmission of diarrheal disease agents. In addition, poor nutrition contributes to poor immunity and increases the frequency and severity of diarrhea.

Diarrheal disease mortality has decreased significantly since the 1980s from an estimated 4.6 million deaths to the 1.8 million estimated today, which is about 17% of all childhood deaths. The decline is due to improved nutrition of infants, better disease recognition, improved care seeking, and appropriate use of oral rehydration therapy. Nonetheless, the burden of diarrheal disease remains very substantial. Diarrhea is a major cause of death and sickness for children younger than five years. Children suffer about 3.2 episodes of diarrhea annually but rates vary worldwide.[13] It is estimated that there are 113 million episodes of bloody diarrhea in children under 5 each year caused by *Shigella*.[12]

Neglected Diseases

Another set of diseases, which are increasingly referred to as neglected diseases, are associated with significant morbidity and economic loss. About 4.2 billion people are at risk of these diseases in 142 countries. These diseases account for 24% of total DALYs lost annually from communicable diseases, and 20% of the communicable disease deaths.[14] Those most affected are children. Ascaris, trichuris, and hookworm infect 1.2 billion, 800 million, and 740 million people worldwide, respectively.[14] As with other tropical infectious diseases, Africa bears the brunt of morbidity and mortality.

Neglected diseases include helminthic worm, protozoan, and bacterial infections, a few of which are discussed here.

Helminth Infections:

Soil-transmitted Helminth infections:

Ascariasis-Trichuriasis-Hookworm
Lymphatic Filariasis (Elephantiasis)
Onchocerciasis (River Blindness)
Schistosomiasis
Dracunculiasis (Guinea Worm)

Protozoan Infections:

Leishmaniasis (Kala-azar)
African Trypanosomiasis (Sleeping Sickness)
Chagas' Disease

Bacterial Infections:

Leprosy
Trachoma
Buruli Ulcer

The life cycles of the soil transmitted helminth infections are similar. The worms live in the gastrointestinal tract of humans. They produce eggs, which are passed out with the human feces. Those who ingest them are at risk of becoming infected. Hookworms can produce anemia in their human hosts. In addition, children with the heaviest burden of worms are at risk of impaired mental and physical development.[15] The burden of worms varies, with 20% of those infected harboring 80% of the worms.[15]

The most important risk factors for soil-transmitted helminths are:

- being an agricultural worker
- poverty, poor sanitation, lack of clean water
- living near wet, warm areas[15]

Lymphatic filariasis is caused by a nematode worm that is carried from an infected to an uninfected person with the bite of a mosquito. The nematode *Wucheria bancrofti*, which is the cause of this illness, is present in many of the humid and tropical parts of the world. Female worms produce microfilariae that enter the bloodstream and can cause a variety of manifestations. Among the most disabling of these problems are swelling of the genitalia and of the limbs, which are both debilitating and stigmatizing.[16]

Schistosomiasis is another neglected disease of importance. It is caused by the liver fluke, a trematode. People with schistosomiasis release fluke eggs in their urine or their feces. The flukes enter into fresh water snails, from which they emerge into the water. The flukes penetrate the skin of a human when they are wading, bathing, or working in water that has been infected. One form of the fluke causes manifestations in the intestinal tract and liver. Another form causes problems in the urinary tract. Over time, these can lead to severe disease of the urinary tract or liver, among other things.[17]

The burden of some of the most important neglected diseases in Africa is shown in Table 8-8.

THE COSTS AND CONSEQUENCES OF COMMUNICABLE DISEASES

The economic and social costs of the enormous burden of communicable diseases are very high. First, these diseases constrain the health and development of infants and children, often by having an impact on their schooling and on their productivity as adult workers. Second, stigma and discrimination against people with HIV, those with TB, and those with a variety of other debilitating communicable diseases, such as leprosy and lymphatic filariasis, are strong and pervasive. Third, adults who suffer from the diseases discussed in this chapter suffer substantial losses in productivity and incomes. Fourth, families spend considerable sums of money trying to treat these illnesses. Fifth, high rates of infectious diseases in any country reduce investments in that country's development. Some of the economic and social consequences that relate more specifically to AIDS, TB, malaria, and the neglected diseases are discussed briefly here.

HIV/AIDS

HIV/AIDS has enormous social and economic consequences, especially in high prevalence countries in Sub-Saharan African countries, which go beyond the usual impact of diseases on morbidity and mortality. Rather, HIV/AIDS affects family cohesion, business, trade, labor, the armed forces, agricultural production, education systems, governance, public services, and even national security.

In the absence of treatment, the person infected with HIV will eventually become sicker, progress to full blown AIDS, and suffer from a variety of opportunistic infections, as noted previously. As this happens, the person becomes less able to work, loses part or all of his or her income, and becomes dependent on others for care. The caretaker may also lose his or her income.

This cycle has caused enormous economic losses to individuals and their families, especially in Sub-Saharan Africa. A

TABLE 8-8 Burden of Selected Helminthic and Protozoan Infections in Africa, by Percent of Global Burden of Condition

Condition	Cases in Africa	% of Global Burden of Condition
Hookworm	198 million	27–34%
Ascariasis	173 million	14–22%
Schistosomiasis	166 million	89%
Trichuriasis	162 million	20–26%
Trachoma	33 million	40%
Lymphatic Filariasis	46 million	38%
Onchocerciasis	18 million	99%
Afr. Trypanosomiasis	0.5 million	100%
Dracunculiasis	< 0.1 million	100%

Source: Reprinted with permission from The World Bank. Hotez PJ, Bundy DAP, Beegle K, et al. Helminth infections: soil-transmitted helminth infections and schistosomiasis. In: Jamison DT, Breman JG, Measham AR, et al., eds. *Disease Control Priorities in Developing Countries.* 2nd ed. New York: Oxford University Press; 2006:467–482.

study done in Tanzania, for example, indicated that men with AIDS lost an average of 297 days of work over an 18-month period and women lost an average of 429 days of work over that same period, which implies that these women were essentially unable to attend to any of their normal tasks.[18] A study in Thailand showed that families that suffered from AIDS lost an average of 48% of their income as a result of their illness.[18]

Another important consequence of HIV/AIDS is the creation of an exceptional number of orphans. When speaking of HIV/AIDS, an orphan is defined as an individual 15 years old or younger who has lost one or both parents to the disease. It is estimated that there are 15 million HIV/AIDS orphans and that this number could rise to 25 million by 2010.[5] Despite efforts by many families to care for their relatives, many orphans do not have anyone with whom to live and may resort to living on the street, where they fall into commercial sex and crime.

HIV/AIDS is a highly stigmatized condition, as are a number of other communicable diseases. HIV/AIDS, however, has a special stigma because people in many societies believe that people acquire HIV/AIDS because they engage in behaviors that society does not sanction, such as men who have sex with men, commercial sex work, or injecting drug use. Understanding the notion of stigma and discrimination against people with HIV is central to understanding the HIV/AIDS epidemic.

In fact, stigmatization of HIV in many societies has led to unwillingness to allow people with HIV to attend schools or be employed, get health care, live in certain places, or even live with their families. Stigma has also been a major constraint to people's getting tested or treated for HIV. It has also complicated prevention efforts in some settings by driving underground some of the very people it is important to reach, such as sex workers and injecting drug users.

For the poorest developing countries, the direct cost of AIDS treatment is very expensive compared to per capita income and per capita health expenditure, even at the reduced prices for those drugs that have been agreed upon globally. In fact, the cost of providing drugs and related laboratory and clinical services costs is generally at least $300 per patient, per year. Yet, many of the low-income countries that are providing AIDS drugs to people living with HIV/AIDS normally spend only about $5 per person per year on health. It will be difficult for low-income countries with high HIV prevalence to support the treatment of a large share of people living with HIV/AIDS without considerable and sustained external assistance.

The increasing attention paid to HIV has been positive in many ways. However another cost of HIV/AIDS is the extent to which attention to it diverts human and financial resources away from other health priorities, such as child health or the neglected diseases. Striking an effective and equitable balance between HIV/AIDS and other public health priorities is a challenge for many countries.

Many studies of the impact of HIV/AIDS have been used to help convince governments that failure to address HIV early could result in lower economic growth of their country. Overall, the studies suggest that HIV/AIDS will have a large impact on the economic growth of high-prevalence countries in Africa, largely because it tends to strike people in their most productive years.[19] The higher the prevalence and the more families that use their savings to help pay for the costs of illness, the more likely HIV is to have a negative impact on the growth of per capita income.[20]

TB

The cost of TB to families, communities, and countries is very high, given the large number of people who are sick with TB, the relatively long course of the illness, and the losses people face when they do have TB. A study of TB in India suggested that those sick with TB lost about 3 months of wages, spent an amount equal to about one quarter of national income per capita on care and treatment, and took on debts to pay for this care that were equal to about 10% of per capita income.[21] A similar study in Bangladesh indicated that those sick with TB lost 4 months of wages.[22] A Thai study showed that TB patients spent more than 15% of their annual wages on TB, that 12% of them took out bank loans to help make up for the costs of their illness, and that 16% sold part of their property to finance the costs of dealing with their illness.[23]

There are also significant social costs associated with TB. Because of the stigma associated with TB, females who get infected are often shunned by their families. In one Indian study, 15% of the women with TB faced familial rejection.[24] In another Indian study, 8% faced rejection.[21]

A study of the macroeconomic impact of TB suggested that the economic growth of a country is inversely correlated with the rate of TB. Every increase of 10% in the incidence of TB was associated with lower annual economic growth of 0.2–0.4%.[25] A study of the economic costs of TB in the Philippines indicated that the annual economic loss due to morbidity and premature mortality from TB was equal to almost $150 million. In addition, the cost to the Philippines of treating all of the expected cases of TB would be between $8 million and $29 million.[26]

Malaria

The cost of malaria at the family level is significantly less than the costs of HIV/AIDS and TB but is still substantial because individuals often have malaria up to five times per year. In one study in Ghana, for example, there were 11 cases of malaria per household, per year, on average.[18] These same studies showed that individuals lost one to five work days per episode of malaria, that the indirect cost of dealing with their illness was greater than the direct costs of treatment, and that each episode of malaria probably cost an adult about 2% of his annual income.[18] In many African countries, malaria typically accounts for 20–40% of outpatient visits at health facilities and 10–15% of hospital admissions.[27]

Over $3.5 billion is lost annually due to malaria in Africa alone.[27] Roll Back Malaria suggests that the economic costs of malaria in countries with a high malaria burden is about 1.3% per year loss of GDP. One study suggested that a 10% reduction in malaria was associated with a 0.3% higher increase in economic growth. Clearly, malaria in Sub-Saharan Africa is a deterrent to trade, business development, tourism, and foreign investment.[28,29]

Neglected Diseases

As noted earlier, neglected diseases cause over 500,000 deaths and 57 million DALYs annually. They also cause a great deal of long-term disability, disfigurement, and suffering.[30] Studies of the economic costs of these diseases have been limited. However, an extensive study done in Kenya indicated that deworming improved school attendance better than any other investment, which should ultimately lead to higher earnings for the students than they would otherwise have.[31] A study of hookworm in the southern part of the United States in the early part of the 20th century showed that hookworm infection was associated with a 23% reduction in school attendance.[32] It has already been noted that parasitic infections are associated with reduced weight gain, lower height, anemia, and lower productivity and capacity for wage earning.

ADDRESSING THE BURDEN OF DISEASE

HIV/AIDS

Despite considerable and increasing efforts, there is not yet either a preventive or therapeutic vaccine for HIV/AIDS. In the absence of such a vaccine, halting the spread of HIV will have to focus on the prevention of new infections. Yet, despite 25 years of efforts to prevent HIV, there is little rigorous evidence about the most cost-effective approaches to prevention. Nonetheless, some evidence is emerging, as discussed below.

The few successful prevention efforts that have occurred, such as in Thailand and Uganda, have consistently been associated with a number of factors related to strong political leadership and commitment and open communications including:

- Sustained political leadership at the highest levels
- Involvement of a broad range of civil society efforts to address HIV/AIDS, including opinion leaders and religious leaders
- Broad-based programs to change social norms in the population
- Open communication about HIV/AIDS and related sexual matters
- Programs to reduce stigma and discrimination[33]

In addition, we also know that to be successful, prevention efforts need to include:

- Good epidemic surveillance
- Information, education, and communication
- Voluntary counseling and testing
- Condom promotion
- Screening and treatment for sexually transmitted infections
- Prevention of mother-to-child-transmission through avoiding pregnancy, antiretroviral treatment, and breast milk substitutes
- Interventions that target populations that transmit the virus from high-risk to low-risk populations
- Prevention of blood-borne transmission through blood safety, harm reduction for injecting drug users, and universal precautions in healthcare settings.[34]

Some additional comments on prevention efforts follow.

First, the approach to prevention will need to vary with the nature of the epidemic. In low-level and concentrated epidemics, the focus can be on changing the behaviors of those who engage in high-risk behaviors. The approach to prevention in a more generalized epidemic, however, will need to be much broader.[34]

Second, there is an emerging consensus globally that an integrated "ABC" approach to HIV/AIDS prevention is needed but that the weights given to different parts of the approach must vary depending on the nature of the epidemic and the cultural background of each country. "ABC" stands for abstinence, being faithful, and correct and consistent condom use. Major elements of this approach include the promotion of safe sexual behavior, correct and consistent use of condoms for those practicing high-risk behaviors, delay of sexual debut for youth, abstinence until marriage, partner reduction, and fidelity. There is a concern globally, however, to ensure that such an approach, and the weights given to different parts of it, is evidence-based, especially relating to the promotion of abstinence.

There has been a considerable degree of discussion in recent years of appropriate approaches to testing and counseling. From the inception of the HIV/AIDS epidemic, concern for stigmatization of HIV-positive people has caused governments to undertake testing and counseling with complete confidentiality of the person being tested and only on a voluntary "opt in" basis. Recently, however, there has been an increasing concern that it is important to raise the share of people who are tested, particularly in high prevalence settings, because most people do not know their status and most infections are spread at the early stages of infection. Therefore, a number of countries, led by Botswana, now offer an HIV test whenever people have contact with the health system, with the possibility of "opting out" of testing. The advocates of this approach hope that it will lead to more people knowing their HIV status as early as possible, thereby enabling them to avoid infecting others.

There has also been increasing attention to trying to stem maternal-to-child transmission of HIV. The most cost-effective measure to reduce maternal-to-child transmission of HIV is to avoid unwanted pregnancies of HIV positive women through contraception. Providing antiretroviral therapy to pregnant women infected with HIV is also cost-effective because this may prevent about one third of the women from having a baby who is HIV-positive. Little information is available on the cost-effectiveness of breast milk substitutes. However, if a women is going to breastfeed her baby, the baby is less likely to be HIV-positive if the mother exclusively breastfeeds, weans early, and then provides food to the baby because mixing breast milk and food raises the risk that the baby will become HIV-positive.[35]

The promotion, distribution, and social marketing of condoms encourages correct and consistent use of condoms and lowers the rates of sexually transmitted infections (STIs) and HIV. However, there are limited data on the cost-effectiveness of these approaches. At least in the early stages of an HIV epidemic, it appears that screening for and treatment of STIs can be a cost-effective way of preventing HIV.[36]

There is good evidence that needle exchanges are effective in high-income countries, but there are little data on such programs in low- and middle-income countries. There is widespread agreement that blood safety is cost-effective and must be a high priority in all settings. There is evidence that circumcised males are 40–60% less likely to be infected with HIV than uncircumcised males;[37] however, there are little data about how one can manage a cost-effective program for adult circumcision, especially in the face of cultural obstacles in many settings.[38] Thus, a number of efforts are now underway to design programs for adult circumcision as a component of HIV/AIDS prevention activities.

There is also considerable support for linking treatment and prevention programs. The question of what is the most cost-effective approach to treatment, however, is complicated by the limited available evidence. It appears that community-based approaches to palliative care of people who are HIV-affected are likely to be highly cost-effective, and certainly more cost-effective than care provided by healthcare professionals in the homes of the affected. Community-based food supplementation programs can also be cost-effective.[39] In addition, there is good evidence that putting people who are affected with HIV on the antibiotic cotrimoxazole can be a cost-effective way to reduce the risk and delay the onset of opportunistic infections.[40]

Widespread use of antiretroviral therapy has only begun in the developing world, outside of a small number of countries such as Thailand and Brazil, in the last several years. It is too early, therefore, to have definitive evidence about the most cost-effective regimens for treatment of HIV infection. Calculating cost-effectiveness of these drugs will not be simple because there are many different regimens, each drug has different side effects, and patients have to change regimens when they develop side effects or resistance. Nonetheless, evidence needs to be gathered continuously on the cost-effectiveness of various regimens.

As a rule of thumb, low-income countries should aim to place about 15% of those infected on drug therapy, because they will be the ones most in need clinically and because these countries are unlikely to be able to place all of their patients with HIV on treatment as soon as they are diagnosed. Once the patient is under treatment, it is exceptionally important that they take all of their drugs exactly as prescribed in order to avoid developing resistance. If the drugs are discontinued because of interrupted supply, poor compliance by the patient, or poor performance of the health system, then resistance may develop and the patient may require more expensive second-line drugs. Drug resistant strains of HIV also pose risks to others, who can become infected with them directly from others and then face difficulties finding effective drug regimens for their strain of HIV.

Overall, effective HIV/AIDS therapy depends on individuals accessing counseling and testing, a definitive HIV test, a clinical diagnosis of the patient, a laboratory assessment of the individual's immune status with a CD4 cell count, patient adherence to their drug regimen, sound nutrition of the patient, and sound and continuous monitoring and evaluation of the patient. About 1.6 million people in the developing world are now receiving antiretroviral therapy.[5] The world has set a goal of universal access to treatment for HIV by 2010.

TB

There is a vaccine for TB called BCG that is a standard part of the Expanded Program of Immunization for Children. The vaccine reduces severe TB in children but because children are not important transmitters of TB, the vaccine has little impact on the overall incidence or prevalence of TB.[41] Rather, the control of TB depends on effective treatment of active tuberculosis. In many respects, implementing a poor TB program is worse than not having a TB program at all because a poor TB program can give rise to drug-resistant TB.

The treatment strategy for TB is called DOTS: Directly Observed Therapy, Short-Course. DOTS consists of a 6-month regimen that normally includes four drugs—isoniazid, rifampin, pyrazinamide, and ethambutol—for the first 2 months—and then isoniazid and rifampin for the following 4 months. DOTS is just what it says—a relatively short course of therapy directly observed by a local care provider or community member, compared to the longer course that had previously been given without such observation.

The DOTS strategy has five essential components:

- Sustained political commitment to a national TB program;
- Access to quality-assured sputum smears and microscopy;
- Standardized regimens of short-course chemotherapy under direct observation;
- Regular uninterrupted supply of quality-assured anti-TB drugs; and,
- Monitoring and evaluation for program supervision.[6]

Once an active case of TB is identified, appropriate drugs are required in adequate supply for 6 months. Patient compliance with the TB regimen is required for effective therapy and direct observation is meant to ensure appropriate treatment for the entire course. Healthcare workers, NGO staff, community volunteers and leaders, such as teachers, religious leaders, and other community members, provide observation. They are sometimes the holders of the medicine, as well as the persons who observe TB patients taking their medicines.

The TB drugs needed to cure a single case of active TB can be purchased in low- and middle-income countries for as little as $15. Treating active TB with DOTS is very cost-effective and ranges from $5 to $50 per DALY gained in most regions.[41] BCG is cost-effective in reducing severe cases of childhood TB in high prevalence settings. Treating multidrug-resistant TB is also relatively cost-effective.

HIV and TB

There is a direct relationship between HIV in adults who are 15 to 49 years old and TB. In many countries with high HIV prevalence, 60% or more of those with active TB are HIV-positive, as noted earlier. TB control programs can help to identify HIV-positive patients and AIDS programs should always determine if an HIV-positive person has TB. Unfortunately, the treatment of a person who is co-infected with HIV and TB is complicated. Efforts are underway to see if DOTS or a "DOTS-like" approach to antiretroviral therapy can be helpful to ensuring high patient adherence with their HIV drug regimen, even if HIV drugs need to be taken for a lifetime.

Malaria

Despite many years of effort, there is still no vaccine against malaria. However, there is widespread agreement on the key interventions required to "roll back" malaria. These include:

- Prompt treatment of those infected
- Intermittent preventative therapy for pregnant women
- Insecticide-treated bed nets for people living in malarial zones
- Indoor residual spraying of the homes of people in malarial zones

The Abuja Declaration of 2000 has three objectives for reducing malaria mortality and morbidity in Africa, with the understanding that their achievement by 2005 will be challenging. The Declaration states that 60% of children should receive prompt and effective treatment, 60% of pregnant women should receive intermittent preventive therapy, and 60% of children and pregnant women should sleep under an insecticide-treated bed net.[42] Each intervention holds great promise but a great deal remains to be done before these goals can be realized.

Appropriate treatment of malaria is essential to reduce malaria morbidity and mortality. If people with malaria are treated promptly, then mosquitoes that bite them will not carry malaria to another person. Drugs such as chloroquine, fansidar, and mefloquine are being used but face growing levels of drug resistance.

Artemisinin, a new drug for malaria, is now being used in combination with other anti-malarial drugs in areas where malaria is resistant to other drugs. Efforts are also underway to get artemisinin into use as soon as possible in all malarial areas, so that the advent of resistance can be delayed. Treatment with artemisinin plus other anti-malarial drugs is referred to as ACT, which stands for artemisinin-based combination therapy. Effective therapy depends on accurate laboratory diagnosis and appropriate case management. In addition, pregnant women are being treated with intermittent preventive therapy from between 18 and 24 weeks of their pregnancy through delivery to reduce complications and deaths from malaria among this group of people.

The use of bed nets and eliminating mosquito breeding sites represent additional means of malaria control. Bed nets, impregnated with a biologically safe insecticide, are being widely distributed and sold by governments, donors, and the private sector. Spraying the inside of homes, or indoor residual spraying, is also to be carried out. Reducing the number of mosquitoes that carry malaria at the community level relies on effective communication and commitment by local leaders, the identification of breeding sites, and the availability of appropriate larvicides and/or tools to drain potential breeding sites. However, reducing the number of mosquitoes, called source reduction, is particularly difficult in Africa because the vector, *Anopheles gambiae*, is ubiquitous and breeds in all types of standing water.

Diarrhea

There are five major disease prevention strategies for diarrhea. Perhaps most effective is the promotion of exclusive breastfeeding for 6 months. This is advantageous to the child and mother because the child receives both maternal antibodies and a nutritious and uncontaminated meal. Mothers benefit from an increased birth interval and a healthier child. The second prevention intervention is improved complementary feeding, introduced with breastfeeding after 6 months. Third, is rotavirus immunization, which will be increasingly cost-effective as the vaccines are more affordable in low- and middle-income countries. Diarrhea from rotavirus kills about 600,000 children under five years each year.[43] The next strategy is increased measles immunizations. Data indicate a clear link between measles immunization and reduced incidence and deaths from diarrhea. If measles coverage is increased, especially in Africa, then the burden of diarrheal disease will decline. The fifth prevention strategy is improving access to safe water supply and sanitation. Clean water and appropriate sanitation will reduce diarrheal disease incidence. Furthermore, hand washing can reduce diarrhea incidence by 3%.[44]

Three case management interventions can significantly reduce the severity and mortality of diarrheal disease. The use of oral rehydration therapy (ORT) is the most cost-effective case management intervention, especially if homemade solutions are administered. Although the use of ORT has expanded globally, only about 49% of the diarrhea cases worldwide are managed with ORT or home fluids.[12] Second, it is estimated that zinc supplementation during an acute diarrhea episode for 10 to 14 days during and after diarrhea could prevent 300,000 deaths per year.[45] Third, antibiotics can be given for bloody diarrhea, primarily caused by *Shigella* infection. However, delivering this intervention where it is most needed may depend on careful training of non-physician healthcare personnel because most low-income and many middle-income countries do not have enough physicians living in places where they are most needed.

Neglected Diseases

Many poor people in low- and middle-income countries suffer from more than one of the neglected diseases. A "rapid-impact" package can simultaneously treat seven of the major neglected diseases including ascariasis, hookworm, trichuriasis, lymphatic filariasis, onchocerciasis, schistosomiasis, and trachoma. For less than $1 per person per year, plus donations of five key drugs, scaling-up a rapid-impact package is feasible. Integrating the control of neglected diseases and malaria control in Africa is also feasible. This package, aimed at a large and underserved population, could reduce disease burden significantly and could enhance productivity in many African nations.

Many policy makers have ignored neglected tropical diseases in favor of HIV/AIDS, TB, and malaria. However, the geographic overlap of many neglected diseases with HIV/AIDS, TB, and malaria makes an integrated control effort possible. Drugs for neglected diseases could be deployed through existing health systems and communities and linked to other disease control efforts. In this case, the burden of neglected diseases could be reduced for over 500 million people at an estimated cost of $0.40 per person treated, including the donated drugs, which would be extremely cost-effective.

CASE STUDIES

The control of communicable diseases remains challenging. However, important progress has been made against some of these diseases. Given the exceptional importance of communicable diseases in low-income countries, this chapter includes five case studies. One of them examines the efforts of Thailand to address sexually transmitted diseases and HIV/AIDS. Another discusses China's attempt to control TB through DOTS. The third reviews the exceptional global effort to eradicate polio. The last two cases concern neglected diseases, one on Chagas disease in Latin America and another on trachoma in Morocco. Those interested in more detail on the cases can consult *Case Studies in Essential Health: Millions Saved.*[46]

HIV/AIDS in Thailand

Preventing HIV/AIDS and Sexually Transmitted Infections in Thailand

Background

In Thailand, approximately 1 in every 60 persons is infected with HIV/AIDS and 75,000 children have been orphaned by AIDS.[47,48] Between 1989 and 1990, HIV among sex workers tripled, from 3.1% to 9.3% and a year later reached 15%. Over the same period, the proportion of male conscripts already infected with HIV when tested on entry to the army at age 21 rose six-fold, from 0.5% in 1989 to 3% in 1991.[48]

The Intervention

In 1989, Dr. Wiwat Rojanapithayakorn, director of a regional office in Communicable Disease Control in Thailand's Ratchaburi province, sought to curb AIDS by making sex in brothels safe, going well beyond the government's approach of raising awareness through mass advertising and education campaigns. Knowing that he could only be effective with political support, he sought the cooperation of the provincial governor. The steep rise in AIDS persuaded the governor to acquiesce, even though prostitution is illegal in Thailand and the government's intervention could imply that it tolerated or even condoned it.

A program was launched with one straightforward rule for all brothels in Ratchaburi: no condom, no sex. Until then, brothels had been reluctant to insist that their clients use condoms for fear of losing them to other establishments where condoms were not required. However, with condoms mandatory in all brothels, the competitive disincentive to individual workers and brothels was removed. Health officials, with the help of the police, held meetings with brothel owners and sex workers to provide them with information and free condoms. Men seeking treatment for sexually transmitted infections (STIs) were asked to name the brothel they had last visited and health officials would then visit the establishment to provide more information. This pilot program had dramatic results, bringing down STIs in Ratchaburi within just a few months.[49] In 1991, the National AIDS Committee, chaired by Prime Minister Anand Panyarachun, adopted this "100% condom program" at the national level.

The Impact

Condom use in brothels nationwide increased from 14% in early 1989 to more than 90% by June 1992.[50] An estimated 200,000 new infections were averted between 1993 and 2000. New STI cases fell from 200,000 in 1989 to 15,000 in 2001, while the rate of new HIV infections fell fivefold between 1991 and 1993–1995.[51] Such dramatic results have raised questions about their accuracy, as well as about their real causes, but independent studies have found the program to be genuinely effective.

The program did little to encourage the use of condoms in casual but noncommercial sex. Interventions among injecting drug users also did not expand to the national level, and the prevalence of HIV among this group is now as high as 50%.[52]

Costs and Benefits

Total government expenditure on the AIDS program has remained steady at approximately $375 million from 1998 to 2001, representing 1.9% of the health budget. Of this, 65% was spent on treatment and care.

Lessons Learned

The success of the program is due, in part, to the sheer scale and level of organization of the sex industry in Thailand, assisting officials in tracing and co-opting brothel owners. Thailand also had a good network of STI services within a well-functioning health system, providing treatment and advice, as well as crucial data for decision makers both at the baseline and when the program took effect. Cooperation between health authorities, governors, and the police was critical to success. Strong leadership from the prime minister, backed by significant financial resources, also made swift action possible. Maintaining Thailand's remarkable results in slowing the AIDS epidemic needs continued vigilance. Due to the high cost of treating STIs, the HIV prevention budget declined by two thirds between 1997 and 2004.[53] Although the Thai experience provides no blueprint for other countries with very different starting conditions, it does demonstrate that targeted strategies and political courage can effect change in deeply entrenched behaviors.

TB in China

Background

Although China established a National Tuberculosis Program in 1981, inadequate financial support hindered its success. In 1991, with $58 million from the World Bank, China embarked on the largest informal experiment in TB control in history: a 10-year Infectious and Endemic Disease Control project in 13 of its 31 mainland provinces.[54] The project adopted the DOTS strategy. Individuals demonstrating TB symptoms were referred to county dispensaries, where they received free diagnosis and treatment. Village doctors were given financial incentives for enrolling patients and completing their treatment. Efforts were also made to strengthen the institutions involved with the establishment of a National Tuberculosis Project Office and a Tuberculosis Control Center. Quarterly reports were submitted by each county to the province, the central government, and the National Tuberculosis Project Office, which strengthened monitoring and quality control.

Impact

China achieved a 95% cure rate for new cases within 2 years of adopting DOTS, and a remarkable cure rate of 90% for those who had previously undergone unsuccessful treatment.[55] The number of people with TB declined by over 37% between 1990 and 2000, and 30,000 TB deaths have been prevented each year. More than 1.5 million patients have been treated, leading to the elimination of 836,000 cases of pulmonary TB.[56]

Costs and Benefits

The program cost $130 million. The World Bank and the WHO estimated that successful treatment was achieved at a cost of less than $100 per person. One healthy life was saved for an estimated $15 to $20, with an economic rate of return of $60 for each dollar invested.[57]

Lessons Learned

The success of China's program can be attributed to strong political commitment, leadership, adequate funding, and a sound technical approach delivered through a relatively strong health system. It was found that DOTS could be scaled up rapidly without sacrificing quality. Free diagnosis and treatment served as an effective incentive for patients and incentives for doctors to diagnose and complete treatment also worked well. However, the overall rate of case detection proved disappointing, mainly due to the inadequate referral of suspected TB cases from hospitals to TB dispensaries; hospitals charging for services had no incentive to refer patients to dispensaries where services were provided for free.[58] In addition, patients at hospitals often abandoned treatment prematurely. Despite the program's success, TB remains a deadly threat in China and efforts continue to maintain cure rates as well as to expand DOTS coverage to the remaining population.

Controlling Chagas Disease in the Southern Cone of South America

Background

Chagas disease, or American trypanosomiasis, was Latin America's most serious parasitic infection in the early 1990s. Endemic in all seven countries of the southern cone, it caused an estimated 16 million to 18 million infections and 50,000 deaths each year. In Brazil alone, it was estimated that over a 2-year period the economic costs of the disease were almost $240 million and that $750 million would have been needed to treat its main health effects.[65]

The Intervention

The disease is named after Carlos Chagas, the Brazilian doctor who first described it in 1909 and subsequently discovered its cause: the parasite *Trypanosoma cruzi*. The parasites are found in the feces of "kissing bugs" that live within house walls in poor, rural areas and emerge at night to suck human blood. The parasites enter the bloodstream when insect bites are rubbed or scratched, or when food is contaminated. They can also enter via infected blood, or be transmitted from mother to fetus.

The first phase of the disease, the acute phase, is marked by fever, malaise, and swelling, and can sometimes be fatal, especially in young children. But most cases enter the second, chronic phase when the parasite damages vital body organs, resulting in heart failure, stomach pain, constipation, and swallowing difficulties that can lead to malnutrition.[66] A third of the cases are fatal.

In the absence of a vaccine or cure, control efforts needed to focus on eliminating the vector and screening the blood supply. Early attempts at control entailed methods such as dousing house walls with kerosene or scalding water, or enclosing and filling houses with cyanide gas.[67] The introduction of synthetic insecticides offered a more plausible solution, and spraying campaigns began in several countries in the 1950s and 1960s. Brazil launched a national eradication campaign in 1983, involving nationwide spraying and volunteer schemes. Brazil's early success demonstrated the technical feasibility of vector control. However, it also highlighted the need for regional efforts against border-crossing insects, and the need for sustained political commitment.[67]

In 1991 a new control program called INCOSUR (Southern Cone Initiative to Control/Eliminate Chagas) was launched to bolster national resolve and prevent cross-border reinfestations. Led by the Pan American Health Organization (PAHO), the initiative was jointly adopted by Argentina, Bolivia, Brazil, Chile, Paraguay, Uruguay, and later, Peru. The countries financed and managed their own programs but met annually to share operational aims, methods, and achievements. Intercountry technical cooperation agreements fostered the sharing of information among regional scientists and governments, with additional scientific support from a network of researchers in 22 countries. Between 1992 and 2001, more than 2.5 million homes were sprayed. Canisters that release insecticidal fumes when lit were also provided. Houses were improved to eliminate hiding places for insects, adobe walls were replaced with plaster, and metal roofs were constructed. The screening of blood donors for the parasite is now virtually universal in 10 South American countries.[68]

Impact

Incidence in the seven INCOSUR countries fell by an average of 94% by 2000. Overall, the number of new cases on the continent fell from 700,000 in 1983 to fewer than 200,000 in 2000.[69] The number of deaths each year from the disease was halved from 45,000 to 22,000. By 2001, disease transmission was halted in Uruguay, Chile, and large parts of Brazil and Paraguay. Surveys indicate an improved sense of well-being, domestic pride, and security. Central America and the Amazon region remain the next major challenges.

Costs and Benefits

Financial resources for INCOSUR, provided by each of the seven countries, have totaled more than $400 million since 1991. The intervention is considered among the most cost-effective interventions in public health, at just $37 per DALY saved in Brazil.[69]

Lessons Learned

Chris Schofield, a researcher at the London School of Hygiene and Tropical Medicine, attributes INCOSUR's success to three factors: it was big and designed to reach a definitive end point; it had a simple, well-proven technical approach; and, it gained political continuity from a close coordination between researchers and governments. Alfredo Solari, Uruguay's former minister of health, mentions four elements: peer pressure from neighboring countries in an exercise dealing with border-crossing insects; commitment by all participating countries, backed by international organizations like PAHO and WHO; an international technical secretariat at PAHO that verified surveillance, shared information about progress, processed certification requests and organized annual meetings; and, a favorable economic and institutional environment that allowed resources for expensive national health programs. Sustaining the achievements of INCOSUR will require vigilance, since premature curtailment of active surveillance against the disease could lead to disease resurgence.

Controlling Trachoma in Morocco

Background

Trachoma is the second leading cause of blindness, after cataract, and the number one cause of preventable blindness in the world. Although it has been eliminated in North America and Europe, trachoma still afflicts more than 150 million people in 46 countries, especially in hot, dry regions where access to clean water, sanitation, and health care is limited.[70] In Morocco, trachoma was once widespread, but in the 1970s and 1980s, treatment with antibiotics lowered its incidence in urban areas. A 1992 survey found that 5.4% of Moroccans still suffered from trachoma, mainly in five rural provinces in the southeast, where 25,000 people showed a serious decline in vision, 625,000 needed treatment for inflammatory trachoma, and 40,000 urgently required surgery.

The Intervention

Caused by the bacterium *Chlamydia trachomatis*, trachoma is highly contagious, spreading mainly among children through direct contact with eye and nose secretions, infected clothing, and fluid-seeking flies. Transmission of the disease is rapid in overcrowded conditions of poor hygiene and poverty. In endemic areas, prevalence rates in children aged 2 to 5 years can reach 90%.[71] Women are infected at a rate two to three times that for men because of their close contact with children. Repeated trachoma infections can lead to a painful in-turning of the eyelash which can cause blindness.

In 1991, Morocco formed the National Blindness Control Program (NBCP) with several international and other agencies to eliminate trachoma by 2005. Between 1997 and 1999, this program implemented a pilot strategy to treat trachoma, developed by the Edna McConnell Clark Foundation, called SAFE (surgery, antibiotics, face washing, and environmental change). SAFE differed from earlier approaches by emphasizing behavioral and environmental change, in addition to medication. Under this four-part strategy, a quick and inexpensive surgery to prevent blindness was provided for large numbers of patients in small towns and villages. Antibiotics were used to treat infection and prevent scarring. Face washing, especially among children, was promoted through an education campaign. Living conditions and community hygiene were improved by constructing latrines, drilling wells, storing dung away from flies, and providing health education.[72]

In the mid-1990s, Pfizer discovered Zithromax®, a one-dose cure to replace the six-week course of tetracycline that had been used for treatment, ensuring a higher compliance rate. Pfizer pharmaceutical company donated the drug for Morocco, as well as for other poor countries, through the International Trachoma Initiative (ITI), a private-public partnership that it forged along with the Clark Foundation.

Impact

Between 1999 and 2003, the SAFE strategy led to a 75% decline in trachoma in Morocco. Overall, the prevalence of active disease in children under 10 was reduced by 90% since 1997.[71]

Costs and Benefits

The Moroccan government provided most of the financing for the program. ITI supplemented this with several grants, while UNICEF contributed $225,000. Pfizer's donation of tens of millions of dollars worth of Zithromax® to Morocco and other countries represents one of the largest donations of a patented drug in history.

Lessons Learned

Government commitment to the program was critical to its success, in addition to the array of effective interventions. Four key factors were also listed by ITI: the program was based on solid scientific evidence; it was locally organized and therefore responded well to local circumstances; it fit within a broader agenda of health promotion, disease control, and health equity; and, treatment was closely linked with prevention and the development of a strong public health infrastructure. ITI and its many partners have helped ensure that Morocco's success with SAFE, like the disease that it has nearly eliminated, is contagious.

AVIAN INFLUENZA

Prevention and control of communicable diseases face a number of significant challenges. One of these challenges relates to the spread of existing communicable diseases to places that had previously not seen them. This has been the case, for example, in the last decade with the spread of the West Nile virus and dengue fever to and within some countries.

Another issue relates to the spread of resistant forms of disease. Comments were made earlier about strains of TB that have emerged in Southern Africa that appear to be resistant to most first- and second-line TB drugs and that have had unusually high case fatality rates. Will equally difficult strains of HIV emerge? There are a number of hospital-based infections that are very difficult to treat. Will they become more difficult to treat as they become increasingly resistant to the available antibiotics? Will the development of new antibiotics stay ahead of the development of new resistant forms of bacteria?

Finally, there is the possibility that new diseases will emerge that previously had been unknown, such as Legionnaire's disease, the Ebola virus, and Sudden Acute Respiratory Syndrome (SARS). New and emerging diseases are the subject of much discussion and study. Some comments will be offered here on only one disease, avian influenza, before returning to a discussion of the challenges faced in addressing HIV/AIDS, TB, malaria, diarrhea, and the neglected diseases.

One challenge of extreme importance is the risk of a major influenza pandemic and the influenza of greatest concern is avian flu. Most of those involved in global work on communicable diseases believe it is not a question of "if" there will be a major global outbreak of avian flu, but only a question of "when" it will occur and how severe it will be.

Avian influenza is caused by the H5N1 strain of the influenza virus. It is transmitted bird-to-bird mainly through fecal contact and from bird-to-human by aerosol transmission. H5N1 is a virus of birds and infects humans irregularly. However, when humans do become infected, severe disease develops. Coughing and fever are the symptoms of the disease in humans, and these symptoms can develop rapidly after initial infection. The development of an avian influenza pandemic among humans would require the emergence of a variant of the H5N1 virus that would be able to replicate in humans, cause serious disease in humans, and be efficiently transmitted from one human to another.

Human influenza pandemics have occurred in the past and will continue to occur in the future. There were three major influenza pandemics is the 20th century, the great Spanish flu of 1918–1919 that killed 40 to 50 million people, the Asian Flu of 1957, and the Hong Kong flu of 1968 that together killed an estimated 4.5 million people. In 1918, two epidemic "waves" occurred. The first wave was contagious, but not very deadly. The second wave spread rapidly as well, and took only 2 months to circle the globe, but had a 10 fold greater mortality. In 3 weeks, two million people died in Africa and an estimated 30% of the world's population fell ill, with most mortality occurring in the 15 to 35 year age group.

Although the 1918 pandemic was extraordinary, influenza continues to cause substantial mortality and morbidity annually. In the United States, in a typical influenza year, about 30 million people are infected and 50,000 are hospitalized with 20,000 to 40,000 deaths occurring, mostly in the elderly.[73] Worldwide, between 250,000 and 500,000 die annually from non-pandemic influenza. It is expected that deaths from a new influenza virus would dwarf those numbers. If 30% of the world were infected, with a case fatality rate of 5%, then about two billion people would be infected and potentially ill, with deaths approaching 100 million.[74]

In addition, this scenario would completely overwhelm health systems in most, if not all, countries. It would also cause incalculable economic loss due to absenteeism, medical expenses, business closings, and the disease control strategies that would keep people, workers, and students at home until transmission and risk of infection subsided. In the United States, the severe epidemic scenario implies 90 million will fall ill, 45 million will require outpatient care, 10 million will need hospitalization, and two million will die.[74]

The key to controlling the risk from a new virus is to prepare carefully for it, and that preparedness depends on four elements: accurate perception of risk, problem identification, rapid response to mitigate impacts, and sustained access to services for recovery. In addition, preparedness requires sound and executable plans, communication, surveillance and case detection, comprehensive situation analyses, and containment. Time is a limiting factor in preparedness and response because a pandemic virus could spread rapidly and overwhelm health systems within 40 days after its appearance. Global preparedness planning is now underway, under the auspices of the United Nations.

Developing a vaccine to address a virus that might cause a pandemic of avian influenza is also a challenging problem and there is a fear that a new avian influenza virus will spread before a vaccine for it could be developed, produced, and distributed. It usually takes 5 to 6 months for a new influenza vaccine to be developed, tested, produced, and distributed and a vaccine can not be produced until a new influenza virus emerges and is identified. In hopes of being more ready for avian influenza, vaccines based on existing strains of H5N1 are being developed collaboratively by governments and industries.

While vaccines are clearly part of the solution to an avian influenza pandemic, laboratory studies suggest some prescription antiviral medicines for human influenza should help to treat avian influenza.[75] With this in mind, governments are stockpiling medicines in order to deliver a comprehensive response to a pandemic if it should occur.

FUTURE CHALLENGES TO THE CONTROL OF COMMUNICABLE DISEASES

A number of challenges constrain efforts to address the burden of the most important communicable diseases. Some of these relate to the need for countries to cooperate to combat communicable diseases. Some concern the ability of weak health systems in low- and middle-income countries to tackle communicable disease problems effectively. Others relate to the issues raised by specific diseases.

First, it is imperative to enhance political commitment to the prevention and control of these diseases. You read earlier that sustained political support at the highest levels is essential if progress is to be made against HIV/AIDS, and this is also true for the other leading causes of communicable disease. Countries will only be successful in acting against these diseases if they make them a real priority both politically and financially.

Second, the underlying causes of communicable diseases in low- and middle-income countries relate to poverty, people's lack of empowerment, people's lack of knowledge of appropriate health behaviors, and a lack of access to basic infrastructure such as safe water, sanitation, and health services. These issues will take many years to address in most low-income countries. Thus, in the short- and medium-run, success against some communicable diseases will depend on community-based efforts.

It is likely that health systems in many low- and middle-income countries will continue to be weak for many years, as well. This suggests that efforts to address communicable diseases will also have to be based on partnership with a variety of actors. This includes communities, religious groups and other non-governmental organizations, the private sector, and government. The great successes in the control of infectious diseases to date have all been built on the foundation of public-private partnerships. The polio eradication effort includes, for example, a remarkable amount of public-private collaboration, as does, for example, the campaign against onchocerciasis. It is especially important that these actors work together in the future across an array of diseases and health systems issues and not just on individual diseases.

Strengthening the surveillance of disease at the local, national, and global levels is also fundamental to effective disease control. A competent body of public health professionals need to be responsible for managing surveillance networks. Appropriate laboratory infrastructures must be an essential part of any improved surveillance efforts. Continuous sharing of surveillance information within and across countries is necessary to prepare for special problems, to know when they arise, and to respond to them effectively.

The lack of adequately trained and appropriately deployed human resources for health will also remain an issue, especially in lower-income countries. There will not be enough personnel, the incentives for their performance will be lacking, and the personnel that do exist will largely be available only in the larger cities. Thus, it will be important to have the lowest level of worker possible handle various health services so that scarce higher-level workers can focus on those things they alone can do. In addition, many services can be devolved to community-based workers. This will be an important point, for example, in countries with high HIV/AIDS prevalence but few trained doctors and nurses, as they spread AIDS treatment beyond the largest cities.

Another important issue will be the balance that needs to be struck between prevention and treatment. This will be especially challenging in the field of HIV/AIDS. There is considerable commitment in the world today to ensuring that all people needing treatment with antiretroviral therapy get it as soon as possible. There are many reasons why this is important. However, it is unlikely to stop transmission because people are most infective early in the disease and usually infect others before they know they have it. Prevention must remain at the core of efforts to address HIV/AIDS.

The challenge of financing enhanced efforts in the control of communicable diseases will also be formidable. Without major changes in their spending patterns and rapid economic growth, many low- and middle-income countries will not be able to pay for the stepped up efforts they need to combat the major communicable diseases. Rather, they will have to depend for some time on financial assistance from the developed countries and private sector partners.

Scientific and technical challenges also remain. There is no effective vaccine for any of the diseases that have been the focus of this chapter, except for rotavirus for some forms of diarrhea. Drug resistance is a constant issue in HIV, a threat in the control of diarrhea and some parasitic infections, and a major issue in the control of TB and malaria. It will be imperative that new drugs are developed that can prevent or overcome such resistance. In HIV, it will be important to continue to have new drugs that are easier to take, easier to transport and store, have fewer side effects, and are less likely to allow resistance to emerge than the present drugs.

Another challenge will be the need to develop models in low- and middle-income countries to provide chronic care of people with HIV. Most health service efforts in low-income countries focus on acute care. The treatment of HIV with antiretroviral therapy creates the possibility that people who are HIV-positive can have full and productive lives for many years. However, it also means that countries with very weak health systems that are mostly accustomed to treating acute illnesses will have to develop effective and efficient models for treating some people for many years of their life.

Another important issue is how low-income and resource-poor countries will be able to financially sustain the progress that they do make in AIDS treatment and several other areas related to the prevention and control of communicable diseases. Successful efforts to prevent and control these diseases will reduce prevalence and, ultimately, reduce the demands on the health system. As the prevalence of hookworm declines, for example, countries will be able to spend less money for hookworm treatment programs. However, the demands on health systems for treatment for HIV/AIDS will continue to be great for many years to come. Low- and middle-income countries with high HIV/AIDS prevalence will have to plan carefully how AIDS treatment can be financed in the future. This is especially important because once people start taking antiretroviral therapy, it is imperative that they continue to take it.

Monitoring and evaluation is an essential tool of public health programming. If the world is to make progress against the most important communicable diseases and continue to learn what is most cost-effective in addressing these diseases, then it is important to enhance the quality of monitoring and evaluation of health investments. All activities require a monitoring and evaluation component to track project progress, estimate cost-effectiveness of the effort, and assess the impact of the activities that are being financed.

MAIN MESSAGES

Communicable diseases account for about 44% of total deaths and 40% of DALYs in low- and middle-income countries. Among the communicable diseases, HIV/AIDS and malaria take an enormous toll on Sub-Saharan Africa. The neglected diseases are also a relatively more important burden of disease in Sub-Saharan Africa than in any other region. The toll from communicable diseases is similar for men and women, but the AIDS epidemic is taking an increasing toll on women, and TB generally affects men more than women.

HIV is an especially important burden. About 40 million people are now infected with HIV; in 2005 about 2.3 million people died from the disease, and another 4.3 million were infected with it that same year. Besides concerns for the African region, there are major concerns that the epidemic will grow in India, China, and the former Soviet Union.

The AIDS epidemic is helping to fuel TB. About one third of the world is infected with TB and there are about nine million people in the world with active TB disease. Both HIV/AIDS and TB mostly affect people in their productive years.

Malaria kills more than one million people a year, mostly young children in Africa. It also causes a huge burden of morbidity because cases of malaria are so common and people may get more than one case a year. Malaria also poses very substantial risks to pregnant women. Diarrhea is an especially important burden of disease for children, as well, and is also responsible for about 1.8 million child deaths a year. A number of parasitic and infectious diseases are often called the neglected diseases and they pose an exceptional burden of disease, again largely in Sub-Saharan Africa and South Asia. The worm *Ascaris*, for example, infects more than one billion people worldwide. Trichuris and hookworm infect 800 million and 740 million, respectively.

The economic and social consequences of the communicable diseases are very considerable. Diarrhea and worms can cause children to fail to develop properly, delay their entry into and performance in school, and lessen their productivity as adults. HIV/AIDS, TB, and malaria also greatly affect adult productivity. The direct and indirect costs of these diseases to individuals and families are very high and often cause people to borrow money, sell their limited assets, and fall below the poverty line. There is good evidence that high levels of malaria are an important impediment to economic growth in low-income countries in Africa.

Addressing HIV/AIDS will require redoubled efforts on prevention and continued efforts to learn what can prevent transmission in the most cost-effective ways. There is an increasing understanding that strong political leadership, focusing on the groups most at risk, and addressing the needs of "bridge populations" are parts of successful prevention efforts. Other key parts of prevention are maintaining a clean blood supply, testing and counseling, and condom promotion, in connection with efforts to delay sexual debut and reduce the number of sexual partners. It is also important to stem the transmission of HIV from mother to child. There are an increasing number of people on treatment for HIV worldwide, and efforts are underway to ensure that all people who need treatment get it, although meeting this goal will be very challenging in low-income countries.

Although TB incidence and the presentation of TB are being dramatically affected by HIV, the mainstay of efforts to address TB has been DOTS, which stands for Directly Observed Therapy, Short-Course. This is a very cost-effective way of treating TB. Malaria can be addressed through prompt diagnosis and treatment, intermittent treatment of pregnant women, the use of insecticide-treated bed nets, and indoor residual spraying. Proper treatment to avoid the development of resistance is central to efforts in TB, HIV/AIDS, and malaria.

The burden of diarrhea can be reduced through immunization against rotavirus and measles and supplementation with zinc. Oral rehydration therapy is a cost-effective way of managing diarrhea in infants and children. The best approach to diarrhea, of course, would be to try to avoid it through improved hygiene. Better access to safe water and sanitation will help to reduce the burden of some of the parasitic and bacterial infections that make up the neglected diseases. In the short-run, however, there is a package of drug therapy that can be integrated with other disease control efforts to reduce the burden of the neglected diseases in a cost-effective way.

The challenge of addressing the burden of communicable diseases effectively is enormous. They are mostly diseases of poverty that also reflect a lack of access to safe water and sanitation, poor knowledge of appropriate health behaviors, and a lack of health services that are geared to meet the highest priority needs. In addition, several of these diseases are highly stigmatized, efforts to control them must be carried out in countries with weak health systems, and considerably more financing is needed for these efforts than has been available. Nonetheless, there has been major progress in the last 40 years in addressing smallpox, onchocerciasis, and a number of vaccine-preventable diseases in children. The lessons from those experiences suggest that it is possible through concerted efforts and partnerships and greatly enhanced disease surveillance efforts to continue making such progress.

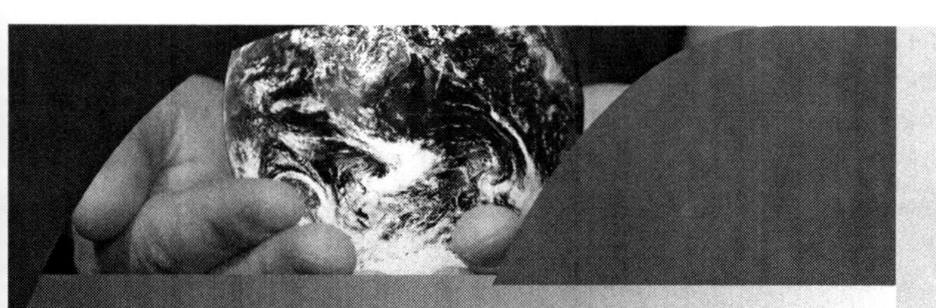

Discussion Questions

1. What are the most important infectious diseases in terms of deaths in low- and middle-income countries? In terms of DALYs?
2. In what regions will the deaths from HIV/AIDS be most important? In what regions will malaria be most important?
3. What is driving the HIV epidemic in Russia? In Sub-Saharan Africa?
4. In Sub-Saharan Africa, what would be the most cost-effective measures to try to prevent further transmission of the HIV virus? What approach would you take to prevention in South Asia, and why would it differ from what you would do in Sub-Saharan Africa?
5. What groups are especially at risk for malaria? What steps would you take to try to reduce the burden of malaria?
6. What is DOTS? What are the key focuses of this approach? Why has it been more effective than previous approaches to TB control?
7. If relatively few people die as a direct result of parasitic diseases, why are they so important?
8. What are the concerns about drug resistance for malaria and TB? How can resistance be kept to a minimum?
9. Why is it important to develop a vaccine for HIV?
10. What risks would the world face in a pandemic of avian influenza, and how can the world prepare for it?

REFERENCES

1. Lopez AD, Mathers CD, Ezzati M, Jamison DT, Murray CJL. Measuring the global burden of disease and risk factors, 1990-2001. In: Lopez AD, Mathers CD, Ezzati M, Jamison DT, Murray CJL, eds. *Global Burden of Disease and Risk Factors*. New York: Oxford University Press; 2006:8.

2. Bertozzi S, Padian NS, Wegbreit J, et al. HIV/AIDS Prevention and Treatment. In: Jamison DT, Breman JG, Measham AR, et al., eds. *Disease Control Priorities in Developing Countries*. 2nd ed. New York: Oxford University Press; 2006:331–370.

3. Chin J, ed. *Control of Communicable Diseases Manual.* 17th ed. Washington, DC: American Public Health Association; 2000.

4. Bertozzi S, Padian NS, Wegbreit J, et al. HIV/AIDS Prevention and treatment. In: Jamison DT, Breman JG, Measham AR, et al., eds. *Disease Control Priorities in Developing Countries*. 2nd ed. New York: Oxford University Press; 2006:353.

5. UNAIDS. 2006 Report on the Global AIDS Epidemic Available at: http://www.unaids.org/en/HIV_data/2006GlobalReport/default.asp. Accessed November 15, 2006.

6. World Health Organization. Fact Sheet No. 104: Tuberculosis. Available at: http://www.who.int/mediacentre/factsheets/fs104/en/. Accessed November 20, 2006.

7. Stop TB. Fact Sheet—Socioeconomic Impact of TB—Impact of TB on Women and Families. www.stoptb.org/stop_tb_initiative/amsterdam_conference_documents/pfs-imp. Accessed November 15, 2006.

8. Stop TB. TB—A Leading Killer of Women. Available at: http://www.searo.who.int/LinkFiles/Tuberculosis_right5.pdf. Accessed November 15, 2006.

9. Centers for Disease Control and Prevention. Extensively Drug-Resistant Tuberculosis (XDR TB)—Update. Available at: http://www.cdc.gov/nchstp/tb/xdrtbupdate.htm. Accessed November 19, 2006.

10. Lopez AD, Mathers CD, Murray CJL. The burden of disease and mortality by condition: data, methods, and results for 2001. In: Lopez AD, Mathers CD, Ezzati M, Jamison DT, Murray CJL, eds. *Global Burden of Disease and Risk Factors*. New York: Oxford University Press; 2006:70.

11. Breman JG, Mills A, Snow RW, Mulligan J-A. Conquering malaria. In: Jamison DT, Breman JG, Measham AM, Alleyne G, eds. *Disease Control Priorities in Developing Countries*. 2nd ed. New York: Oxford University Press; 2006:413–432.

12. Keusch GT, Fontaine O, Bhargava A, Boschi-Pinto C. Diarrheal Diseases. In: Jamison DT, Breman JG, Measham AM, Alleyne G, eds. *Disease Control Priorities in Developing Countries*. 2nd ed. New York: Oxford University Press; 2006:371–388.

13. Parashar UD. Global illness and deaths caused by rotavirus disease in children. *Emer Infect Dis*. 2003;9(5):565–572.

14. Hotez P, Molyneux DH, Fenwick A, Ottesen E., Sachs SE, Sachs JD. Incorporating a rapid-impact package for neglected tropical diseases with programs for HIV/AIDS, tuberculosis and malaria. *PLos Medicine*. 2006;3(5):576–584.

15. Hotez PJ, Bundy DAP, Beegle K, et al. Helminth infections: soil-transmitted helminth infections and schistosomiasis. In: Jamison DT, Breman JG, Measham AR, et al., eds. *Disease Control Priorities in Developing Countries*. 2nd ed. New York: Oxford University Press; 2006:467–482.

16. Chin J, ed. *Control of Communicable Diseases (Manual)*. 17th ed. Washington, DC: American Public Health Association; 2000.

17. Chin J, ed. *Control Of Communicable Diseases (Manual)*. 17th ed. Washington, DC: American Public Health Association; 2000.

18. Russell S. The economic burden of illness for households in developing countries: a review of studies focusing on malaria, tuberculosis, and human immunodeficiency virus/acquired immunodeficiency syndrome. *Am J Trop Med Hyg*. 2004;71(2 Suppl):147–155.

19. Brown LR. The potential impact of AIDS on population and economic growth rates. Available at: http://ideas.repec.org/p/fpr/2020br/43.html. Accessed November 22, 2006.

20. Ainsworth M, Over M. AIDS and African Development. *The World Bank Research Observer*. 1994:9(2)203–240.

21. Chand N, Singh T, Khalsa JS, Verma V, Rathore JS. A study of socio-economic impact of tuberculosis on patients and their family. *CHEST*. 2004:126(4)832S.

22. Croft RA, Croft RP. Expenditure and loss of income incurred by tuberculosis patients before reaching effective treatment in Bangladesh. *Int J Tuberc Lung Dis*. 1998;2(3):252–254.

23. Kamolratanakul P, Sawert H, Kongsin S, et al. Economic impact of tuberculosis at the household level. *Int J Tuberc Lung Dis*. 1999;3(7):596–602.

24. Rajeswari R, Balasubramanian R, Muniyandi M, Geetharamani S, Thresa X, Venkatesan P. Socio-economic impact of tuberculosis on patients and family in India. *Int J Tuberc Lung Dis*. 1999;3(10):869–877.

25. Grimard F, Harling G. The Impact of Tuberculosis on Economic Growth. Available at: http://neumann.hec.ca/neudc2004/fp/grimard_franque_aout_27.pdf. *World Bank Res Observer*. Accessed November 22, 2006.

26. Peabody JW, Shimkhada R, Tan C, Jr., Luck J. The burden of disease, economic costs and clinical consequences of tuberculosis in the Philippines. *Health Policy Plan*. 2005;20(6):347–353.

27. Lynch M. Malaria Presentation. 2005.

28. Roll Back Malaria Partnership. Economic Costs of Malaria. Washington: USAID; Available at: http://www.rbm.who.int/cmc_upload/0/000/015/363/RBMInfosheet_10.htm. Accessed November 22, 2006.

29. Gallup JL, Sachs JD. The economic burden of malaria. *Am J Trop Med Hyg*. 2001;64(1-2 Suppl):85–96.

30. Sachs JD, Hotez PJ. Fighting tropical diseases. *Science*. 2006;311(5,767):1521.

31. Miguel EA, Kremer M. Worms: identifying impacts on education and health in the presence of treatment externalities. *Econometrica*. 2003;71(1):159–217.

32. Bleakley H. Disease and development: evidence from hookworm eradication in the American South. *Eur Econ Assoc*. 2003;1(2–3):376–386.

33. Bertozzi S, Padian NS, Wegbreit J, et al. HIV/AIDS Prevention and treatment. In: Jamison DT, Breman JG, Measham AR, et al., eds. *Disease Control Priorities in Developing Countries*. 2nd ed. New York: Oxford University Press; 2006:332.

34. Bertozzi S, Padian NS, Wegbreit J, et al. HIV/AIDS Prevention and treatment. In: Jamison DT, Breman JG, Measham AR, et al., eds. *Disease Control Priorities in Developing Countries*. 2nd ed. New York: Oxford University Press; 2006:331–170.

35. Bertozzi S, Padian NS, Wegbreit J, et al. HIV/AIDS Prevention and treatment. In: Jamison DT, Breman JG, Measham AR, et al., eds. *Disease Control Priorities in Developing Countries*. 2nd ed. New York: Oxford University Press; 2006:345–346.

36. Bertozzi S, Padian NS, Wegbreit J, et al. HIV/AIDS Prevention and treatment. In: Jamison DT, Breman JG, Measham AR, et al., eds. *Disease Control Priorities in Developing Countries*. 2nd ed. New York: Oxford University Press; 2006:345.

37. Centers for Disease Control and Prevention. Male Circumcision and Risk for HIV Transmission: Implications for the United States. Available at: http://www.cdc.gov/hiv/resources/factsheets/circumcision.htm. Accessed March 6, 2007.

38. Bertozzi S, Padian NS, Wegbreit J, et al. HIV/AIDS Prevention and treatment. In: Jamison DT, Breman JG, Measham AR, et al., eds. *Disease Control Priorities in Developing Countries*. 2nd ed. New York: Oxford University Press; 2006:344–346.

39. Bertozzi S, Padian NS, Wegbreit J, et al. HIV/AIDS Prevention and treatment. In: Jamison DT, Breman JG, Measham AR, et al., eds. *Disease Control Priorities in Developing Countries*. 2nd ed. New York: Oxford University Press; 2006:351–353.

40. Bertozzi S, Padian NS, Wegbreit J, et al. HIV/AIDS Prevention and treatment. In: Jamison DT, Breman JG, Measham AR, et al., eds. *Disease Control Priorities in Developing Countries.* 2nd ed. New York: Oxford University Press; 2006:355.

41. Dye C, Floyd K. Tuberculosis. In: Jamison DT, Breman JG, Measham AR, et al., eds. *Disease Control Priorities in Developing Countries.* 2nd ed. New York: Oxford University Press; 2006:289–312.

42. The Abuja Declaration and the Plan of Action. Available at: http://www.rbm.who.int/docs/abuja_declaration_final.htm. Accessed November 15, 2006.

43. Centers for Disease Control and Prevention. Rotavirus. Available at: http://www.cdc.gov/ncidod/dvrd/revb/gastro/rotavirus.htm. Accessed October 15, 2006.

44. Huttly SR, Morris SS, Pisani V. Prevention of diarrhoea in young children in developing countries. *Bulletin of the World Health Organization.* 1997;(75):163–174.

45. Black RE. Zinc deficiency, infectious disease, and mortality in the developing world. *J Nutr.* 2003;133 (5 Suppl 1):1485S–1489S.

46. Levine R. *Millions Saved.* Washington, DC: Center for Global Development; 2004.

47. UNAIDS. *AIDS Epidemic Update (December).* Geneva: UNAIDS; 2002.

48. U.S. Centers for Disease Control and Prevention. Global AIDS Program, Country Profiles: Thailand. www.cdc.gov/nchsp/od/gap/countries/thailand.htm. Accessed February 6, 2004.

49. UNAIDS. *Evaluation of the 100% Condom Programme in Thailand.* Geneva: UNAIDS, in collaboration with the Ministry of Public Health, Thailand; 2000. Document 00.18E.

50. Rojanapithayakorn W, Hanenberg R. The 100% Condom Programme in Thailand. *AIDS.* 1996;10(1):1–7.

51. Celentano D, Nelson K, Lyles C, et al. Decreasing incidence of HIV and sexually transmited diseases among young Thai men: evidence for success of the HIV/AIDS control and prevention program. *AIDS.* 1998;12(5): F29-F36.

52. Chitwarkorn A. HIV/AIDS and sexually transmitted infections in thailand: lessons learned and future challenges. In: Narain JP, ed. *AIDS in Asia: The Challenge Continues.* New Delhi: Sage Publications; 2004.

53. UNAIDS. *Report on the Global AIDS Epidemic.* Geneva: UNAIDS; 2004.

54. China Tuberculosis Control Collaboration. Results of directly observed short-course chemotherapy in 112,842 Chinese patients with smear-positive tuberculosis. *Lancet.* 1996;347:358–362.

55. World Health Organization Regional Office for the Western Pacific. *DOTS for All: Country Reports.* Geneva: World Health Organization; 2002.

56. Zhao F, Zhao Y, Liu X. Tuberculosis control in China. *Tuberculosis.* 2003;85:15–20.

57. The World Bank. *Implementation Completion Report for the China Infectious Diseases Control Project.* Washington, DC: The World Bank; 2002.

58. Chen X, Zhao F, Duanmu H, Wan L, Wang X, Chin DP. The DOTS strategy in China: results and lessons after 10 years. *Bulletin of the World Health Organization.* 2002;80(6):430–436.

59. Musgrove P. Is the eradication of polio in the western hemisphere economically justified? *Bulletin of the Pan American Sanitary Bureau.* 1988;22(1):1–16

60. Henderson DA, de Quadros CA, Andrus J, Olive J-M, Guerra de Macedo C. Polio eradication from the western hemisphere. *Ann Rev Public Health.* 1992;13:239–252.

61. de Cuadros CA. Polio. *Encyclopedia of Microbiology 3.* 2000:762–772.

62. Gawande A. The Mop-Up: Eradicating Polio from the Planet. *The New Yorker.* January 12, 2004:34–40.

63. Jamison DT, Torres AM, Chen LC, Melnick JL. Poliomyelitis. In: Jamison DT, Mosley H, Measham A, Bobadilla JL, eds. *Disease Control Priorities in Developing Countries.* Oxford: Oxford Univesity Press; 1993.

64. Global Polio Eradication Initiative. Afghanistan, Egypt, India, Niger, Nigeria, and Pakistan, Progress Report. www.polioeradication.org/content/publication/2003-progress.pdf. Accessed August 10, 2004.

65. World Health Organization. *Control of Chagas Disease. Report of a WHO Expert Committee. WHO Technical Report Series: 811.* Geneva: World Health Organization; 1991.

66. U.S. Centers for Disease Control and Prevention. Fact Sheet: Chagas Disease. Available at: http://www.cdc.gov/ncidod/dpd/parasites/chagasdisease/factsht_chagas_disease.htm. Accessed July 29, 2003.

67. Dias JCP, Silveira AC, Schofield CJ. The impact of Chagas disease control in Latin America—a review. *Memorias do Instituto Oswaldo Cruz.* 2002;97:603–612.

68. Schmunis GA, Zicker F, Cruz J, Cuchi P. Safety of blood supply for infectious diseases in Latin American countries, 1994–1997. *Am J Trop Med Hygiene.* 2001;65:924–930.

69. Moncayo A. Chagas disease: current epidemiological trends after interruption of vectorial and transfusional transmission in the southern cone countries. *Memorias do Instituto Oswaldo Cruz.* 2003;98(5):577–591.

70. Kumaresan J, Mecaskey J. The global elimination of blinding trachoma: progress and promise. *Am J Trop Med Hygiene.* 2003;69(Supplement 5):S24-S28.

71. Mecaskey J, Knirsch C, Kumaresan J, Cook J. The possibility of eliminating blinding trachoma. *Lancet.* 2003;3:728–734.

72. West S. Blinding trachoma: prevention with the SAFE strategy. *Am J Trop Med Hygiene.* 2003;69(Supplement 5):S18-S23.

73. Centers for Disease Control and Prevention. Key Facts about Influenza and the Influenza Vaccine. Available at: http://www.cdc.gov/flu/keyfacts.htm. Accessed November 15, 2006

74. United States Government. Pandemic Planning Assmptions. Available at: http://www.pandemicflu.gov/plan/pandplan.html. Accessed November 15, 2006.

75. United States Government. Pandemic Flu—General Information. Available at: http://www.pandemicflu.gov/general/. Accessed November 15, 2006.

CHAPTER 9

The Environment and Health

Learning Objectives

By the end of this chapter the reader will be able to:

- Discuss the most important environmental threats to health in low- and middle-income countries
- Review the burden of disease from indoor and outdoor air pollution and unsafe water and sanitation
- Examine the contribution of personal hygiene to reducing the burden of environmentally-related health problems
- Comment on the costs and consequences of these environmental burdens
- Describe some of the most cost-effective ways of reducing the global burden of environmental health problems

VIGNETTES

Rashmi lived in the eastern part of Nepal in a modest home. Rashmi often had difficulty breathing. This was linked to the way Rashmi cooked, with a stove inside the house that was not vented outside. She used cow dung or wood as fuel. She cooked two meals a day on the stove and she often held her new baby on her back as she did so. She heard about different stoves and about using kerosene for fuel. However, she lacked the money to buy a new stove or to fuel it with kerosene.

Sunisa was a young mother in a rural area in northern Laos. She had two children, a 1 year old and a 3 year old. Sunisa was not wealthy. Her house was simple and had no water supply. She collected water daily from the stream about half a mile from her house in containers she carried on her head. She stored the containers at the edge of her house, covered by cloth. Sunisa was not an educated woman and did nothing to purify the water. Her two daughters regularly had bouts of diarrhea, partly the result of drinking unsafe water.

Juan had lived in Mexico City his whole life and was now 70 years old. He remembered a time when the city was not so crowded, had few cars, and when the views from the city were magnificent. He lamented the fact that today the city was too crowded to enjoy, the traffic was overwhelming, and the air was often unbreathable. It was so polluted that on many days there was no view at all. Juan had a very hard time breathing, as he suffered from chronic obstructive pulmonary disease (COPD). Juan suspected that air pollution contributed to his illness.

Raj and his family lived in a slum at the edge of Patna, India. The slum was the size of a small city. Most of the houses were made of scrap wood with scrap metal roofing. The houses had no water connection and people had to walk to the edge of the slum to get their water from a standpipe or to buy it from a tanker if the standpipe did not work. There were no private toilets either. There were a few communal toilets that were shared but they were always dirty. For this reason, many people in the slum, especially the women, waited until dark and then went to defecate in fields near the slum.

THE IMPORTANCE OF ENVIRONMENTAL HEALTH

Environmental health issues are major risk factors in the global burden of disease. Using a somewhat narrow definition of what is an "environmental" cause of disease, a recent study of the global burden of disease[1] suggests that about 8.4% of the total burden of disease in low- and middle-income countries is the result of three environmental conditions: unsafe water, hygiene, and excreta disposal; urban air pollution; and indoor smoke from household use of solid fuels. Another study, which took a broader view of "environmental" risk factors, concluded that between 25–33% of the global burden of disease can be attributed to environmental risk factors.[2]

The importance of environmental risk factors to the global burden of disease should not be a surprise. The third leading cause of death in low- and middle-income countries is lower respiratory infections, the sixth is chronic obstructive pulmonary disease, and the seventh is diarrheal disease. As you know, each of these is closely linked with environmental factors. In addition, environmental risk factors are even more important when considering the causes of death of children 0 to 14 years of age in low- and middle-income countries. Lower respiratory conditions are the second leading cause of death for them and diarrheal diseases third. Together, they account for about 30% of all deaths in this age group.

Environmental health matters are also of special importance because addressing them effectively is central to the achievement of the MDGs, as shown in Table 9-1.

TABLE 9-1 Environmental Health and the MDGs

Goal 1—Eradicate Poverty and Hunger
Link—Reducing environmental risk factors is central to eradicating poverty by reducing the burden, which falls largely on the poor, of environmentally-related morbidity and mortality.

Goal 2—Achieve Universal Primary Education
Link—Children that do not have access to clean water and sanitation are more likely to suffer from undernutrition due to a vicious cycle of diarrheal disease and malnutrition. There is a correlation between nutritional status and learning. Children with poor nutritional status are not as likely to stay in school or learn as much as healthy children.

Goal 3—Promote Gender Equality and Empower Women
Link—Improving access to water can improve the lives of poor women in the developing world by reducing the amount of time required to get water. Reducing indoor air pollution can also substantially improve the lives of women since they suffer a disproportionate burden when they are cooking.

Goal 4—Reduce Child Mortality
Link—Addressing environmental risk factors can reduce the two leading causes of death in children—diarrheal diseases and pneumonia. Diarrheal disease is reduced through improved access to clean water and sanitation. Pneumonia can be reduced through improvements in indoor air quality.

Goal 5—Improve Maternal Health
Link—Diarrheal disease associated with poor sanitation and unsafe water can harm the nutritional status of the mother.

Goal 6—Combat HIV/AIDS, malaria, and other diseases
Link—Environmental improvements can reduce the breeding grounds for malarial mosquitoes and vectors of some other disease, such as schistosomiasis and dengue fever.

Goal 7—Ensure environmental sustainability
Link—Measures to improve water supply, sanitation, and personal hygiene promote sustainability, especially when they are carried out in community-based ways.

Source: Author commentary on the UN Millennium Goals. Available at: http://www.un.org/millenniumgoals/ goals. Accessed July 11, 2006.

As you can see in the table, reducing environmental risk factors is critical to meeting the poverty and hunger goal, given the large share of ill health and resulting economic losses from these risk factors. Improving access to water can be a major improvement to the lives of poor women in the developing world, given the amount of time they have to spend getting water. Enhancing sanitation produces important social gains for women, as well, because in the absence of improved sanitation, they face major discomforts, inconveniences, and sometimes illness. Addressing environmental risk factors can clearly make a major contribution to reducing child mortality by reducing two of the leading causes of death in children. As you will read about later, reducing indoor air pollution can also lead to major improvements in the health of women and children. Finally, environmental improvements can reduce the breeding grounds for malarial mosquitoes, and many measures that reduce the health risks of the environment will increase environmental sustainability.

This chapter aims to introduce you to some of the most important links between health and the environment. Environmental health is a very broad topic. Given the introductory nature of this book, this chapter will focus largely on only three of the most important risk factors in terms of the burden of environmentally-related diseases in low- and middle-income countries. Following the recent burden of disease study, these will include unsafe water, sanitation, and hygiene; outdoor air pollution; and indoor air pollution that comes from the use of solid fuels.[3] These factors are also the focus of attention of this chapter because the risk factors that will be examined take a disproportionate toll on the health of low-income people in the developing world and the enhancement of their health status will require important gains in environmental health.

The chapter begins by covering some of the most important terms and concepts that relate to environmental health. It then explores the burden of disease related to the three risk factors noted previously. After that, it briefly reviews the costs and consequences of the selected environmental risk factors. The chapter concludes by discussing some of the most cost-effective ways to address these risk factors in low- and middle-income settings. Much has been written about environmental health. Those readers who wish to explore environmental health in greater detail are encouraged to pursue some of those writings. They might wish to begin with an introductory text on environmental health.[4,5]

KEY CONCEPTS

It is important to understand how the word "environment" will be used in this chapter. In some cases, the word environment in a health context is defined very broadly, meaning everything that is not genetic. In other cases, when considering health, the word environment includes only physical, chemical, or biological agents that directly affect health. For the purposes of this chapter, the environment will largely be defined as "external physical, chemical, and microbiological exposures and processes that impinge upon individuals and groups and are beyond the immediate control of individuals."[6] The chapter, however, also looks at some behavioral matters related to water and sanitation and indoor air pollution.

It is also valuable to understand the meaning of "environmental health." This generally refers to a set of public health efforts that "is concerned with preventing disease, death, and disability by reducing exposure to adverse environmental conditions and promoting behavior change. It focuses on the direct and indirect cases of disease and injuries and taps resources inside and outside the healthcare system to help improve health outcomes."[7]

The World Health Organization takes a broad view of the environment and says,

> Environmental health comprises those aspects of human health, including quality of life, that are determined by physical, chemical, biological, social, and psychosocial factors in the environment. It also refers to the theory and practice of assessing, correcting, controlling, and preventing those factors in the environment that can potentially affect adversely the health of present and future generations.[8]

Table 9-2 highlights some examples of environmental health issues, their determinants, and their consequences. It organizes these examples by their level of impact: the household, the community, the region, or global.

TABLE 9-2 Typical Environmental Health Issues: Determinants and Health Consequences

Underlying Determinants	Selected Adverse Health Consequences
Household	
Unsafe water, inadequate sanitation and solid waste disposal, improper hygiene	Diarrhea, and vector-related diseases, such as malaria, schistosomiasis, and dengue
Crowded housing and poor ventilation of smoke	Respiratory diseases and lung cancer
Exposure to naturally occurring toxic substances	Poisoning from arsenic, manganese, and fluorides
Community	
Improper water resource management, including poor drainage	Vector-related diseases, such as malaria and schistosomiasis
Exposure to vehicle emissions and industrial air pollution	Respiratory diseases, some cancers, and reduced IQ in children
Global	
Climate change	Injury/death from extreme heat/cold, storms, floods, and fires Indirect effects: spread of vector-borne diseases
Ozone depletion	Aggravation of respiratory diseases, population dislocation, water pollution from sea level rise, etc. Skin cancer, cataracts Indirect effects: compromised food production, etc.

Source: Adapted with permission from The World Bank. Environmental Health. Available at: http://web.worldbank.org/WBSITE/EXTERNAL/TOPICS/EXTHEALTHNUTRITIONANDPOPULATION/EXTPHAAG/0,,contentMDK:20656146~menuPK:2175463~pagePK:64229817~piPK:64229743~theSitePK:672263,00.html. Accessed October 27, 2006.

KEY ENVIRONMENTAL HEALTH BURDENS

The next section very briefly examines the most important health conditions that relate to the environmental issues that are discussed in this chapter. The section after that will examine the burden of disease from those conditions.

Indoor Air Pollution

WHO estimates that about half of all of the people in the world depend on solid fuel for their cooking and heating. The indoor air pollution that is discussed here is related to these uses. Such fuels include the fossil fuel coal, and the biomass fuels of cow dung, wood, logging wastes, and crop waste.[9,10] In the cases that most concern us, cooking and heating are done on open stoves that are not vented to the outside. These are generally used by poorer segments of society, as people usually move to kerosene or gas for cooking and switch to improved stoves as their family income grows.

Biomass fuels and coal do not completely combust when they are burned. Instead, they leave behind breathable particles of a variety of gases and chemical products. The amount of these substances in a poorly ventilated home can exceed WHO norms by more than 20 times.[10] Smoke from burning biomass inside the home can produce conjunctivitis, upper respiratory irritation, and acute respiratory infection. The carbon monoxide produced can lead to acute poisoning. Other gases and smoke are associated over the long term with cardiovascular disease, chronic obstructive pulmonary disease, adverse reproductive outcomes, and cancer.[11] As discussed further later, women and children are especially vulnerable to the effects of indoor air pollution.

Outdoor Air Pollution

Many pollutants can be found in the urban air. The most common effects of outdoor air pollution are respiratory symptoms, including cough, irritation of the nose and throat, and shortness of breath.[12] Table 9-3 indicates some of the most common pollutants in the outdoor air, examples of their sources, and the most important health effects. Some preexisting health factors make some people susceptible to being harmed by air pollution. Older and younger people are generally most susceptible to the health effects of outdoor air pollution.

There have been a number of instances in which severe air pollution has been associated with considerable excess mortality in a very short time. Among the most famous cases was in London, England, in 1952. Because of what is called a temperature inversion, a dense fog, full of pollutants, hung over the city center for several days. The value of certain particulates in the air was 3 to 10 times the normal value. On December 13, 1952, the city administration reported a death rate per 100,000 people that was more than four times the normal daily death rate for that period.[13]

TABLE 9-3 Selected Urban Air Pollutants

Name of Pollutant	Example of Source	Health Effects
Carbon monoxide (**criteria pollutant**)	Combustion of gasoline and fossil fuels; cars	Reduction in oxygen-carrying capacity of the blood
Lead (**criteria pollutant**)	Leaded gasoline, paint, batteries	Brain/CNS damage; digestive problems
Nitrogen dioxide, nitrogen oxides (**criteria pollutant**)	Combustion of gasoline and fossil fuels; cars	Damage to lungs and respiratory system
Ozone (**criteria pollutant**)	Variety of oxygen formed by chemical reaction of pollutants	Breathing impairment; eye irritation
Particulate matter (**criteria pollutant**)	Burning of wood and diesel fuels	Respiratory irritation; lung damage
Smog	Mixture of pollutants, esp. ozone; originates from petroleum-based fuels	Irritation of respiratory system, eyes
Sulfur dioxide (**criteria pollutant**)	Burning of coal and oil	Breathing problems; lung damage
Volatile organic compounds (VOCs)	Burning fuels; released from certain chemicals (e.g., solvents)	Acute effects similar to those of smog; possible carcinogen

Source: Adapted from US Environmental Protection Agency. The Plain English Guide to the Clean Air Act: The Common Air Pollutants. Available at: http://www.epa.gov/oar/oaqps/peg_caa/pegcaa11.html. Accessed March 28, 2005; and US Environmental Protection Agency. The Plain English Guide to the Clean Air Act: Glossary. Available at: http://www.epa.gov/oar/oaqps/peg_caa/pegcaa10.html. Accessed January 28, 2007.

Sanitation, Water, and Hygiene

Only about 65% of the people in the world have access to safe excreta disposal. This ranges from about 80% in the Latin America region to only slightly above 50% in the Africa region.[14] Many of the large cities in Africa have no modern sanitation system, and in Asia large shares of the populations in some areas also have no access to sanitary disposal of human waste.

There is good evidence that improved disposal of human waste is associated with reductions in diarrheal disease, intestinal parasites, and trachoma. Failure to dispose properly of human waste contaminates water and food sources and leads to an increase in transmission of pathogens through the oral-fecal route. Failure to improve sanitation is also associated with the spread of parasitic worms, such as ascaris and hookworm.[15] Improved sanitation reduces the burden of trachoma, because the flies that are significantly involved in the spread of that disease breed, among other places, in human waste.[16]

More than one billion people, mostly in low- and middle-income countries, lack access to safe water sources within a reasonable distance of their home.[17] Access to improved water sources ranges from below 50% in Sub-Saharan Africa to about 70% in Asia to almost universal access in developed countries.[18] It is estimated that about 400 million children lack access to safe water.[19] In addition, even the water that people do have access to and that is deemed safe in official statistics is often of low bacteriological quality and contains important pathogens. Many diseases relate to water in one of a variety of ways.

Waterborne diseases are among the most important in terms of the burden of disease and they are numerous in low- and middle-income countries. Some of the most important waterborne pathogens are shown in Table 9-4.

These pathogens are associated with diarrhea and a host of other gastrointestinal problems, and they can be deadly when they lead to severe diarrhea and dehydration. Such diseases are especially risky for the very young, the very old, and people who have compromised immune systems, such as people living with HIV/AIDS.

THE BURDEN OF ENVIRONMENTALLY-RELATED DISEASES

As noted earlier, it is estimated that about 8.4% of the total burden of disease in low- and middle-income countries is due to water, sanitation, and hygiene; urban air pollution; and indoor air pollution. The relative share of each of these factors is:

- Indoor smoke from household use of solid fuels—3.7%
- Unsafe water, sanitation, and hygiene—3.2%
- Urban air pollution—1.5%[3]

These are explored more fully later.

Many people believe that the most important environmental risk factor in low- and middle-income countries is outdoor air pollution; however, this is not true. Rather, indoor air pollution is the third most important risk factor in high mortality developing countries, exceeded only by malnutrition and unsafe sex, and similar in importance to water, sanitation, and hygiene.[9] It is estimated that indoor air pollution from the use of solid fuels is responsible for 1.6 million deaths annually from pneumonia, chronic respiratory disease, and lung cancer. It is thought, in fact, that indoor air pollution is responsible for about 700,000 of the 2.7 million annual deaths from chronic obstructive pulmonary disease (COPD) and about 15% of all deaths from lung cancer.[9]

These figures include only those diseases for which there is solid evidence of a link with indoor air pollution from the use of solid fuels. However, this may be an underestimate of the real burden of disease from indoor air pollution because there is some evidence that indoor air pollution of this type is also associated with asthma, cataracts, and TB. There is also tentative evidence of links with adverse pregnancy outcomes,

TABLE 9-4 Classification of Water-Related Infections

Transmission	Water-Related infections
Waterborne	The pathogen is in water that is ingested
Water-washed (or water-scarce)	Person-to-person transmission because of a lack of water for hygiene
Water-based	Transmission via an aquatic intermediate host
Water-related insect vector	Transmission by insects that breed in water or bite near water

Source: Data with permission from The World Bank. Cairncross S, Valdmanis V. Water supply, sanitation, and hygiene promotion. In: Jamison DT, Breman JG, Measham AR, et al., eds. *Disease Control Priorities in Developing Countries.* 2nd ed. New York: Oxford University Press; 2006:775.

especially low birthweight, ischemic heart disease, and two types of cancer other than lung cancer.[9]

Almost all the burden of disease from indoor air pollution from the use of solid fuels is in the developing world. Women do most of the cooking in low- and middle-income countries and they are most subject to the health risks from indoor air pollution. Indeed, it is estimated that 59% of all of the deaths attributable to indoor air pollution are among females.[9] Young children in developing countries are often carried by their mothers on their backs as they attend to household and work chores, such as cooking. They also tend to spend long hours at home with their mothers. Therefore, they are also exposed more than others to indoor air pollution and it is estimated that 56% of all deaths attributable to indoor air pollution are among children younger than five years.[9]

Urban Outdoor Air Pollution

One study of the global burden of disease attributed 1.5% of annual deaths and 0.5% of the total burden of disease to outdoor air pollution.[20] The study further indicated that 81% of the deaths and 49% of the DALYs attributable to outdoor air pollution occur among people 60 years of age or more. Three percent of the deaths and 12% of the DALYs occur in children younger than five years.[20] It has also been estimated that outdoor air pollution by urban particulate matter causes about 5% of the global cases of lung cancer, 2% of the deaths from cardiovascular and respiratory conditions, and 1% of respiratory infections.[21]

India and China have major burdens of disease that relate to outdoor air pollution from particulate matter. In fact, about two thirds of the global burden of disease from outdoor air pollution is in the developing countries of Asia.[22] A number of countries in Eastern Europe also face a high burden of disease from outdoor air pollution. In some countries of that region, between 0.6–1.4% of the burden of disease is attributable to outdoor air pollution from particulate matter.[22]

Sanitation, Water, and Hygiene

Unsafe disposal of human waste, unsafe water, and poor hygiene are associated with 3.2% of the total deaths in low- and middle-income countries and 3.7% of the DALYs.[3] Studies that have been done suggest that within the African region, about 85% of the DALYs from these risk factors are related to the oral-fecal route of disease transmission and to diarrheal disease, primarily among young children. These studies also suggest that schistosomiasis, in the water-based group, has the second largest loss of DALYs related to these risk factors in Africa.

We should expect globally that the burden of disease related to these risk factors will fall disproportionately on children, who suffer such a large share of the global burden of disease from diarrhea. The burden of these risk factors will also fall overwhelmingly on poor and less well-educated people in the poorer countries of South Asia and of Sub-Saharan Africa. They have less access than others to improved water supply and sanitation and to the knowledge of good hygiene they need to avoid illness in the face of unsafe water and sanitation.

It is very complicated to try to assess individually the relative contribution of unsafe sanitation, unsafe water, and poor hygienic practices to the burden of diarrheal disease, partly because they are all so closely linked with each other. Nonetheless, both historical experiences in what are now the developed countries and a number of studies in developing countries suggest that improving water supply alone will not reduce diarrheal disease as needed. This seems to stem from the large amount of diarrhea that is associated with food that is unsafe and the way in which people use water if they are not knowledgeable about and do not practice good personal hygiene. More will be said about this later.

Separate from any impact on the reduction of diarrheal disease, improvements in water supply are associated with important reductions in the burden of disease from dracunculiasis, schistosomiasis, and trachoma, as shown in Table 9-5.[23]

THE COSTS AND CONSEQUENCES OF KEY ENVIRONMENTAL HEALTH PROBLEMS

The social and economic consequences of the environmental health issues that have been discussed are enormous. First, they constitute 8.4% of the total deaths in low- and middle-income countries and 7.2% of their total burden of disease. Taken together, the burden of disease from these causes is about 25% more than unsafe sex and about twice as much as tobacco use.[3] The magnitude of their burden itself suggests substantial social and economic costs related to these issues.

Second, as indicated earlier, the burden of these causes falls disproportionately on relatively poorer people. It is the poorer people who cook with biomass fuels and coal, not the better-off people. These burdens also fall on low- and middle-income countries more than on high-income countries. People in high-income countries do not customarily cook with biomass fuel or coal and they do not have to contend with the problems of unsafe water and sanitation that people in the lower- and middle-income countries face. Their knowledge of good hygiene practices is also superior to the level of knowledge of most people in the developing world.

Third, these environmental health burdens have very negative consequences on productivity. It is women who suffer the ill effects of indoor air pollution the most. The results of this are very costly to women in terms of morbidity and disability and days of reduced productivity from both acute and chronic illnesses. In addition, the economic and social consequences of ill health for women in many low- and middle-income countries go considerably beyond the poor health of the women. Rather, they spillover onto the health of the rest of her family, especially young children, whose own health and survival depend in important ways on the health of the mother.

Young children are especially at risk to all three forms of the environmental issues discussed in this chapter. They are especially vulnerable to unsafe water and diarrheal disease can put them into a cycle of infection and malnutrition, ultimately retard their growth and development, or be deadly. Indoor air pollution can also lead to a cycle of illness and respiratory infection, death from pneumonia, or disability from asthma. To a lesser extent, outdoor air pollution can do the same. The elderly face particular risks from outdoor air pollution. This can exacerbate chronic health problems they already have, leading to additional disability and its attendant reduction in productivity.

TABLE 9-5 Selected Waterborne Pathogens

Waterborne Pathogens

Enteric protozoal parasites
- *Entamoeba histolytica*
- *Giardia intestinalis*
- *Cryptosporidium parvum*
- *Cryptosporidium cayetanensis*

Bacterial enteropathogens
- *Salmonella*
- *Shigella*
- *Escherichia coli*
- *Vibrio cholerae*
- *Campylobactor*

Viral Pathogens
- Enteroviruses
- Adenoviruses
- Noroviruses

Source: Adapted with permission from Friis RH. "Water Quality." *Essentials of Environmental Health.* Sudbury, MA: Jones and Bartlett Publishers, Inc.; 2007:211.

REDUCING THE BURDEN OF DISEASE

Important progress has been made in some settings in addressing the environmental health issues discussed here. The next section examines some of the lessons learned to date and some of the most cost-effective measures that can be taken to enhance health in low- and middle-income countries by addressing selected environmental health issues.

Outdoor Air Pollution

Outdoor air pollution is a very broad topic, and there is very little published data on the cost-effectiveness of approaches to addressing outdoor air pollution in developing countries. The studies that have been done on developed countries, however, suggest that developing countries could take a number of cost-effective steps to reduce the health burden of outdoor air pollution.[24]

A number of cities, including Jakarta, Manila, Kathmandu, and Mumbai, participated in a World Bank assisted effort to assess their outdoor air pollution and take measures to reduce it. They examined:

- the amount and type of pollution
- how it was being dispersed
- the health impacts of reductions in particulate matter
- time and cost to implement reductions
- health benefits
- the value of those health benefits
- how the benefits compared to the costs of the intervention[24]

Some of the first measures that these cities and some other large cities in the developing world have taken to reduce outdoor air pollution have included:

- the introduction of unleaded gasoline
- low smoke lubricant for two stroke engines
- the banning of two stroke engines
- shifting to natural gas to fuel public vehicles
- tightening emissions inspections on vehicles
- reducing the burning of garbage[24]

It would also be reasonable to ensure that governments use their regulatory authority to incorporate information about outdoor air pollution in their policies on transportation and industrial development.[24] In line with this, many of the low-income countries do not yet have a significant problem of outdoor air pollution. It will be much more cost-effective for those countries to put in place cost-effective approaches now to minimizing outdoor air pollution and its health effects than it will be to try later to mitigate those effects. In doing so, they should take account of vehicular and industrial pollution.

Indoor Air Pollution

There are a number of areas in which actions could be taken to reduce indoor air pollution from the burning of solid fuels for cooking and heating. In terms of the source of pollution, cooking devices can be improved, less polluting fuels can be used, and families can reduce their need for these fuels by using solar cooking and heating. Some changes can also be made to the living environment. Mechanisms for venting smoke can be built into the house, for example, or the kitchen can be moved away from the main part of the house. People can also change their behaviors to reduce pollution or exposure to it by using dried fuels, properly maintaining their stoves and chimneys, and keeping children away from the cooking area.[25]

Public policy can also play a helpful or hurtful role in trying to reduce indoor air pollution. The public sector, for example, can promote information and education about indoor air pollution and how to reduce it in schools, in the media, and in communities. The government can also use tax policy to reduce the cost of cooking appliances and fuels that will reduce pollution. If necessary, it could subsidize the cost of improved fuels and appliances for those below a certain income level. Governments could also undertake surveillance of the problem and if possible, set standards for indoor air pollution, although this will certainly be beyond the capacity of most low-income countries.[25]

Calculating the cost-effectiveness of different approaches to reducing the health effects of indoor air pollution is a very complicated matter and requires many assumptions. Nonetheless, the conclusions of the analyses that have been done are instructive. The main findings are that the most cost-effective approach to reducing indoor air pollution in Sub-Saharan Africa and South Asia, where the needs are greatest, would be to promote the use of improved stoves. The most cost-effective approach in East Asia would be to promote the use of better fuels, such as kerosene and gas. Of course, these conclusions presume that the stoves get maintained and the fuels are of good quality, which may not always be the case and which would detract from the effectiveness of these approaches.[26]

In addition, a number of lessons have been learned about how to encourage the uptake of better stoves and better fuels, some drawn from extensive experiences in China and India. These include:

- Involve end users, especially women, in helping to assess needs and design approaches
- Promote demand for better stoves and fuels to encourage the development of competitive suppliers and market choice
- Consider subsidies and microcredit for selected interventions to help defray the cost of improvements for the poor
- Establish national and local policies that encourage the needed changes in stoves and fuels[27]

Sanitation

There are a number of different levels of technology associated with excreta disposal, many different forms of toilets, and a wide array of costs associated with them. Sanitation could range from the simple technology of bucket latrines to modern urban sewage systems. Table 9-6 lists the different approaches to excreta disposal. Although we usually think of toilets as owned by individuals, they can also be public and shared by many individuals and families.

The cost per person for methods of sanitary removal of human waste varies considerably. At the bottom levels of service, it appears that pour-flush latrines, ventilation improved latrines, and simple pit latrines can be constructed in low- and middle-income settings for about US$60. Assuming that these last approximately 5 years, the annual cost per capita would be about US$12. The construction cost of conventional sewage systems in some countries is more than 10 times that amount. In addition, they need water to function properly and water is often in short supply.[28] Work is ongoing to develop more cost-effective toilets, and in Bangladesh a simple pour-flush pan has been developed that only costs about US$0.27 per household to construct.[28]

Contrary to what we might normally believe, all of these systems can be operated in a hygienic manner that addresses health concerns. A very important review that was done in the early 1980s, for example, concluded that from the point of view of health, pit latrines would be just as hygienic as modern sewage systems, even if they were considerably less convenient.[29]

Given the relatively low cost of simple methods of sanitation and their relative effectiveness, it might be surprising that such a small share of households in low- and middle-income countries have a sanitary means of excreta disposal. Yet, besides the cultural constraints to their use, there are some other important constraints, as well:

- Lack of knowledge of options—especially the poor may not understand the options available to them and may believe that toilets cost more to install than they do
- Cost—even at relatively low prices, the poor may not have the money to pay for the up-front costs of the toilet

- Construction—there may be a lack of skills to help install the toilets
- Local laws—particularly in urban areas, local laws may forbid low-cost sanitation, even if the area has no modern sewage system[30]

There are some countries in which the public sector leads the effort to build low-cost sanitation systems. In some places, the public sector also subsidizes the cost of toilets for the poorest families, given what can be seen as the benefits to society as a whole of toilets being used by individual families. In addition, the public sector can try to enforce regulations to require the use of toilets. Although such regulatory authority is weak in most low-income and many middle-income countries, one of the main cities in Burkina Faso was able to promote toilet construction by taking away the title of homes if their owners did not install a toilet within a specific period of time.[31]

It is also possible, if the private sector believes that there is a market for low-cost sanitation, for such efforts to be handled in the private sector. In this case, the public sector may confine its role to areas needed to encourage private sector involvement and public demand for the toilets. This would include, for example, promoting the use of toilets, encouraging private sector involvement, setting standards, and helping to train people in installation and maintenance techniques.[31]

Promotion of improved sanitation can also be done with a public and private partnership and led by NGOs. Two of the most successful cases of improving low-cost sanitation were led by NGOs in Zimbabwe and Bangladesh. In Zimbabwe, an NGO was able to help communities construct 3400 latrines for about $13 per unit, or only about $2.25 per person served.[32] In Bangladesh, an NGO has helped to make 100 villages free of open defecation for a cost of only about $1.50 per person served.[33] In both of these cases, the families in the communities served paid for the latrines themselves.

The largest impact of improved sanitation is in the reduction of diarrhea and studies that have been done suggest that this impact may be on the order of about 35% overall. Some studies, such as one in Brazil suggested that children living in slum homes with a toilet suffered only one third the number of cases of diarrhea as children in homes without a toilet. It is very important to note that having a toilet seems to also increase the hand washing habits of families, which itself brings benefits, as discussed later.

Finally, the benefits of sanitary excreta removal go beyond diarrhea. Improving sanitation should reduce the prevalence of several worms, including Ascaris, Trichuris, and hookworm.[34] Given the low-cost of some forms of latrines, they would be cost-effective approaches to reducing the prevalence of these worms. As noted earlier, the same would be true in terms of the positive impact and low costs of reducing trachoma through improved sanitation.[35]

TABLE 9-6 Selected Sanitation Technologies

- Simple pit latrine
- Small bore sewer
- Ventilation-improved latrine
- Pour-flush
- Septic tank
- Sewer connection

Source: Data with permission from The World Bank. Cairncross S, Valdmanis V. Water supply, sanitation, and hygiene promotion. In: Jamison DT, Breman JG, Measham AR, et al., eds. *Disease Control Priorities in Developing Countries.* 2nd ed. New York: Oxford University Press; 2006:780.

Water Supply

There are many analogies between water supply and sanitation. For water, as well as for sanitation, there are many different levels of technology and the costs vary considerably according to the level of technology employed. One could get water, for example from the following types of improved water sources:

- House connection
- Standpost
- Borehole
- Dug well
- Rainwater collection

The section below examines the relative cost-effectiveness of different approaches to achieving health benefits from improved water supply. In considering these costs and benefits, reasonable access to water was considered to be access to at least 20 liters per day from one of these sources from not more than 1 kilometer distance.[36]

Improving water supply can lead to a variety of health benefits. The most important studies that have been done have shown that providing a continuous supply of water with good bacteriological quality can reduce the morbidity of a number of diseases, as shown in Table 9-7 for the Africa region. Studies showed a median reduction in trachoma, for example, of 27%, schistosomiasis of 77%, and dracunculiasis of 78%.[23]

Other studies have looked at the health benefits from different combinations of investments in water quantity, water quality, sanitation, and the promotion of hygiene. The results of these studies are somewhat surprising to those not involved in the environmental field. They suggest that the largest reductions in diarrhea morbidity—approximately 30%—come from investing in sanitation only, water and sanitation, or hygiene only. The lowest reductions, between 15% and 20%, came from investing in water quantity only, or a combination of water quality and quantity, all without complementary investments in hygiene or in sanitation.

As noted earlier, many of the pathogens that are waterborne are also carried on food. Thus, sanitation has a large potential impact on reducing those pathogens. However, water alone may not yield the results that sanitation would. For this, among other reasons, complementary investments for the promotion of hygiene are critical to realizing gains from water and sanitation.[37]

Another important lesson is that the greatest effect of investments in water on health are realized when people have water connections in their homes. Unfortunately, community standpipes, for example, do not produce the level of health gains of individual household water connections.[37] A review in New Guinea, for example, showed that there was 56% less diarrhea in homes with an individual connection than in homes that got their water from standpipes.[37] This may partly be the case because people with individual connections use considerably more water than those without such connections and much of the additional water may be used to engage in better hygiene.

TABLE 9-7 Potential Morbidity Reduction from Excellent Water Supply

Condition	Percentage Reduction
Scabies	80
Typhoid fever	80
Trachoma	60
Most diarrheas and dysentery	50
Skin and subcutaneous infections	50
Paratyphoid, other Salmonella	40

Source: Adapted with permission from The World Bank. Cairncross S, Valdmanis V. Water supply, sanitation, and hygiene promotion. In: Jamison DT, Breman JG, Measham AR, et al., eds. *Disease Control Priorities in Developing Countries.* 2nd ed. New York: Oxford University Press;2006:776.

Hygiene

Unfortunately, there have been relatively few studies of the impact of hygiene promotion on actual health behaviors and on related reductions in the burden of disease. The studies that have been done showed that investing in hygiene promotion led to a 33% reduction in diarrhea. They also found that to be successful and sustainable, hygiene promotion efforts need to focus on simple messages about hand washing and avoid trying to promote too many messages at once. It appears that the messages that families acquire through hygiene promotion do stay with them and that retraining is necessary only once every five years.[38] Studies have also been done on the impact of hand washing on respiratory infections. Hand washing was associated in these studies with a significant reduction in acute respiratory infections.[38]

Integrating Investment Choices about Water, Sanitation, and Hygiene

When the information from the studies previously discussed is reviewed together, it appears that the promotion of hygiene, the promotion of sanitation, and the construction of standposts are all likely to be cost-effective in low- and middle-income countries. Using public funds to provide individual household connections to water supply systems is likely to be above the cut-off for cost-effective investments. This is shown in Table 9-8.

The costs of hygiene and sanitation promotion compare favorably, for example, with the costs per DALY averted of oral rehydration. In addition, such investments might help to reduce the burden of diarrhea and decrease the need for oral rehydration.

On that basis, what would be a sensible approach to improving health through investments in water supply, sanitation, and hygiene in low- and middle-income countries? First would be to promote hygiene. This is necessary both for its own sake and to maximize the value that will accrue from investments in water supply and sanitation. Second, governments should promote low-cost sanitation schemes. In doing this, they should encourage the private sector to invest in this business, encourage demand from consumers, try to ensure that there are skills to install the latrines, and try to set and enforce standards to which they have to be built. Third, low-cost water supply schemes should also be developed. This can often be done best in conjunction with communities and with community-based approaches. Finally, the government should use its regulatory and other authority to be sure that it helps consumers meet the costs of these schemes and also encourages investment in water supply schemes with household connections that families pay for. Much has been written about approaches to water and sanitation. Those interested in how such schemes get designed, built, operated, and financed are encouraged to review some of the literature on those topics, which is beyond the scope of this book.

FUTURE CHALLENGES

There will be many challenges to reducing the burden of disease that is related to hygiene, water supply, and sanitation; indoor air pollution; and outdoor air pollution. One important challenge has to do with population growth. The population is continuing to grow in many developing countries and will do so for some time. As the population grows, and as increasing numbers of people move to cities, for example, will low- and middle-income countries be able to provide the infrastructure needed for improved water supply and sanitation when they already face such substantial gaps in this provision?

At the same time, as the economies of low- and middle-income countries hopefully grow at a relatively rapid and sustained pace, how will they manage the pollution that is related, for example, to increased use of energy and greater use by better-off people of automobiles? In addition, will relatively poorly governed societies be able to manage and regulate industrial forms of pollution that could further harm air and water quality?

Many of the more difficult problems of indoor air pollution and health impacts of unsafe water and sanitation exact a larger tool on rural people than urban people, on the poor rather than the better-off, and on women and children. In this light, many countries will need to explore ways to reduce indoor air pollution and improve the safety of the water supply through community-based approaches that will often have to link the public, private, and NGO sectors with communities and that will have to explicitly focus on women and children.

Reducing the burden of environmentally-related health problems will also require that people be better informed about that burden. At the societal level, people and communities will need to understand more about the links between their health and the environment. At national, regional, local, and family levels, people will also need to be more aware of the solutions to these problems that might be available to them. The need for better and more information about issues and options for addressing them will be especially important among the poor, poorly educated, the rural, and women.

Another challenge of addressing environmental health issues is that efforts to address them generally require action outside the health sector. Urban water supply systems are usually under the control of public or private companies. Urban sanitation is usually managed by individual cities. In rural areas, water supply and sanitation are most likely to be controlled by communities and individuals. Indoor air pollution is an issue that can best be addressed by working with families and communities to change the way they cook and the fuel that they use for cooking. Outdoor air pollution comes, among other things, from industrial plants and vehicles, the control of which depends on an array of economic and policy matters beyond the scope of the health ministry.

TABLE 9–8 Cost per DALY of Selected Investments in Water, Sanitation, and Hygiene

Investment	US$/DALY
Hygiene promotion	3.35
Sanitation promotion only	11.15
Water sector regulation and advocacy	47.00
Hand pump or standpost	94.00
House connection	223.00
Construction and promotion	≤ 270.00

Source: Adapted with permission from The World Bank. Cairncross S, Valdmanis V. Water supply, sanitation, and hygiene promotion. In: Jamison DT, Breman JG, Measham AR, et al., eds. *Disease Control Priorities in Developing Countries.* 2nd ed. New York: Oxford University Press; 2006:791.

MAIN MESSAGES

Environmental health issues have a large impact on the global burden of disease. These impacts occur at the individual, household, community, and global level. Broadly speaking, about one third of the total global burden of disease is related to environmental factors.[39] About 8% of the global burden of disease is associated with the environmental factors discussed in this chapter, including outdoor air pollution, indoor air pollution from the use of sold fuels, and water, sanitation, and hygiene.[3]

The risks of these environmental factors are greatest for poor women and their children due to their exposure to indoor air pollution from the burning of solid fuel and to poor quality water. The risks of environmental impacts on health are greatest in the low-income countries of Africa and Asia. Environmental risk factors are especially important causes of illness and death from diarrhea and acute respiratory infections among young children. They also have a large impact on the burden of disease from certain parasitic infections, such as worms. Given the prominence of these risk factors, it is essential that improvements be made in water, sanitation, and hygiene if the MDGs are to be met.

The burden of indoor air pollution stems largely from cooking on unventilated stoves with solid biomass fuels or coal, as done by a large share of poor people in the world. The sources of outdoor air pollution are many and vehicle emission is among the most important in most cities. Poor sanitation allows pathogens in human waste to spread but only about 40% of the people in the world have access to improved sanitation. Unsafe water carries pathogens. The lack of water prevents people from engaging in appropriate hygiene practices. Poor hygiene practices, including open defecation and the failure to engage in hand washing, are common in the developing world, especially among people who lack education.

Data are weak on cost-effective approaches to reducing outdoor air pollution in the developing countries. However, it appears that there are a number of measures that could be taken to reduce pollution and enhance health including eliminating leaded gasoline, eliminating two stroke engines, strengthening emissions standards, and shifting vehicle fuel to natural gas. In Africa and South Asia, the most cost-effective approach to reducing indoor air pollution will be to promote the use of improved stoves. In Asia, the most cost-effective approach would be to encourage a shift from biomass fuels and coal to kerosene or gas.

The most cost-effective approach to reducing the burden of water-related diseases, especially diarrhea, is to invest in low-cost sanitation and standposts for water and to promote hand washing. Investments in water can have numerous benefits, including saving the time of women who are usually charged with getting water and often have to expend large amounts of energy to do so. The provision of water can also contribute to reduction in certain parasitic diseases. However, in the absence of improved hygiene, the provision of improved access to water alone still fails to address an important share of the burden of diarrheal disease.

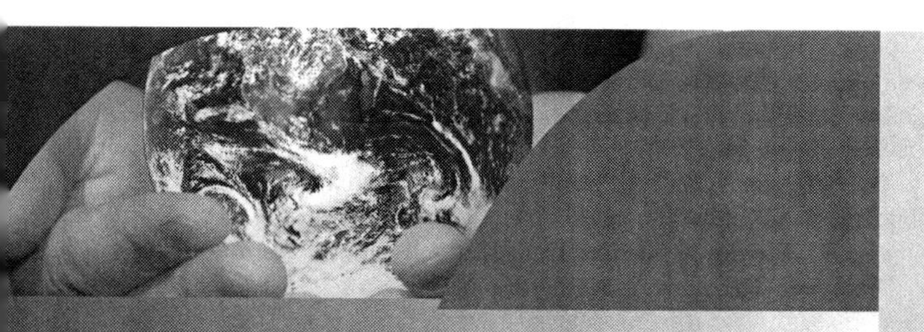

Discussion Questions

1. Why are environmental health issues important in global health? Which of them are the most important and why?
2. Why would the burden of disease from indoor air pollution in low- and middle-income countries be larger than that from outdoor air pollution?
3. In what regions of the world would the burden from indoor air pollution be the greatest? Why?
4. What are the different ways in which unsafe water is related to the spread of disease? Give some examples of specific diseases that are spread in various water-related ways.
5. What are some of the health problems associated with outdoor air pollution?
6. Why is it important to promote hand washing?
7. What approach would you take in a low-income African country to enhancing the access of the poor to better water supplies? Why?
8. How would you try to expand access to low-cost sanitation in Nepal? Why?
9. What would constrain poor people in Nepal from investing their own resources in improved low-cost sanitation? How could those constraints be overcome?
10. How would you help people in Guatemala to adopt the use of better stoves?

REFERENCES

1. Lopez AD, Mathers CD, Murray CJL. *Global Burden of Disease and Risk Factors.* New York: Oxford University Press; 2006.

2. Smith KR, Corvalan CF, Kjellstrom T. How much global ill health is attributable to environmental factors? *Epidemiology.* 1999;10(5):573.

3. Lopez AD, Mathers CD, Ezzati M, Jamison DT, Murray CJL. Measuring the global burden of disease and risk factors 1990–2001. In: Lopez AD, Mathers CD, Ezzati M, Jamison DT, Murray CJL, eds. *Global Burden of Disease and Risk Factors.* New York: Oxford University Press; 2006:10.

4. Friis RH. *Essentials on Environmental Health.* Sudbury, MA: Jones and Bartlett Publishers, Inc.; 2007.

5. Yassi A, Kjellstrom T, de Kok T, Guidotti TL. *Basic Environmental Health.* New York: Oxford University Press; 2001.

6. McMichael AJ, Kjellstrom T, Smith KR. Environmental health. In: Merson MH, Black RE, Mills A, eds. *International Public Health: Diseases, Programs, Systems, and Policies.* Gaithersburg, MD: Aspen Publishers; 2001:379.

7. The World Bank. Environmental Health. Available at: http://web.worldbank.org/WBSITE/EXTERNAL/TOPICS/EXTHEALTHNUTRITIONANDPOPULATION/EXTPHAAG/0,,contentMDK:20656146~menuPK:2175463~pagePK:64229817~piPK:64229743~theSitePK:672263,00.html. Accessed October 27, 2006.

8. World Health Organization. Protection of the Human Environment. Available at: http://www.who.int/phe/en/. Accessed May 19, 2005.

9. World Health Organization. Indoor Air Pollution and Health: Fact Sheet No. 292. Available at: http://www.who.int/mediacentre/factsheets/fs292/en/index.html. Accessed October 29, 2006.

10. Yassi A, Kjellstrom T, de Kok T, Guidotti TL. Health and energy use. *Basic Environmental Health.* New York: Oxford University Press; 2001:315.

11. Yassi A, Kjellstrom T, de Kok T, Guidotti TL. Health and energy use. *Basic Environmental Health.* New York: Oxford University Press; 2001:317.

12. Yassi A, Kjellstrom T, de Kok T, Guidotti TL. Air. *Basic Environmental Health.* New York: Oxford University Press; 2001:188.

13. Yassi A, Kjellstrom T, de Kok T, Guidotti TL. Air. *Basic Environmental Health.* New York: Oxford University Press; 2001:193–194.

14. Yassi A, Kjellstrom T, de Kok T, Guidotti TL. Water and sanitation. *Basic Environmental Health.* New York: Oxford University Press; 2001:233.

15. Cairncross S, Valdmanis V. Water supply, sanitation, and hygiene promotion. In: Jamison DT, Breman JG, Measham AR, et al., eds. *Disease Control Priorities in Developing Countries.* 2nd ed. New York: Oxford University Press; 2006:776.

16. Cairncross S, Valdmanis V. Water supply, sanitation, and hygiene promotion. In: Jamison DT, Breman JG, Measham AR, et al., eds. *Disease Control Priorities in Developing Countries.* 2nd ed. New York: Oxford University Press; 2006:784.

17. World Bank. Access to Safe Water. Available at: http://www.worldbank.org/depweb/english/modules/environm/water/. Accessed November 3, 2006.

18. United Nations. The Millennium Development Goals Report 2005. Available at: www.un.org/Docs/summit2005/MDGBook.pdf. Accessed November 3, 2006.

19. UNICEF. Press Release: 400 Million Children Deprived of Safe Water. Available at: http://www.unicef.org/media/media_31772.html. Accessed November 3, 2006.

20. Ostro B. Outdoor Air Pollution: Assessing the Environmental Burden of Disease at National and Local Levels. Available at: http://www.who.int/quantifying_ehimpacts/publications/ebd5.pdf. Accessed November 3, 2006.

21. Kjellstrom T, Lodh M, McMichael AJ, Ranmuthugala G, Shrestha R, Kingsland S. Air and water pollution: burden and strategies for control. In: Jamison DT, Breman JG, Measham AR, et al., eds. *Disease Control Priorities in Developing Countries.* 2nd ed. New York: Oxford University Press; 2006:820.

22. Cohen AJ, Ross Anderson H, Ostro B, et al. The global burden of disease due to outdoor air pollution. *J Toxicol Environ Health A.* 2005;68(13-14):1301–1307.

23. Cairncross S, Valdmanis V. Water supply, sanitation, and hygiene promotion. In: Jamison DT, Breman JG, Measham AR, et al., eds. *Disease Control Priorities in Developing Countries.* 2nd ed. New York: Oxford University Press; 2006:778.

24. Kjellstrom T, Lodh M, McMichael AJ, Ranmuthugala G, Shrestha R, Kingsland S. Air and water pollution: burden and strategies for control. In: Jamison DT, Breman JG, Measham AR, et al., eds. *Disease Control Priorities in Developing Countries.* 2nd ed. New York: Oxford University Press; 2006:825–826.

25. Bruce N, Rehfuess E, Mehta S, Hutton G, Smith K. Indoor air pollution. In: Jamison DT, Breman JG, Measham AR, et al., eds. *Disease Control Priorities in Developing Countries.* 2nd ed. New York: Oxford University Press; 2006:800.

26. Bruce N, Rehfuess E, Mehta S, Hutton G, Smith K. Indoor air pollution. In: Jamison DT, Breman JG, Measham AR, et al., eds. *Disease Control Priorities in Developing Countries.* 2nd ed. New York: Oxford University Press; 2006:802–808.

27. Bruce N, Rehfuess E, Mehta S, Hutton G, Smith K. Indoor air pollution. In: Jamison DT, Breman JG, Measham AR, et al., eds. *Disease Control Priorities in Developing Countries.* 2nd ed. New York: Oxford University Press; 2006:808–811.

28. Cairncross S, Valdmanis V. Water supply, sanitation, and hygiene promotion. In: Jamison DT, Breman JG, Measham AR, et al., eds. *Disease Control Priorities in Developing Countries.* 2nd ed. New York: Oxford University Press; 2006:780.

29. Feachem R, Bradley D, Garelick H, Mara D. *Sanitation and Disease: Health Aspects of Excreta and Wastewater Management.* Chichester, U.K.: John Wiley & Sons; 1983.

30. Cairncross S, Valdmanis V. Water supply, sanitation, and hygiene promotion. In: Jamison DT, Breman JG, Measham AR, et al., eds. *Disease Control Priorities in Developing Countries.* 2nd ed. New York: Oxford University Press; 2006:780–182.

31. Cairncross S, Valdmanis V. Water supply, sanitation, and hygiene promotion. In: Jamison DT, Breman JG, Measham AR, et al., eds. *Disease Control Priorities in Developing Countries.* 2nd ed. New York: Oxford University Press; 2006:781.

32. Waterkeyn J. Cost-Effective Health Promotion: Community Health Clubs. Abuja, Nigeria: Paper presented at the 29th WEDC Conference; 2003.

33. Allan S. The WaterAid Bangladesh/VERC 100% Sanitation Approach; Cost, Motivation and Subsidy. *M.Sc. dissertation, London School of Hygiene and Tropical Medicine*; 2003.

34. Cairncross S, Valdmanis V. Water supply, sanitation, and hygiene promotion. In: Jamison DT, Breman JG, Measham AR, et al., eds. *Disease Control Priorities in Developing Countries.* 2nd ed. New York: Oxford University Press; 2006:783–784.

35. Emerson PM, Lindsay SW, Alexander N, et al. Role of flies and provision of latrines in trachoma control: cluster-randomised controlled trial. *Lancet.* 2004;363(9415):1093–1098.

36. Cairncross S, Valdmanis V. Water supply, sanitation, and hygiene promotion. In: Jamison DT, Breman JG, Measham AR, et al., eds. *Disease Control Priorities in Developing Countries.* 2nd ed. New York: Oxford University Press; 2006:772.

37. Cairncross S, Valdmanis V. Water supply, sanitation, and hygiene promotion. In: Jamison DT, Breman JG, Measham AR, et al., eds. *Disease Control Priorities in Developing Countries.* 2nd ed. New York: Oxford University Press; 2006:777.

38. Cairncross S, Valdmanis V. Water supply, sanitation, and hygiene promotion. In: Jamison DT, Breman JG, Measham AR, et al., eds. *Disease Control Priorities in Developing Countries.* 2nd ed. New York: Oxford University Press; 2006:784–785.

39. Smith KR, Corvalan CF, Kjellstrom T. How much global ill health is attributable to environmental factors? *Epidemiology.* 1999;10(5):573–584.

CHAPTER 10

Natural Disasters and Complex Humanitarian Emergencies

LEARNING OBJECTIVES

By the end of this chapter the reader will be able to:

- Describe several types of disasters that impact human health
- Discuss the health effects of natural disasters and complex humanitarian emergencies
- Review how those health impacts vary by age, sex, location, and type of disaster
- Describe key measures that can be taken to mitigate the health impacts of natural disasters and complex humanitarian emergencies

VIGNETTES

Javad lived in the Pakistani province of Kashmir when the earthquake hit. All the buildings in his village were destroyed. Hundreds of people in the village were killed, mostly a result of being buried in the rubble. Many other people were badly injured from rubble falling on them. Their injuries were overwhelmingly orthopedic in nature. As the earthquake destroyed the village, it also destroyed wells, a health center, and roads leading to and from the village. Javad feared that many of those injured would soon die.

Samuel was living in the Eastern part of Sierra Leone when the war started. He did all that he could to protect his family, but it was not enough. In the first year of the conflict, as he and his family were getting ready to flee, a band of armed men stormed the village. As Samuel had heard they would do, they used machetes to kill or take limbs off of many village people. They also raped a large number of women. In addition, they kidnapped some of the children in hopes of making them into sex slaves or soldiers.

As the civil war spread in Rwanda, Sarah and her family fled across the border to what was fast becoming a large refugee camp in Zaire, later called the Democratic Republic of Congo. Although the camp workers did what they could to help the refugees, the circumstances at the camp were not good. There was little shelter, water, or food. In addition, a cholera epidemic went through the camp not long after Sarah's arrival there. It hit the camp especially hard and led to a large number of deaths.

A number of international organizations rushed staff to refugee camps, just across the border from intense fighting. Some of the agencies involved had long experience doing such work and had clear guidelines for their staff concerning relief efforts. Other agencies, however, were not so experienced in this work. They brought to the camps medicine that was not appropriate for the health conditions they found and food to which the local people were completely unaccustomed. Although it would have been most efficient if all of the aid agencies worked together, they did not. Many of them had their own way of working and wanted the local government to do it their way.

THE IMPORTANCE OF NATURAL DISASTERS AND COMPLEX EMERGENCIES TO GLOBAL HEALTH

Complex emergencies and natural disasters have a significant impact on global health. They can lead to increased death, illness, and disability and the economic costs of their health impacts can also be very large. Measures can be taken in cost-effective ways, however, to reduce the costs of disasters and conflicts and to address the major health problems that relate to them. These measures would be most effective if those involved in disaster relief would work together according to agreed standards that focused on the most important priorities for action.

This chapter will review the relationships between natural disasters and health and complex humanitarian emergencies (CHEs) and health. The chapter will begin by introducing you to some key concepts and definitions that relate to these topics. The chapter will then review the incidence of natural disasters and CHEs. Following that, the chapter will review their main health impacts. Lastly, the chapter will examine measures that can be taken to prevent and address some of their effects on health in cost-effective ways.

KEY TERMS

Understanding the health impacts of natural disasters and complex humanitarian emergencies requires an introduction to several terms and concepts that are examined briefly here.

A disaster is "any occurrence that causes damage, ecological destruction, loss of human lives, or deterioration of health and health services on a scale sufficient to warrant an extraordinary response from outside the affected community area."[1] Another way to think of this would be as "an occurrence, either natural or man made, that causes human suffering and creates human needs that victims can not alleviate without assistance."[2] Some disasters are natural. These include, for example, the results of floods, volcanoes, and earthquakes. Some, however, are man-made, such as the cloud of poisonous gas that rained over the town of Bhopal, India, in 1984, as a result of an industrial accident. Some disasters are rapid-onset, such as an earthquake, while others are slow-onset, such as a drought or famine. Although the long-term effects of these natural and man-made disasters can be substantial, they are often characterized by an initial event and then its aftereffects. Some examples of recent natural disasters that caused a significant loss of life are listed in Table 10-1.

TABLE 10-1 Selected Natural Disasters, 2004 and 2005

2004

March—Typhoon Gafilo, with 160-mile-per-hour winds, kills 295 people in Madagascar

May—Flooding and mudslides from heavy rains in the Dominican Republic and Haiti kill 3000 people

June—Monsoon floods in Bangladesh, India, and Nepal leave more than 5 million people homeless and kill 1800

December—Tsunamis after a 9.0 magnitude earthquake kill more than 225,000 people in India, Indonesia, Sri Lanka, and Thailand

2005

February—Flooding from snow and rain killed 460 people in Pakistan with thousands of people missing

March—An 8.7 magnitude earthquake in Indonesia killed more than 1300 people

July—The heaviest rains in Indian history killed more than 1000 people

July—Famine stemming from drought and locusts put more than 3.6 million people at risk of starvation in Niger

August—Hurricane Katrina kills 1800 people in the United States

October—Rains from Hurricane Stan killed more than 2000 people in Central America and caused many people to evacuate their homes

Source: Data from Infoplease. World Disasters—2004 and 2005 Disasters. Available at: http://www.infoplease.com/ipa/A0001437.html. Accessed February 25, 2007.

In response to the large number of civil conflicts that have taken place, the term "complex emergency" or "complex humanitarian emergency" has been established. A complex emergency can be defined as a "complex, multi-party, intra-state conflict resulting in a humanitarian disaster which might constitute multi-dimensional risks or threats to regional and international security. Frequently within such conflicts, state institutions collapse, law and order break down, banditry and chaos prevail, and portions of the civilian population migrate."[3] CHEs have also been described as: "situations affecting large civilian populations which usually involve a combination of factors, including war or civil strife, food shortages, and population displacement, resulting in significant excess mortality."[4]

Such emergencies include war and civil conflict. They usually affect large numbers of people and often include severe impacts on the availability of food, water, and shelter. Linked to these phenomena and the displacement of people that often go with them, complex humanitarian emergencies usually result in considerable excess mortality, compared to what would be the case without such an emergency.[5] Some of the better known complex humanitarian emergencies are listed in Table 10-2.

Complex emergencies create "refugees." Under international law, a refugee is a person who is outside his/her country of nationality or habitual residence; has a well-founded fear of persecution because of his/her race, religion, nationality, membership in a particular social group or political opinion; and is unable or unwilling to avail himself/herself of the protection of that country, or to return there, for fear of persecution. They are a subgroup of the broader category of displaced persons.[6] It is important to note that there are a number of international conventions that define refugees and that accord them rights according to international law, as well. Table 10-3 notes a number of countries with significant refugee populations and the countries they fled. A United Nations Agency, the United Nations High Commissioner for Refugees (UNHCR), is responsible for protecting the rights of refugees.

Some of the people who flee or are forced to migrate during a disaster or complex humanitarian emergency leave their homes but stay in the country in which they were living. These are called internally displaced people (IDP). These are more formally defined as "someone who has been forced to leave their home for reasons such as religious or political persecution or war, but has not crossed an international border."[7] The term is a subset of the more general "displaced person." There is no legal definition of internally displaced person, as there is for refugee, but the thumbnail rule is that "if the person in question would be eligible for refugee status if he or she crossed an international border then the IDP label is applicable."[7] Table 10-4 shows selected examples of countries with large numbers of internally displaced persons. It is important to note that the legal status of IDPs is not as well defined as that for refugees.[8] It is also important to understand that, unlike the case for refugees, no agency or organization is responsible for IDPs. Rather, their own government is responsible for them, but that government is often part of the problem as to why these people are fleeing.

One of the indicators of significance of the health impact of a complex humanitarian emergency is the "crude mortality rate." This is the proportion of people who die from a population at risk over a specified period of time.[9] For addressing CHEs, the crude mortality rate is generally expressed per 10,000 population, per day. The extent to which diseases might spread in a refugee camp depend partly on the "attack rate" of a disease, which is "the proportion of an exposed

TABLE 10-2 Selected Complex Humanitarian Emergencies of Importance

Angola—A civil war lasted 27 years and ended in 2002.

Armenia/Azerbaijan—Conflict between the two countries has created almost 250,000 refugees and 600,000 IDPs.

Bosnia and Herzegovina—Between 1992 and 1994, war with various parts of the former Yugoslavia led to more than 100,000 deaths and 1.8 million people displaced.

Burma—Government offensives against a number of ethnic groups have gone on for more than 20 years and produced between 500,000 and 1,000,000 IDPs.

Democratic Republic of Congo—Fighting since the mid-1990s between government forces and rebels have led to more than 2 million displaced people.

Liberia—Civil war from 1990–2004 led to almost 500,000 IDPs and more than 125,000 refugees in Guinea alone.

Nepal—Conflict between the government forces and Maoist rebels from 1996 to 2006 has led to 100,000 to 200,000 IDPs.

Rwanda—More than 800,000 people were killed in the 1994 genocide, which also produced more than 2 million refugees who fled to Burundi, what is now the Democratic Republic of Congo, Tanzania, and Uganda.

Sudan—Internal conflicts since the 1980s, including a war with groups in the South and genocide against people in the Darfur region, have displaced 5–6 million people.

Uganda—Rebellion by the Lord's Resistance Army in the North for almost 20 years has led to between 1 and 2 million displaced people.

Source: Data from CIA. The World Fact Book. Available at: http://www.cia.gov/cia/publications/factbook/. Accessed February 25, 2007.

TABLE 10-3 Internally Displaced People—Selected Countries of Importance, 2006

Country	Number of IDPs
Sudan	5,300,000–6,200,000
Colombia	2,900,000–3,400,000
Democratic Republic of Congo	2,330,000
India	600,000
Burma	550,000–1,000,000
Azerbaijan	528,000
Ivory Coast	500,000–800,000
Indonesia	500,000
Liberia	464,000
Algeria	400,000–600,000
Somalia	400,000
Russia	339,000
Bosnia and Herzegovina	309,000

Source: Data from CIA. The World Fact Book. Field Listing Refugees and Internally Displaced People. Available at: http://www.cia.gov/cia/publications/factbook/fields/2194.html. Accessed October 8, 2006.

TABLE 10-4 Selected Refugee Populations and Source of Refugees, 2006

Country	Number of Refugees	Source Countries
Jordan	1,828,000	Palestinian Refugees
Iran	1,040,000	Afghanistan, Iraq
Gaza Strip	990,000	Palestinian Refugees
Pakistan	960,000	Afghanistan
West Bank	700,000	Palestinian Refugees
Tanzania	597,000	Burundi, Democratic Republic of Congo
Syria	446,000	Palestinian Refugees, Iraq
Lebanon	404,000	Palestinian Refugees
China	350,000	Vietnam, North Korea
Serbia	275,000	Croatia, Bosnia, and Herzegovina
Uganda	258,000	Sudan, Rwanda, Democratic Republic of Congo
Chad	255,000	Sudan, Central African Republic
Armenia	235,000	Azerbaijan
Kenya	229,000	Somalia, Ethiopia, Sudan
India	157,000	Tibet/China, Sri Lanka, Afghanistan
Zambia	151,000	Angola, Democratic Republic of Congo, Rwanda
Guinea	141,000	Liberia, Sierra Leone, Ivory Coast
Sudan	139,000	Eritrea, Chad, Uganda, Ethiopia
Ethiopia	125,000	Sudan, Somalia, Eritrea
Thailand	121,000	Myanmar
Nepal	105,000	Bhutan

Source: Data from CIA. The World Fact Book. Field listing refugees and internally displaced people. Available at: http://www.cia.gov/cia/publications/factbook/fields/2194.html. Accessed October 8, 2006.

population at risk who become infected or develop clinical illness during a defined period of time."[3] Finally, it is important to understand **case fatality rate**, which is "the number of deaths from a specific disease in a given period, per 100 episodes of the disease in the same period."[10]

THE CHARACTERISTICS OF NATURAL DISASTERS

There are several types of natural disasters. Some of these are related to the weather, including droughts, hurricanes, typhoons, cyclones, and heavy rains. Tsunamis, like the one that occurred in 2004, can also cause extreme devastation, injuries, and death. In addition, earthquakes and volcanoes can have important impacts on the health of various communities. Despite the exceptional nature of the 2004 tsunami and the deaths associated with that, among the natural disasters it is earthquakes that generally kill the most people.

It appears that the number of natural disasters is increasing, affecting larger numbers of people, causing more economic losses than earlier, but causing proportionately fewer deaths than before. In addition, the biggest relative impact of natural disasters is in developing countries. More than 90% of the deaths from these disasters occur in low- and middle-income countries.[11] The relative impact of natural disasters on the poor, of course, is greater than on the better-off because the share of the poorer people's total assets that are lost in these disasters is greater than that lost by higher-income people. Moreover, the poor are often the most vulnerable to losses from natural disasters because they often live in places at risk from such disasters or have housing that can not withstand such shocks.[12]

Natural disasters can cause significant harm to infrastructure, such as water supply and sewage systems, that are needed for safe water and sanitation, and roads that may be needed to transport people requiring health care. Natural disasters can also damage the health infrastructure itself, such as hospitals, health centers, and health clinics. People can die directly as a result of the natural disaster, such as from falling rubble during an earthquake or drowning during a flood. However, they may also die as an indirect result of the disaster because of epidemics linked to the lack of safe water or sanitation, food, or access to health services.[12] In addition, people affected by the disaster could wind up living in camps, which pose a range of health hazards.

THE CHARACTERISTICS OF COMPLEX EMERGENCIES

Over the 10-year period from 1975 to 1985, there were on average about five complex emergencies per year, according to the International Committee of the Red Cross. However, it is estimated that at the end of the 1990s there were about 40 such emergencies per year in countries in which more than 300 million people live.[8] It is also estimated that in 2001 there were more than 14 million refugees and more than 20 million internally displaced people in the world.[13] Although natural disasters have been associated with considerable death and economic loss, the impact of complex emergencies on health over the last decade has been considerably greater than that of natural disasters.

Complex humanitarian emergencies have a number of features that particularly relate to their health impacts. First, these emergencies often go on for long periods of time. The strife in Sudan, for example, has gone on for more than a decade.[14] In addition, these emergencies are increasingly civil wars, as in Bosnia, Liberia, Sierra Leone, Rwanda, and the Democratic Republic of Congo. As a result of the nature of the conflict, it is quite common that one or more of the groups that are fighting will not allow humanitarian assistance to be provided to other groups. In fact, humanitarian workers have increasingly been the targets of those who are fighting, despite what should be their protected status.

During complex emergencies, combatants often intentionally target civilians, as well, for displacement, injury, and death. Many fighters also engage in systematic abuse of human rights, including torture, sexual abuse, and rape "as a weapon of war." Those same fighters often intentionally destroy health facilities. Given the nature of some of the fighting and its impact on civilians, large numbers of people have been displaced by some of these conflicts, as noted above. Sometimes they choose to flee, but sometimes they are forced to flee.[15]

Unfortunately, these are not the only characteristics of complex humanitarian emergencies. The disruption of society often leads to food shortages. Besides the loss of some health facilities, it is also common that the publicly supported health system may break down entirely, as it did, for example, in the civil war in Liberia. Damage may also be done to water supply and sanitation systems.[16] In El Salvador, for example, the shortage of safe drinking water for the poor was seen as a significant health threat.[14]

It is important to understand that the migration of large numbers of people, some of whom will live in camps, brings with it a number of problems, as well. Migrants carry diseases with them, sometimes into areas that did not previously have that disease. When Ethiopian refugees who were living in Sudan returned home, for example, they brought malaria from Sudan. Diseases can also spread faster among refugee populations than they would normally, given the large number of people living in crowded conditions, often without appropriate hygiene and sanitation. In addition, large numbers of migrants, sometimes suddenly, need care from health systems that were weak before and which may now be almost nonexistent after suffering the effects of civil conflict. Finally, one should note that many factions in civil conflicts use landmines and their health effects on individuals can be devastating.[14]

THE HEALTH BURDEN OF NATURAL DISASTERS

In the 1990s, about 62,000 people per year died on average during natural disasters. There are very few data available on the morbidity and disability associated with natural disasters. The direct and indirect health effects of natural disasters depend on the type of disaster. Earthquakes can kill many people quickly. In addition, they can cause a substantial number of injuries in a very short period of time. In the longer term, earthquake survivors face increased risks of permanent orthopedic disabilities, mental health problems, and possibly an increase in the rates of heart disease and other chronic disease. The indirect effect of earthquakes on health depends on the severity and location of the earthquake and the extent to which it damages infrastructure and forces people out of their homes.[17]

In the popular imagination, people are thought to die from the lava flows of volcanoes. In fact, this is rarely the case. About 90% of the deaths from volcanoes are due to mud and ash or from floods on denuded hillsides affected by the volcano.[18] In addition, volcanoes can harm health by displacing people, rendering water supplies unsafe, and causing mental health problems among the affected population.[18]

Tsunamis take most of their victims immediately by drowning and cause relatively few injuries, compared to the number of deaths.[18] In storms and flooding, most fatalities occur from drowning and few deaths result from trauma or wind-blown objects. These flood-related events generally lead to an increase in diarrheal disease, respiratory infections, and skin diseases. Most of these problems that relate to natural disasters are relatively short-lived, except for drought-related famine. Epidemics do not often spring up as a result of them, except in drought-related famine and when health systems are completely destroyed for long periods of time.

There are few data on the distribution by age and sex of morbidity, disability, and death related to natural disasters. It appears, however, that being very old, very young, or very sick makes one more vulnerable to disasters in which one has to flee for survival. These groups were disproportionately affected by the 1970 tidal wave in Bangladesh and the 2004 Tsunami in Asia. Whether men or women suffer the effects of a natural disaster may depend on when and where it occurs and be most related to the kind of work men or women are doing. Women, however, face considerable risks in the aftermath of natural disasters if housing has been harmed and people are living in camps, as will be discussed further later.[12]

THE HEALTH EFFECTS OF COMPLEX HUMANITARIAN EMERGENCIES

The burden of illness, disability, and death related to complex humanitarian emergencies is large and probably underestimated, given the difficulties of collecting such data. Some of the effects of these CHEs are direct. It has been estimated for, example, that between 320,000 and 420,000 people are killed each year as a direct result of these CHEs.[8] In addition, it is estimated that between 500,000 and 1 million deaths resulted from trauma during the genocide in Rwanda in 1994.[19] It is thought that about 4–13% of the deaths during CHEs in Northern Iraq, Somalia, and the Democratic Republic of Congo were the direct result of trauma.

Other illness, disability, and death, however, come about as an indirect result of the emergencies. These stem from malnutrition, the lack of safe water and sanitation, shortages of food, and breakdowns in health services. They are exacerbated by the crowded and difficult circumstances in which people have to live when they are displaced. One estimate, for example, suggested that almost 1.7 million people more died in a 22-month period of conflict in the Democratic Republic of Congo, than would have died in a "normal" 22-month period in that country.[8]

The burden of deaths related to wars is also hard to estimate. Another estimate suggests that about 200,000 people died in war in 2001 in low- and middle-income countries. Just over 10% of these deaths occurred in the South Asia Region. Almost 70% of these deaths, however, took place in Sub-Saharan Africa.[20] About 6.5 million DALYs were lost in 2001 due to war in low- and middle-income countries. That was about one third as much as was lost due to other forms of violence. It was about two thirds as much as the number of DALYs lost from all sexually transmitted diseases and about the same as those lost due to maternal sepsis or breast cancer.[20] Other estimates suggest that between 1975 and 1989 more than five million people died in civil conflicts.[21] In terms of deaths from CHEs, some of the most severely affected countries in the last two decades have been the Democratic Republic of Congo, Afghanistan, Burundi, and Angola.[8]

The data on the breakdown of deaths by age in CHEs suggests that child mortality rates early in the CHE are two to three times the rates of adults but that they slowly decline to those of the rest of the population. The data on deaths by sex are limited.[22] About 20% of the non-fatal injuries in the Bosnian conflict were among children. Almost 50% of the deaths in the Democratic Republic of Congo were among women and children younger than 15 years of age.[19] UNICEF estimates that more than 1.5 million children have been killed in war since 1980.[23] In European conflicts, the overwhelming majority of those who died have been men between 19 and 50 years of age.[19]

Causes of Death in CHEs

In the early stages of dealing with large numbers of displaced people in CHEs, most deaths occur from diarrheal diseases, respiratory infections, measles, or malaria.[19,24] Generally, diarrheal diseases are the most common cause of death in refugee situations. Major epidemics of cholera occurred in refugee camps in Malawi, Nepal, and Bangladesh, among others, and the case fatality rates from cholera have ranged from 3–30% in settings such as these. Dysentery, which refers to severe diarrhea caused by an infection in the intestine, has also commonly occurred in such situations over the last 15 years, including in camps in Malawi, Nepal, Bangladesh, and Tanzania. The case fatality rate for dysentery has been highest among the very old and very young, in whom it reaches about 10%.[19,24] In one of the most significant humanitarian crises in the last few decades, tens of thousands of Rwandan refugees poured into the Democratic Republic of Congo during the genocide in Rwanda. Between July and August 1994, 90% of the deaths among the refugees in Goma, Democratic Republic of Congo, were from cholera spread by the contamination of a lake from which the refugees got their water.[19,24]

Measles has also been a major killer in camps for displaced persons. This is especially significant in populations that are malnourished and have not been immunized against measles. The risk of a child dying of measles is increased substantially if the child is vitamin A deficient, as would be the case for many refugees. Up to 30% of the children who get measles in these situations may die from it.[24]

Malaria is also a significant contributor to death in refugee camps. This is especially the case when refugees move from countries in which there is relatively little malaria to places in which it is endemic. The risk of malaria in such cases is highest in Sub-Saharan Africa and a few parts of Asia.[24,25] Acute respiratory infections are also major causes of death in refugee camps. This is to be expected because the camps are crowded, housing is inadequate, and refugees could remain in the camps for many years. Although less common than the problems noted previously, there have also been outbreaks of meningitis in some refugee camps in areas in which that disease is prevalent, such as Malawi, Ethiopia, and Burundi. These outbreaks have generally been contained by mass immunization, as it became clear that there was a risk of epidemic.[26] However, an outbreak in Sudan in 1999 led to almost 2400 deaths.[25] Outbreaks of hepatitis E have occurred in Somalia, Ethiopia, and Kenya. These led to high case fatality rates among pregnant women, in particular.[26]

The populations that are affected by CHEs are generally poor and not well nourished, and nutritional issues are always of grave concern during CHEs, when there may also be problems of food scarcity. In addition, the relationship of infection and malnutrition also poses risks to displaced populations. In CHEs in Sub-Saharan Africa, the rates of acute protein-energy malnutrition during at least the early period of a CHE have been very high, particularly among young children. Reported rates of such malnutrition varied from around 12% among internally displaced Liberians[27] to as high as 80% among internally displaced Somalis.[25] In CHEs in Bosnia and Tajikistan, the elderly were the group that was the worst affected by acute protein-energy malnutrition.[25]

The underlying nutritional status of the refugees or internally displaced people is often poor, and micronutrient deficiencies can also be very important in CHEs. Vitamin A deficiency can be very important among these populations, given their low stores of vitamin A, the fact that some of the diseases most prevalent in camps, such as measles, further deplete the stores they have of vitamin A, and the fact that food rations in camps have historically been deficient in vitamin A. There have also been epidemics of pellagra, which is a deficiency of niacin that causes diarrhea, dermatitis, and mental disorders. One such case affected more than 18,000 Mozambican refugees in Malawi, whose rations in the camp were deficient in niacin. Scurvy, from a lack of vitamin C, has also occurred in a number of settings, such as Ethiopia, Somalia, and Sudan. Iron deficiency anemia has also been a problem in some camps and affects primarily women of childbearing age and young children. It appears that women and children who are in the camps without a male adult are at particular risk of not getting enough food in camps and of suffering acute protein-energy malnutrition and micronutrient deficiencies.[24]

Violence Against Women in CHEs

The security conditions during CHEs put women at considerable risk of sexual violence. Rape may be used as a "weapon of war." In addition, the chaos and economic distresses of conflict situations place women at risk of sexual violence and sometimes force them to "trade" sex for food or money, what people call "survival sex." Such women are often very young.

The data on sexual violence against women during CHEs are not good. However, some recent data suggest that the rates of violence against women are very high in these circumstances. A survey carried out in East Timor indicated that 23% of the women surveyed after the crisis there reported that they had been sexually assaulted. 15% of the women in Kosovo who were surveyed reported sexual violence against them during the conflict period. It is estimated that between 50,000 and 64,000 women in Sierra Leone were sexually assaulted during the conflict there, and 25% of Azerbaijani women reported sexual violence against them during a 3-month period in 2000.[28]

Mental Health

Those who study CHEs agree that they are associated with a range of social and psychological shocks to affected people due to changes in their way of living, their loss of livelihoods, damaged social networks, and physical and mental harm to them, their families, and their friends. Nonetheless, there is considerable disagreement among those working with CHEs about the validity of defining the impact on people affected by CHEs through the framework of a "Western" medical model of mental health.[29,30]

Some studies have focused on post-traumatic stress disorder (PTSD) and shown rates of prevalence for PTSD among adults that ranged from 4.6% among Burmese refugees in Thailand to 37.2% among Cambodian refugees in Thailand. The rate of post-traumatic stress disorder is about 1% in the population of the United States. Similar studies showed rates of depression in Bosnian refugees of 39%, Burmese refugees of almost 42%, and Cambodian refugees of almost 68%. By comparison, one estimate of the baseline rate of depression in the U.S. population is 6.4%.[31]

Other studies have looked at the mental health impacts of CHEs on children and the extent to which they suffer from both post-traumatic stress and depression. The studies that have been done on such populations have been small ones that can not be used to draw major conclusions on this question. However, they suggest that children who have been through conflict situations do suffer from high rates of both PTSD and depression. A survey of 170 adolescent Cambodian refugees, for example, indicated that almost 27% of them suffered from PTSD. A survey of 147 Bosnian children refugees suggested that almost 26% of them suffered from depression.[32]

It should be noted, however, that a number of those involved with the mental health impacts of CHEs believe that the stress placed by some on PTSD is not valid. Rather, they believe that while a small minority of those affected may need psychotropic medication, the most important issue is to help people as rapidly as possible to rebuild their lives and their social networks. This requires a variety of forms of social assistance and help in reuniting families, finding families a place to live, rebuilding social networks, and restoring livelihoods.[22,29,30]

ADDRESSING THE HEALTH EFFECTS OF NATURAL DISASTERS

The health effects of rapid-onset natural disasters occur in phases, starting with the immediate impact of the event and then continuing for some time until displaced people can be resettled. It is very important that the health situation be assessed immediately after the disaster has occurred. This assessment will set the basis for the initial relief effort. At the same time, care must begin of those injured in the disaster. Once the immediate trauma cases are taken care of, relief workers and health service providers can turn their attention to other injured people who are in need of early care and treatment. This would include urgent psychological problems. In the earliest stages of the disaster, some important public health functions also need to be carried out, including the establishment of continuous disease surveillance among the affected populations and provision of water, shelter, and food.[18]

Many countries do not have all of the resources needed to cope with the health impacts of the disaster, and they will depend on assistance from other countries to address their health problems. Unfortunately, there have been many instances when such help was poorly coordinated and did not effectively match the conditions on the ground. It has become clear over time, however, that to be most helpful in addressing the impact of natural disasters, external assistance will have to:

- Include all of the external partners
- Be based on a cooperative relationship among the partners
- Have partners working in ways that are complementary to each other
- Be evidence-based and transparent
- Involve the affected communities[33]

In some respects, it is easier to predict places that are at risk of natural disasters than it is to predict where CHEs will occur. There are certain countries that are vulnerable to earthquakes, volcanoes, hurricanes, typhoons, and flooding during major rains. In this light, much can be done to prepare for natural disasters and to reduce their health impact. Disaster preparedness plans can be formulated to:

- Identify vulnerabilities
- Develop scenarios of what might happen and its likelihood
- Outline the role that different actors will play in the event of an emergency
- Train first responders and managers to deal with such emergencies[34]

It is also possible when constructing water systems and hospitals, for example, to take measures that will make them less vulnerable to damage during natural disasters.

Given the way that the health impacts of natural disasters unfurl, what would be the most cost-effective ways for external partners to help in addressing the disaster? There are at least several lessons that have emerged on this front. First, although many countries send search and rescue teams to assist the victims of natural disasters, the efforts of such teams are not cost-effective. Most people who are freed from the rubble of an earthquake, for example, are saved by people in their own community immediately after the event. By the time foreign search and rescue teams arrive, most victims of falling rubble will already have been saved or will be dead. It cost about $500,000 for the United States search and rescue team to carry out its work after an earthquake in Armenia in 1988, but they were only able to save two people.[35]

It is also common that countries will send field hospitals to disaster areas. The cost of each hospital is about $1 million, and they generally arrive two to five days after the initial event. Unfortunately, by the time they arrive, they are of little value in addressing the most urgent trauma cases. It appears to be more cost-effective to have fewer field hospitals but to have a few that will remain in place for some time, in addition to building some temporary but durable buildings that can also serve as hospitals.[35]

Countries send different kinds of goods to disaster-affected places. Unfortunately, these goods can be inappropriate to the needs of the problem. This has often been the case, for example, for drugs. Better results occur when the impacted country clearly indicates what it needs and other countries send only those goods. Large camps of tents are often established after natural disasters. This is generally also not a cost-effective approach to helping the affected community to rebuild. Providing cash or building materials to affected families allows them to rebuild as quickly as possible, in a manner in line with their cultural preferences. The lack of income, even beyond the cost of rebuilding their home, can be a major impediment to the reconstruction of affected areas. Although it must be managed carefully to avoid abuse, cash assistance to families appears to be a cost-effective way of helping communities rebuild.[35]

ADDRESSING THE HEALTH EFFECTS OF COMPLEX HUMANITARIAN EMERGENCIES

It is difficult to take measures that can prevent complex humanitarian emergencies from occurring and harming human health because these emergencies so often relate to civil conflict. Thus, the key to avoiding such problems lies in the political realm and in the avoidance of conflict, rather than by taking measures that are directly health related. "Primary prevention in such circumstances, therefore, means stopping the violence."[36]

However, if such conflicts continue to occur, are there measures of "secondary prevention" that can be taken to detect health-related problems as early as possible and take actions to mitigate them? To a large extent, the early warning systems that exist for natural disasters do not exist for political disasters. Although some groups do carry out analyses of political vulnerability in countries, corruption, and the risk of political instability, these analyses are not used to prepare contingency plans for civil conflict.

Given the extent of conflict, however, it would be prudent if organizations, countries, and international bodies would cooperatively establish contingency plans for areas of likely conflict. It would also be prudent to stage near such areas the materials needed to address displacement and health problems that would occur if conflict breaks out. This would be similar to what is done for disaster preparedness in some places, such as those regularly exposed to hurricanes.[37] You read earlier that complex humanitarian emergencies are characterized by:

- Potentially massive displacement of people
- The likelihood that these displaced people will live in camps for some time
- The need in those camps for adequate shelter, safe water, sanitation, and food
- The importance of security in the camps, especially for women
- The need to address early in the crisis the potentially worst health threats, which are malnutrition, diarrhea, measles, pneumonia, and malaria
- The need to avoid other epidemic diseases, such as cholera and meningitis
- The need as one moves away from the emergency phase of a CHE to dealing with longer-term mental health issues, primary health care, TB, and some non-communicable diseases

Some of the most important measures that can be taken to address these points are discussed briefly hereafter. As you review these, it is important to keep in mind that the aim of these efforts is to establish a safe and healthy environment, treat urgent health problems and prevent epidemics, and then to address less urgent needs and establish a basis for longer-term health services among the displaced people.[38]

Assessment and Surveillance

As with natural disasters, among the first things that needs to be done during the emergency phase of a CHE is to carry out an assessment of the displaced population and establish a system for disease surveillance. Such an assessment would try to immediately gather information on the number of people who are displaced, their age and sex, their ethnic and social backgrounds, and their state of health and nutrition. Although it is difficult to get this information in the chaotic moments of an emergency, it is impossible to rationally plan services for displaced people without this information.

There are a number of health indicators that guide services in CHEs and a surveillance system needs to be established at the start of the emergency phase of a CHE. Given the difficulties of the emergency, the surveillance system must be simple but still give a robust sense of the health of the affected community. Given the importance of nutrition and the likelihood that a large part of the population will be undernourished, it is essential that the weight for height of all children younger than 5 be checked.[39] It is also important to have surveillance for diseases that cause epidemics among displaced persons, such as measles, cholera, and meningitis.

In general, the daily crude mortality rate is used as an indicator of the health of the affected group and one goal is to keep that rate below 1 death per 10,000 persons in the population per day. Where the daily rate is twice the normal rate, it signifies that a public health emergency is occurring. Say, for example, that the baseline crude mortality rate for Sub-Saharan Africa is 0.44/10,000 per day. Thus, if the rate in an affected population were to get to 0.88/10,000 per day, it would signal a public health emergency that would require urgent attention. For children younger than five years, the crude mortality rate for Sub-Saharan Africa is 1.14/10,000 per day. The goal in a public health emergency, therefore, would be to keep that rate below about 2.0/10,000 per day.[40] Death rates in a large camp are not always easy to get and sometimes people have resorted to "creative" ways of getting such data, such as daily reports by grave-diggers.

A Safe and Healthy Environment

It is critical in camps and other situations with large numbers of displaced people that efforts be made to ensure that environmental and personal hygiene are maintained. This will be the key to avoiding the potentially serious effect of diarrheal disease. It is recommended that 15 liters of water per person per day should be provided, that people should not have to walk more than 500 meters to a water source, and that people should not have to wait more than 15 minutes to get their water when they get to a source. Of the 15 liters per day that are recommended, about 2.5 to 3 liters are considered the minimum essential for drinking and food. Another 2 to 6 liters are needed for personal hygiene and the remainder is needed for cooking.[41]

Providing appropriate sanitation in situations of displaced people is also very challenging. Ideally, every family would have their own toilet. This, however, is certainly impossible in the acute phase of an emergency. The goal instead is one toilet for every 20 people. These should be segregated by sex to provide the most safety to women. They should not be more than 50 meters from dwellings, but must be carefully situated to avoid contamination of water sources.[41]

Many of the people who have been displaced will be poor people with little education and, often, poor hygiene practices. It is very important in these circumstances that efforts be made to make the community aware of the importance of good hygiene and to see that soap is available to all families and used.

Of course, people will also need shelter. The long-term goal is to help them return as quickly as possible to their homes. In the short term, if possible, the goal is to have families be sheltered temporarily with other families. Nonetheless, it is obvious from the tables shown earlier that many displaced people do end up living in camps, often for very long periods of time. When shelter is needed, the goal is to provide 3.5 square meters of covered area per person, with due attention paid in the construction of the shelter to the safety of women. Whenever possible, local and culturally appropriate building materials should be used. In the short-run, the aim is to get people into covered areas. When the emergency phase has passed, the need to enhance some of the structures can be prioritized.[42]

Food

It is suggested that each adult in a camp should get at least 2000 kilocalories of energy from food per day. Food rations should be distributed by family unit, but special care has to be taken, as noted earlier, to ensure that female-headed households and children without their families get their rations. Vitamin A should be given to all children, and the most severely malnourished children may also need urgent nutrition supplementation.[43]

Disease Control

As suggested earlier, "The primary goals of humanitarian response to disasters are to 1) prevent and reduce excess morbidity and mortality, and 2) promote a return to normalcy."[40] Along these lines, the control of communicable diseases is one of the first priorities in the emergency phase of a disaster, especially a complex humanitarian emergency.

An important priority in the emergency phase of a complex humanitarian emergency is to prevent an epidemic of measles. This starts with vaccinating all children from 6 months to 15 years. Another important priority is to ensure that children up to 5 years get vitamin A. Systems also need to be put in place so that other epidemics that sometimes occur in these situations, such as meningitis and cholera, can be detected and then urgent measures can be taken to address them. Other priorities will include the proper management of diarrhea in children and the appropriate diagnosis and treatment for malaria, in zones where that is prevalent. Of course, health education and hygiene promotion must take place continuously to try to help families prevent the onset of these diseases in the first place.[40]

Unfortunately, preventing the outbreak of communicable diseases is not the only effort that needs to be taken in the emergency phase of a CHE. Measures need to be in place to handle injuries and trauma, first to stabilize people and then to refer them to where they can receive the additional medical help they need. There will almost certainly be pregnant women among the displaced people, and there will be an immediate need for some reproductive health services. This will generally have to focus on the provision of a minimum package of care that would include safe delivery kits, precautions against the transmission of HIV, and transport and referral in case of complications of pregnancy.[40–44]

The care of non-communicable diseases will be a lower priority in emergency situations than addressing communicable diseases. However, some psychiatric problems will require urgent attention and will need to be treated as far as possible with counseling, the continuation of medicines people were taking, and the provision of new medications, if needed. As the emergency recedes, greater attention can be paid to long-term treatment, counseling, and psychosocial support for dealing with mental health problems and the many disruptions that people have faced in their lives.[31] At that time, one can also turn additional attention to ensuring the appropriate medication of people with other non-communicable diseases.

CASE STUDIES

This chapter does not contain any case studies that have been based on careful review of the evidence about specific interventions. However, some comments follow on two CHEs of importance. One concerns the genocide in Rwanda and the plight of Rwandan refugees in Goma, in what is now the Democratic Republic of Congo. The other concerns a major earthquake that hit Pakistan in 2005. Both cases suggest some lessons for enhancing the global response to CHEs in the future.

Rwanda

In mid-July 1994, nearly one million Rwandan Hutus tried to escape persecution from the newly established government of Rwanda that was led by the Tutsis. The border town of Goma, in what is now the Democratic Republic of Congo, situated in the North Kivu region, became the entry point for the majority of the refugees. Many of them settled on Lake Kivu.[45]

Almost 50,000 people died in the first month after the start of the influx, largely as a result of an epidemic of cholera, which was followed by an epidemic of bacillary dysentery. In the first 17 days of the emergency, the average crude mortality rate of Rwandans was 28.1–44.9 per 10,000 per day, compared to the 0.6 per 10,000 per day in pre-war conditions inside Rwanda. This crude mortality rate is the highest by a considerable margin over the rate found in any previous CHE. In addition, in Goma, diarrheal disease affected young children and adults alike, whereas normally young children are much more severely affected than adults.[45]

Humanitarian assessments began in the first week of August, 3 weeks after the initial flow of refugees. Rapid surveys conducted in the three refugee camps of Katale, Kibumba, and Mugunga indicated that diarrheal disease contributed to 90% of deaths, that food shortages were prevalent, especially among female-headed households, and that acute malnutrition afflicted up to 23% of the refugees. In early August, a meningitis epidemic arose.[45]

The circumstances were complicated by the large numbers of people who fled to Goma in such a short period of time. In addition, the lake represented an easy source of water, but one from which disease could be spread. The soil around Goma was very rocky and it made it very difficult to construct an appropriate number of latrines. In addition, Hutu leaders were given control over distribution of relief but this did not provide for the equitable distribution of food that was hoped for.[45]

By early August, the response of the international community was beginning to have the desired effect, under the coordination of the UNHCR. A disease surveillance network was established. An information system was set up for the camps. 5 to 10 liters of safe water per day was distributed. Measles immunization was carried out, vitamin A supplements were distributed, and disease problems were attacked using standard protocols.[45]

Despite the exceptional efforts made by many people to deal with the crisis, the events in Goma highlighted a number of shortcomings of the response. First, there was a general lack of preparedness for dealing with this type of emergency, despite the well-known political instability of Rwanda. Second, the medical teams on the ground did not have the physical infrastructure or the experience needed for a task of this magnitude. Many of these staff, for example, were not as knowledgeable about oral rehydration as they needed to be, even though this is fundamental to treating diarrheal disease. Third, the work of the military forces that joined the effort was not integrated into the planning of the other work.[45]

Although the Goma crisis was exceptional in many ways, it does suggest a number of lessons for enhancing the response to CHEs in the future. These include the need to:

- Establish early warning systems for CHEs
- Prepare in advance for CHEs
- Strengthen the existing non-governmental groups with capability to respond to CHEs

The Earthquake in Pakistan

In early October 2005, Pakistan experienced an earthquake measuring 7.6 on the Richter scale. The epicenter was in Kashmir but the earthquake also devastated the North-West Frontier Province (NWFP). Within a matter of minutes, homes and livelihoods were destroyed, leaving over 3 million people homeless and many individuals buried under the rubble or injured by debris.[46]

It is estimated that 76,000 people, many of whom were children, lost their lives either from instantaneous death, such as severe head injury or internal bleeding, rapid death, such as asphyxia due to dust, or delayed death, such as wound infections. An additional 80,000 people were injured.[46] Moreover, 84% of the infrastructure in Kashmir, including 65% of all previously existing healthcare facilities, failed to withstand the seismic forces and collapsed. Thus, the immediate needs of the population included "winterized shelter, medical care, food and water, and sanitation facilities."[46]

To respond to the earthquake, the government of Pakistan created the Federal Relief Commission (FRC) and the Earthquake Rehabilitation and Reconstruction Authority (ERRA) that offered short- and long-term recovery efforts. Furthermore, a week after the initial earthquake, the government presented a plan for relief that included compensation for survivors. The World Bank, along with the Asian Development Bank, conducted assessments to identify vulnerable groups and areas that might hinder early recovery, such as unsanitary environments. Moreover, the South Asia Earthquake Flash Appeal (SAEFA) was created to receive donations for the recovery effort.

Doctors Without Borders (MSF) was an integral part of the interventions, as it provided emergency relief within a day of the earthquake, given that MSF medical teams were already on the ground in Kashmir. These teams focused initially on hygiene promotion, distributing tents, cookware and mattresses, and treating the injured. They administered 30,000 measles vaccines and later redirected attention to rebuilding medical infrastructure. In NWFP, MSF created hospitals with beds to house patients, as well as developed medical villages that were used to treat the overwhelming number of injured.

Despite national and international efforts to mobilize an effective response, injured individuals flooded hospitals that were still intact but which did not have the personnel or the equipment to respond effectively. Thus, many patients suffered more severe secondary complications due to prolonged waiting for medical treatment, a common characteristic when earthquakes significantly affect the medical system.[46,47]

Furthermore, small, remote villages remained inaccessible because of significant road damage. Given the impending winter, therefore, the Pakistani military, MSF, and UN agencies used helicopters to distribute basic relief. In addition, the government pledged the provision of tents. People inside and outside of Pakistan responded very generously with donations to help those affected by the disaster. However, many of the donations did not fit what was most needed.[46]

Several valuable lessons emerge from the efforts of the government and military of Pakistan and Pakistan's foreign partners to assist in the rescue and recovery from the earthquake. First, buildings in rural areas in seismic zones should be built or designed to decrease human injury. Second, governments should analyze existing risks to their ability to rapidly respond to emergencies and prepare emergency plans in advance that take those risks into account. Third, donations of materials and supplies should be managed carefully so that they fit real needs. Lastly, NGO expertise, like that provided by MSF in Pakistan, can be very helpful in addressing natural disasters, particularly if the involved organizations already have a presence in the affected country.[46,47]

FUTURE CHALLENGES IN MEETING THE HEALTH NEEDS OF DISASTERS

A number of critical challenges confront efforts to address the health effects of natural disasters and complex humanitarian emergencies. One such challenge for the future is how to prevent these from having such negative health impacts. It is difficult in resource-poor settings, many of which are poorly governed, to focus attention on the prevention of disasters and their impacts. Nonetheless, through better mitigation measures, such as water control, greater education of the community about how to deal with disasters, and having a disaster preparedness plan for which people are trained, it should be possible, even for very poor countries, to reduce deaths from natural disasters. If these steps are coupled with the development of standard approaches for dealing with health issues when they do arise and the forward staging of medicines, equipment, and materials near to disaster prone areas, it should be possible to reduce deaths from natural disasters, even in very low-income settings. Bangladesh, which is subject to annual flooding, has reduced the annual deaths from such floods, for example, with a series of the previously mentioned measures.[48]

There has been considerable progress among the international community in the establishment of common standards and protocols for responses to disasters. There remains, however, the need to enhance these further. Ideally, the organizations involved in responding to natural disasters and CHEs will:

- subscribe to a common set of norms, such as the Sphere Project
- have common protocols for dealing with key issues
- train their staff to work with those protocols
- work in close conjunction with the affected communities and local governments[49]

In addition, it is important that responses to disasters focus on cost-effective approaches to the provision of healthcare services in emergencies. We have already seen that search and rescue assistance from abroad is not cost-effective. The same is true for most field hospitals. Moreover, many agencies have provided health services in emergencies that did not focus on immediate needs and that could have waited. Morbidity and mortality can be prevented and reduced more quickly if the agencies involved in disaster relief carefully set priorities for action that would be based on the principle of cost-effectiveness analysis, taking appropriate account of concerns for social justice and equity.[24,50,51]

The continued refinement of indicators that can be used to measure performance of services in disasters will be helpful to gauging the performance of local and international relief efforts.[50]

MAIN MESSAGES

Natural disasters and complex humanitarian emergencies are important causes of illness, death, and disability. They affect large numbers of people, have huge economic impact, and their aftereffects can go on for some time. Their biggest relative impact is on the poor, who are generally more vulnerable to the effects of these disasters than are better-off people. Some of these disasters are man-made. Some are slow-onset and some are rapid-onset.

Natural disasters, such as droughts, famines, hurricanes, typhoons, cyclones, and heavy rains have important health impacts. Earthquakes and volcanoes are also natural disasters with large potential effects on health. It appears that the number of natural disasters is increasing but the number of deaths from them is decreasing. More than 90% of deaths from natural disasters occur in low- and middle-income countries.

Some deaths are a direct result of natural disasters. However, the impact of those disasters on water supply and sanitation systems, health services, and availability of food can also, indirectly, lead to many more deaths. There are also special health problems associated with living in camps, which sometimes happen to those who survive natural disasters that displace many people from their homes.

In the late 1990s, there were about 40 CHEs each year. There are probably more than 14 million refugees in the world and more than 20 million internally displaced people. Overall, CHEs are associated with considerably larger health impacts than natural disasters. In addition, they may have an acute phase when large numbers of people flee and they generally go on for long periods of time.

Complex humanitarian emergencies have increasingly been linked to civil conflict. Like natural disasters, they also have direct and indirect impacts on health. They not only take lives directly through war-related trauma, but also they lead to the destruction of infrastructure. The health effects of some of these conflicts have been dramatic, sometimes because civilians have been targeted by combatants. Women are especially vulnerable in CHEs to sexual violence.

In the emergency phase of a CHE when large numbers of displaced persons are coming into camps, there are a number of health risks that have to be addressed. Among the most important are diarrhea, measles, malaria, and pneumonia. Malnutrition is also of exceptional importance. Cholera epidemics can also arise and kill large numbers of people quickly.

Countries at risk can take a number of measures to mitigate vulnerability to damage from natural disasters. This could include preparing a disaster plan, building seawalls and levees, and requiring, for example, that buildings in earthquake prone areas are earthquake proof. It might also be cost-effective to strengthen other infrastructure, such as water supply systems so that they can withstand important threats.

Addressing the health impacts of a natural disaster requires that the health situation be assessed quickly and that urgent cases be handled immediately. Less urgent problems can be handled in the following days, weeks, and months. Long-term support for those psychologically affected by the disaster will also need to be provided in the medium and long term.

The health situation of a CHE also needs to be assessed quickly and continuously. Early attention in dealing with large numbers of displaced people must focus on the environment, shelter, water, and food. The next step is the prevention of disease outbreaks and their treatment if they do occur. Particular attention must be paid to malnutrition, measles, pneumonia, and malaria. Some immediate attention will also have to be paid to a minimum package of reproductive health services and the avoidance of HIV. As the acute phase of the emergency subsides, more attention can be paid to TB, overall primary health care, non-communicable diseases, and longer-term mental health issues.

There has been some important progress in the coordination and standardization of measures to address CHEs and natural disasters. However, there are still gaps in the preparation and training of staff in some organizations. In addition, there has been inadequate attention to the cost-effectiveness of interventions. There is now enough information about the lessons of CHEs and natural disasters that the priority actions that are needed should be clear and organizations active in relief work need to concentrate their efforts on what will prevent the most deaths, disability, and morbidity, at least cost, with due attention to concerns for social justice.

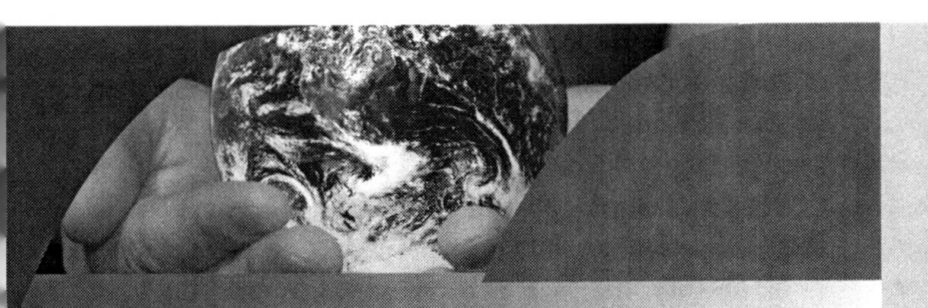

Discussion Questions

1. How does the annual burden of disease from natural disasters and complex humanitarian emergencies compare with other causes of illness, death, and disability?
2. What is a disaster? A natural disaster? A complex humanitarian emergency?
3. What is an internally displaced person? A refugee? What are the differences between them?
4. What have been some of the most significant natural disasters in the last decade? How many deaths were associated with them? How did people die? How did deaths vary for different types of disasters by age and sex?
5. What countries in Sub-Saharan Africa have been the largest sources of displaced people? What countries in Sub-Saharan Africa have received the largest numbers of refugees?
6. In the early stages of a complex humanitarian emergency, what are likely to be the most significant health concerns for the refugees? How do those health concerns change over time? Who are the most affected by malnutrition, measles, pneumonia, and cholera?
7. In what ways are women especially vulnerable during complex humanitarian emergencies? What problems do they face as a consequence of these vulnerabilities?
8. What are key steps that can be taken to reduce the vulnerability of certain places to the potential health threats of natural disasters?
9. What are key steps that need to be taken within the first few days of people fleeing to a refugee camp? How do those concerns change over time?
10. How can one try to ensure that relief agencies work together around a common framework and that they focus on the most cost-effective activities?

REFERENCES

1. National Highway Transportation Safety Authority. Glossary. Available at: Available at: http://www.nhtsa.dot.gov/people/injury/ems/emstraumasystem03/glossary.htm. Accessed September 29, 2006.

2. Pearson Prentice Hall. Glossary. Available at: http://www.nhtsa.dot.gov/people/injury/ems/emstraumasystem03/glossary.htm. Accessed September 29, 2006.

3. ILSI Risk Science Institute. Food Safety Risk Assesment. Available at: http://www.fsra.net/glossary.html. Accessed October 13, 2006.

4. Burkholder BT, Toole MJ. Evolution of complex disasters. *The Lancet.* 1995(346):1012–1015.

5. Toole MJ, Waldman RJ. The public health aspects of complex emergencies and refugee situations. *Annu Rev Public Health.* 1997;18:285.

6. Wikipedia. Refugee. Available at: http://en.wikipedia.org/wiki/Refugees. Accessed September 29, 2006.

7. Wikipedia. Internally Displaced Person. Available at: http://en.wikipedia.org/wiki/Internally_displaced_person. Accessed September 29, 2006.

8. Brennan RJ, Nandy R. Complex humanitarian emergencies: a major global health challenge. *Emerg Med (Fremantle).* 2001;13(2):149.

9. Last JM. *A Dictionary of Epidemiology.* 4th ed. New York: Oxford University Press; 2001:47.

10. The White Ribbon Alliance. Glossary: Case Fatality Rate. Available at: http://www.whiteribbonalliance.org/Resources/default.cfm?a0=Glossary. Accessed November 9, 2006.

11. de Ville de Goyet C, Zapata Marti R, Osorio C. Natural disaster mitigation and relief. In: Jamison DT, Breman JG, Measham AR, et al., eds. *Disease Control Priorities in Developing Countries.* 2nd ed. New York: Oxford University Press; 2006:1148.

12. de Ville de Goyet C, Zapata Marti R, Osorio C. Natural disaster mitigation and relief. In: Jamison DT, Breman JG, Measham AR, et al., eds. *Disease Control Priorities in Developing Countries.* 2nd ed. New York: Oxford University Press; 2006:1149.

13. Brennan RJ, Nandy R. Complex humanitarian emergencies: a major global health challenge. *Emerg Med (Fremantle).* 2001;13(2):149–150.

14. Hansch S, Burkholder B. When chaos reigns. *Harvard Int Rev.* 1996;18(4):10–14.

15. Brennan RJ, Nandy R. Complex humanitarian emergencies: a major global health challenge. *Emerg Med (Fremantle).* 2001;13(2):148–149.

16. Toole MJ, Waldman RJ. The public health aspects of complex emergencies and refugee situations. *Annu Rev Public Health.* 1997;18:283–312.

17. de Ville de Goyet C, Zapata Marti R, Osorio C. Natural disaster mitigation and relief. In: Jamison DT, Breman JG, Measham AR, et al., eds. *Disease Control Priorities in Developing Countries.* 2nd ed. New York: Oxford University Press; 2006:1149–1150.

18. de Ville de Goyet C, Zapata Marti R, Osorio C. Natural disaster mitigation and relief. In: Jamison DT, Breman JG, Measham AR, et al., eds. *Disease Control Priorities in Developing Countries.* 2nd ed. New York: Oxford University Press; 2006:1150.

19. Brennan RJ, Nandy R. Complex humanitarian emergencies: a major global health challenge. *Emerg Med (Fremantle).* 2001;13(2):151.

20. Lopez AD, Mathers CD, Murray CJL. The burden of disease and mortality by condition: data, methods, and results for 2001. In: Lopez AD, Mathers CD, Ezzati M, Jamison DT, Murray CJL, eds. *Global burden of disease and risk factors.* New York: Oxford University Press; 2006:45–240.

21. Zwi AB, Ugalde A. Political violence in the Third World: a public health issue. *Health Policy Plan.* 1991;6:203–217.

22. Personal communication, Waldman RJ to Skolnik R, March 2007.

23. UN Children's Fund. *The State of the World's Children.* New York: United Nations; 1994.

24. Waldman RJ. Prioritising health care in complex emergencies. *Lancet.* 2001;357(9266):1427–1429.

25. Brennan RJ, Nandy R. Complex humanitarian emergencies: a major global health challenge. *Emerg Med (Fremantle).* 2001;13(2):152.

26. Toole MJ, Waldman RJ. The public health aspects of complex emergencies and refugee situations. *Annu Rev Public Health.* 1997;18:295.

27. Toole MJ, Waldman RJ. The public health aspects of complex emergencies and refugee situations. *Annu Rev Public Health.* 1997;18:297.

28. Marsh M, Purdin S, Navani S. Addressing sexual violence in humanitarian emergencies. *Global Public Health.* 2006;1(2):138.

29. Ager A. Psychosocial needs in complex emergencies. *Lancet.* 2003;360:43–44.

30. Almedom A, Summerfield D. Mental well-being in settings of complex emergency: an overview. *JBiosocial Sci.* 2004;36:381–388.

31. Mollica RF, Cardozo BL, Osofsky HJ, Raphael B, Ager A, Salama P. Mental health in complex emergencies. *Lancet.* 2004;364(9450):2058–2067.

32. Mollica RF, Cardozo BL, Osofsky HJ, Raphael B, Ager A, Salama P. Mental health in complex emergencies. *Lancet.* 2004;364(9450):2061.

33. de Ville de Goyet C, Zapata Marti R, Osorio C. Natural disaster mitigation and relief. In: Jamison DT, Breman JG, Measham AR, et al., eds. *Disease Control Priorities in Developing Countries.* 2nd ed. New York: Oxford University Press; 2006:1154.

34. de Ville de Goyet C, Zapata Marti R, Osorio C. Natural disaster mitigation and relief. In: Jamison DT, Breman JG, Measham AR, et al., eds. *Disease Control Priorities in Developing Countries.* 2nd ed. New York: Oxford University Press; 2006:1155.

35. de Ville de Goyet C, Zapata Marti R, Osorio C. Natural disaster mitigation and relief. In: Jamison DT, Breman JG, Measham AR, et al., eds. *Disease Control Priorities in Developing Countries.* 2nd ed. New York: Oxford University Press; 2006:1157.

36. Toole MJ, Waldman RJ. The public health aspects of complex emergencies and refugee situations. *Annu Rev Public Health.* 1997;18:300.

37. Toole MJ, Waldman RJ. The public health aspects of complex emergencies and refugee situations. *Annu Rev Public Health.* 1997;18:302.

38. Brennan RJ, Nandy R. Complex humanitarian emergencies: a major global health challenge. *Emerg Med (Fremantle).* 2001;13(2):153.

39. Toole MJ, Waldman RJ. The public health aspects of complex emergencies and refugee situations. *Annu Rev Public Health.* 1997;18:296.

40. The Sphere Project. Minimum standards in health services. *The Sphere Handbook 2004: Humanitarian Charter and Minimum Standards in Disaster Response.* Geneva: Oxfam Publishing; 2004:249–312.

41. The Sphere Project. Minimum standards in water supply, sanitation, and hygiene promotion. *The Sphere Handbook 2004: Humanitarian Charter and Minimum Standards in Disaster Response.* Geneva: Oxfam Publishing; 2004:51–102.

42. The Sphere Project. Minimum standards in shelter, settlements, and non-food items. *The Sphere Handbook 2004: Humanitarian Charter and Minimum Standards in Disaster Response.* Geneva: Oxfam Publishing; 2004:203–248.

43. Toole MJ, Waldman RJ. The public health aspects of complex emergencies and refugee situations. *Annu Rev Public Health.* 1997;18:303–304.

44. Krasue SK, Meyers JL, Friedlander E. Improving the availability of emergency obstetric care in conflict-afffected settings. *Global Public Health.* 2006;1(3):229–248.

45. Goma Epidemiology Group. Public health impact of Rwandan refugee crisis: what happened in Goma, Zaire, in July 1994? *Lancet.* 1995 1995;345(8946):339–344.

46. Medicins Sans Frontieres. South Asian Earthquake: 6-month Overview of MSF Operations MSF Response to the Disaster. Available at: http://www.doctorswithoutborders.org/news/2006/04-21-2006.cfm. Accessed February 25, 2007.

47. Noji EK. Earthquakes. In: Noji EK, ed. *The Public Health Consequences of Disasters.* New York: Oxford University Press; 1997.

48. ICDDRB Center for Health and Population Research. Documenting effects of the July–August floods of 2004 and ICDDR,B's response. *Health Sci Bulletin.* 2004;2(3).

49. The Sphere Project. *The Sphere Handbook 2004: Humanitarian Charter and Minimum Standards in Disaster Response.* Geneva: Oxfam Publishing; 2004.

50. Spiegel P, Sheik M, Gotway-Crawford C, Salama P. Health programmes and policies associated with decreased mortality in displaced people in postemergency phase camps: a retrospective study. *Lancet.* 2002;360(9349):1927–1934.

51. de Ville de Goyet C, Zapata Marti R, Osorio C. Natural disaster mitigation and relief. In: Jamison DT, Breman JG, Measham AR, et al., eds. *Disease Control Priorities in Developing Countries.* 2nd ed. New York: Oxford University Press; 2006:1147–1162.

CHAPTER 11

Working Together to Improve Global Health

LEARNING OBJECTIVES

By the end of this chapter the reader will be able to:

- Discuss the value of cooperation in addressing health problems
- Discuss the most important types of cooperative action in global health
- Describe the major organizational actors in global health and their focuses
- Discuss the rationale for the creation of public-private partnerships for health
- Outline the key challenges to enhancing cooperative action in global health

VIGNETTES

The world came close to eradicating polio in 2004. However, in 2005, polio spread from Northern Nigeria to a number of other African countries, due to a failure to immunize children in Northern Nigeria by some groups. By July 2005, polio cases had moved from Africa to Saudi Arabia and Indonesia, and then began appearing in Angola, which had not had a case of polio since 2001. By September 2005, cases appeared in Somalia, which had also been free of polio for several years.[1] Stopping new cases of polio and preventing it from spreading from one country to another requires a global effort to correctly identify polio cases and then immediately carry out special immunization campaigns.

About nine million people worldwide suffer from tuberculosis, which is one of the leading causes of deaths of adults in the developing world. The number of TB cases worldwide has grown with the spread of HIV, and 13% of the deaths of people with AIDS are due to TB.[2] Despite the importance of TB, however, no new drugs for TB have been developed since the 1960s.[3] TB is a disease that largely affects poor people in low- and middle-income countries. These people have little money to spend on drugs and there is minimal economic incentive for pharmaceutical companies to develop new TB drugs. Can actors in global health work together to encourage the development of new drugs for TB and other neglected diseases? What would they have to do to encourage public and private sector investment in such drugs? What would they have to do to ensure investors that if they are able to develop such drugs that there will be a market for them?

Vaccines are among the most cost-effective investments in health. For young children in the developing countries, there are six basic vaccines. There are also other vaccines that would be cost-effective in some countries, including the vaccines for hepatitis B and for Haemophilus influenza type B. Yet, throughout the 1990s there were important gaps in coverage of the six basic vaccines in the poorest countries. In addition, the rate of coverage was actually going down in some countries.[4] Although the hepatitis B vaccine began to be widely used in developed countries in the 1980s, almost 20 years later it is still rarely used in developing countries. The main reasons behind this failure include limited money for immunization, a lack of the infrastructure needed to carry out effective immunization programs, and a lack of political interest in immunization. In 2000, a number of governments, foundations, and individuals established the Global Alliance for Vaccines and Immunization (GAVI), the aim of which is to provide financing and technical assistance to dramatically improve vaccine coverage and the spread of new vaccines. So far, GAVI has been involved in enhancing immunization coverage in a number of low-income countries.[5]

INTRODUCTION

This chapter focuses on how different actors work together to enhance global health. First, it discusses the importance of such cooperation. The chapter then has an extensive review of the key organizational actors in global health activities. Third, the chapter examines the roles in cooperation of different types of organizations. The chapter then outlines how the global health agenda is set and how that agenda has evolved historically. The chapter concludes with an assessment of some of the future challenges to cooperative action and a case study on one of the most successful global health efforts to date.

COOPERATING TO IMPROVE GLOBAL HEALTH[6,7]

There are a number of reasons why different actors cooperate in global health activities and why such cooperation is in everyone's interest. First is the value of cooperating to create consensus around and advocate on behalf of different health causes.[6,7] Although health is an extremely important issue for both individuals and societies, it does not always receive the political, economic, and financial support that it should. A good example of this is the lack of attention by many countries to nutrition, despite the poor nutritional status of their people. The impact of advocacy efforts is likely to be much greater if numerous actors, across organizations and across countries, work together to promote important health causes. This has been evident in the field of HIV, for example, where AIDS activists worldwide have been able to work together to promote the treatment of people who are HIV-positive with anti-retroviral drugs.

The need to share knowledge and to set global standards for health activities are other reasons for cooperation in the global health field. It has become clear from trials of different anti-malarial drugs, for example, that some drug regimens for malaria are more effective than others. This knowledge is especially important because some malaria has become resistant to what has been standard treatment. If lessons like this are to be shared globally, then it is important that technical standards be developed and disseminated by an organization that countries believe is technically sound and internationally representative. As you will read later, helping to define and promulgate such standards is one of the main functions of the World Health Organization.

Another important reason for cooperation to achieve global health aims is the fact that many aspects of global health are "global public goods." Thus, it is only through cooperative efforts that the world can ensure that a sufficient amount of these goods are produced and shared. Individual countries, for example, may not have an interest in reducing pollution generated within their borders that causes health problems in adjacent countries, and it is only through collective action that countries will be able to address such problems. A similar issue arises with respect to efforts to reduce the burden of communicable diseases. Individual countries may have little incentive to take the measures needed to effectively address some communicable diseases, despite the fact that the spread of these diseases does not respect national boundaries. Efforts to deal with them, therefore, require cooperative efforts across countries.

The surveillance of disease also has many aspects of a "global public good" and requires cooperation among many actors to be successful. It is important for all countries to work together to monitor the appearance of diseases and to fashion approaches to dealing with them. Surveillance by individual countries, for example, is not sufficient to stem the spread of disease *across* countries. The global effort to address the SARS problem in 2003 is an excellent example of the need for close collaboration among countries on surveillance.[8]

Cooperation to achieve better global health outcomes can also take place to assist in financing health efforts in poorer countries. There are multiple motivations for this aid. In one case, wealthier countries may contribute out of humanitarian concern for the well being of less fortunate people. Richer countries may also wish to assist in addressing these problems because of "enlightened self-interest." In an age of travel and extensive contacts among people of different countries, governments may be concerned that the health problems of developing countries will endanger their own people if not properly tackled. Many low-income countries, for example, have high burdens of TB but may not have the financial, technical, or institutional resources needed to combat TB effectively. Yet, TB can endanger both their population and that of other countries. Thus, it is in everyone's interest for developed countries to provide financial and technical assistance to developing countries to deal effectively with diseases such as TB.

KEY ACTORS IN GLOBAL HEALTH

Besides governments, there are many different actors involved in global health activities. Some of these are international organizations with a global reach. Others are organizations that work globally but are based in individual countries. Some are public organizations. A number are private and for profit, while others are private but operate on a not-for-profit basis. Foundations are also actively involved in global health activities. Increasingly, there are also organizations that bring the public and private sectors together to work cooperatively on a global health problem. The next section discusses some of the most important organizations that are involved in global health and examples of how they operate in that field.

In considering action on global health, it is valuable to remember that actors may play one or more of several possible roles at a time. They could, for example, engage in advocacy. They could also participate in knowledge sharing and technical assistance. In addition, they might provide financing for health efforts. Table 11-1 lists some of the most important actors in the global health field.

The discussion further examines the nature of these actors and their major contribution to the global health agenda. You should note, however, that this discussion is only introductory. It is meant to outline the stated aims in global health of those organizations. It is beyond the scope of this book to examine such work critically. Considerable information is available for those of you wishing to examine global health actors and cooperation in this field more analytically.[9–12]

Agencies of the United Nations

There are a number of United Nations (UN) agencies that work on health and focus on a specific set of public health concerns. Among the most important are the World Health Organization, the United Nations Children's Fund, the United Nations Fund for Population Activities, and the United Nations Development Program. This section will examine the two UN agencies most involved in health, the World Health Organization and the United Nations Children's Fund.

The World Health Organization

The World Health Organization (WHO) was established in 1948 and is the United Nations agency that is responsible for health.[13] The headquarters of WHO is located in Geneva, Switzerland, and WHO employs about 3500 people, including experts on many health topics. The World Health Organization has offices located in each region of the world,

TABLE 11-1 Selected Organizational Actors in Global Health, by Type of Organization

United Nations Agencies	**WHO Related Partnerships**
UNAIDS	Global Alliance for the Elimination of Leprosy
UNDP	Roll Back Malaria
UNFPA	Stop TB
UNICEF	Tropical Disease Research Program
WHO	
	Non-Governmental Organizations
Multilateral Development Banks	CARE
African Development Bank	Catholic Relief Services
Asian Development Bank	Doctors Without Borders
Inter-American Development Bank	OXFAM
World Bank	Save the Children
Bilateral Development Assistance Agencies	**Other Special Programs**
Australian Agency for International Development	Global Alliance for Vaccines & Immunization
Canadian International Development Agency	Global Fund to Fight Against AIDS, TB, & Malaria
Danish International Development Agency	
Department for International Development of the UK	**Public-Private Partnerships for Health**
Dutch Agency for Development Cooperation	Global Alliance for TB Drug Development
United States Agency for International Development	International AIDS Vaccine Initiative
	International Partnership on Microbicides
Foundations	Malaria Vaccine Initiative
The Bill & Melinda Gates Foundation	
The Rockefeller Foundation	

Source: The Author

with special responsibility for work within that geographic area, as shown in Table 11-2. In addition, WHO has a country office in almost all poor countries and in many other countries in which important health efforts or reforms of the health sector are taking place.[13]

The objective of WHO is to promote "the attainment by all peoples of the highest possible level of health."[13] In pursuit of this goal, WHO largely focuses its attention on the following:

- Advocacy and consensus building for various health causes, such as HIV and TB.
- Sharing health knowledge across countries, through studies, reports, conferences, and other forums. The publication of the *World Health Report* on a different topic of global health importance each year is an example of this work.
- Carrying out selected critical public health functions within an international forum, such as the surveillance of epidemics, including influenza, or the outbreak of potentially dangerous diseases, such as Ebola. This also includes, for example, WHO certification of quality standards for the manufacturing of vaccines and pharmaceuticals.
- Setting global standards on key health matters, such as appropriate regimens for drug therapy for leprosy, TB, and HIV.
- Leading the development of international agreements and conventions, such as the Framework Convention on Tobacco Control.
- The provision of technical assistance to its member states, such as helping China to contain the outbreak of SARS or assistance to countries in managing their child vaccine programs.
- Serving as the secretariat of a number of cooperative efforts, such as Stop TB, Roll Back Malaria, and the Global Alliance to Eliminate Leprosy.

TABLE 11-2 WHO Regional Offices

Regional Office	Location
The Americas	Washington, DC, USA
Europe	Copenhagen, Denmark
North Africa and the Middle East	Alexandria, Egypt
Sub-Saharan Africa	Harare, Zimbabwe
Southeast Asia	Delhi, India
Western Pacific	Manila, Philippines

Source: Data from World Health Organization. About WHO. Available at: http://www.who.int/about/en/. Accessed on November 3, 2006.

WHO is primarily a technical agency that engages in advocacy and the sharing of knowledge. Although WHO does have relatively small country budgets to assist in the financing of selected health projects in low- and middle-income countries, it is not a financing agency. Rather, the work that WHO does both globally and in particular countries is largely financed with assistance from the high-income countries.

WHO is governed through its annual World Health Assembly, which sets policy, reviews and approves the budget, and appoints the Director-General of the organization. Voting power at the WHO Health Assembly is based on the principle of "one country–one vote." The overall budget of WHO comes from membership subscriptions and from special donations, again, mostly from better-off countries.

The WHO has helped lead some of the world's most important cooperative efforts in health, including the "Health for All" effort[14] that began with the Declaration of Alma Ata on primary health care. WHO also led the world's smallpox eradication campaign, has played a major role in efforts to expand the coverage of immunization for children in developing countries, and is one of the leaders of the world's global polio eradication program. More recently, WHO has been instrumental in helping to address issues of tobacco control. WHO also leads the global surveillance of disease and has played an active role in work on avian flu, SARS, and other new and emerging diseases, such as the Ebola virus. Additional, more analytical, comments on the work of WHO are cited in the endnotes.[10,11,15,16]

UNICEF

The United Nations Children's Fund was established in 1946 by the UN to respond to the effects of World War II on children in Europe and China. UNICEF is headquartered in New York but has offices in more than 125 countries.[17] The main function of UNICEF is to enhance the health and well being of children. In these efforts, UNICEF has been deeply involved in the promotion of family planning, antenatal care, and safe motherhood practices.

UNICEF is involved in a wide range of activities in support of its mission, including advocacy, knowledge generation and knowledge sharing, and the financing of investments in health. In addition, UNICEF works closely with other development partners such as WHO and the World Bank to help raise the health status of poor women and children globally. UNICEF has carried out significant programs in a number of areas. Traditionally, it has been involved in major ways in nutrition and early childhood development issues, in which it is generally considered the world's leader. Immunization and child survival have also been areas of deep UNICEF involvement. In addition, UNICEF has been a major supporter of primary education, especially for poor girls in low- and middle-income countries. More recently, UNICEF has paid particular attention to child protection, child rights, and HIV/AIDS.[18]

UNICEF has an Executive Board of 36 members who guide all UNICEF work and administration under the leadership of the Executive Director. All of UNICEF's funding is from voluntary contributions; governments provide two thirds of funding while 37 National Committees, consisting of private entities and millions of individuals, raise the remaining third. These National Committees are non-governmental organizations (NGOs) that advocate for children, sell UNICEF products, and fundraise through several well known campaigns, such as "Check out for Children" in grocery stores, "Change for Good" on airplanes, and "Trick or Treat for UNICEF" on Halloween.[19]

UNAIDS

In 1996, six agencies joined forces to launch UNAIDS—the Joint United Nations Program on HIV/AIDS. Today, as shown in Table 11-3, there are 10 co-sponsors for UNAIDS.[20]

UNAIDS is based in Geneva, Switzerland, has offices in more than 70 countries, and is guided by a Program Coordinating Board that consists of 22 representatives from country governments, its co-sponsors, and 5 NGOs.

UNAIDS is the global agency with primary responsibility for dealing with HIV/AIDS. UNAIDS monitors and evaluates the epidemic and the world's response to it. It also advocates on behalf of the epidemic and engages civil society, the private sector, and development partners in the fight against HIV/AIDS. In addition, UNAIDS generates and shares knowledge, sets standards, and mobilizes resources. UNAIDS focuses it attention on the regions of the world most affected by HIV/AIDS, particularly Sub-Saharan Africa.[21]

Another important emphasis of the work of UNAIDS is to assist countries in developing and implementing national AIDS plans. The co-sponsors financially support the preparation of these plans. For instance, in 2002 the World Bank and other UN agencies provided over $1 billion to assist countries with the development and implementation of their national AIDS plans.[22,23] Technical experts from UNAIDS also help countries build their technical and institutional capacity and mobilize resources to fight against HIV/AIDS. UNAIDS, for example, assists countries in preparing applications for funding from the Global Fund to Fight Against AIDS, TB, and Malaria, which is discussed further later.[21]

TABLE 11-3 UNAIDS Co-Sponsors

- International Labor Organization
- Office of the United Nations High Commissioner for Refugees
- UNICEF
- United Nations Development Program
- United Nations Educational, Scientific, and Cultural Organization
- United Nations Population Fund
- United Nations Office on Drugs and Crime
- World Bank
- World Food Program
- World Health Organization

Source: UNAIDS. Available at: http://www.unaids.org/en/AboutUNAIDS/Cosponsors_about/default.asp. Accessed November 3, 2006.

UNAIDS is engaged in a range of HIV/AIDS activities. First, UNAIDS works with countries to strengthen their surveillance of the epidemic. Second, UNAIDS continues to put an important emphasis on prevention of HIV. Third, UNAIDS is also increasingly involved in efforts to increase the number of HIV-positive people worldwide who are treated with anti-retroviral therapy. UNAIDS has a particular concern for the extent to which the epidemic affects females. In addition, UNAIDS cooperates with others in the search for technologies, such as microbicides and vaccines, that might be able to help halt the epidemic.

Multilateral Development Banks

There are a number of development banks that lend or grant money to developing countries and economies in transition to help promote their economic and social development. These banks are owned by all of their member countries and they are referred to as "multilateral." These institutions have some characteristics of real banks. However, these banks do not function to earn money through their lending operations. Rather, their main focus is to serve as a financial intermediary. Essentially, they channel financial resources from more developed countries and their people through bond sales and grants to help finance development activities in low- and middle-income countries and countries that are making the transition to more open, market-based, economies. All of these banks are involved in work on health, to at least some degree, but the ones most involved are the African Development Bank, the Asian Development Bank, the Inter-American Development Bank, and the World Bank.

Among the multilateral development banks, the World Bank is the largest, has the broadest scope of activities, and is the most involved in health.[24] The World Bank is located in Washington, DC, and is "owned" by more than 180 member countries. The stated aim of the World Bank is to assist countries in improving the lives of their people and reducing poverty. It seeks to do this by helping them to strengthen the management of their economy and to finance investments in selected areas, including agriculture, transport, private sector development, health, and education. The World Bank lends money at reduced rates to countries with per capita incomes above a certain point, lends money interest free to the poorest countries, and also provides grants to some countries for special activities that affect the poor, such as HIV/AIDS. The Bank lends about $20 billion per year and has more than 10,000 staff who work in Washington and in the Bank's offices in a large number of other countries that receive development assistance from the World Bank.[25]

In its health work, the Bank carries out a wide range of functions. It advocates on behalf of important causes, generates and disseminates information and knowledge about key health issues, provides technical assistance to countries, and finances specific investments in health and related work in nutrition and family planning. The World Bank focuses its health work largely on the links between health and poverty. It pays considerable attention to the development of health systems. In public health, the Bank has emphasized nutrition, maternal and child health, HIV/AIDS, malaria, TB, and tobacco control.

The Bank is also a partner in a number of global health initiatives, including GAVI, Stop TB, Roll Back Malaria, and UNAIDS. In addition, the World Bank has provided financing to other initiatives, such as the International AIDS Vaccine Initiative (IAVI). The Bank over the last few years has provided about $15 billion of financing for its health related work[26] and, until the advent of the Bill & Melinda Gates Foundation, it has been the largest financier of investments in health in resource poor settings. Those interested in a more analytical assessment of the World Bank's work both generally and in health can consult extensive literature on those subjects.

TABLE 11-4 Selected Bilateral Development Assistance Agencies Involved in Global Health

Australian Agency for International Development
Canadian International Development Agency
Danish International Development Agency
Department for International Development of the United Kingdom
Dutch Agency for Development Cooperation
United States Agency for International Development

Source: The Author

Bilateral Agencies

Another set of organizations that are very actively involved in global health are bilateral agencies. These are mostly the development assistance agencies of developed countries that work directly with developing countries to help them enhance the health of their people. Some of the bilateral development agencies that are most involved in the health sector are shown in Table 11-4.

USAID is the development assistance agency of the U.S. federal government. USAID promotes U.S. foreign policy goals by advancing economic and social development all over the world. USAID works with other governments and with universities, businesses, international agencies, and NGOs to support its development assistance efforts. In the health field, USAID engages in a wide variety of activities, including advocacy for global health, the generation and sharing of knowledge, and the financing of health investments.

USAID is headquartered in Washington, DC, and has regional field offices for Sub-Saharan Africa, Asia and the Near East, Latin America and the Caribbean, and Europe and Eurasia. In addition to these geographic bureaus, USAID has functional bureaus for Economic Growth, Agriculture and Trade, Democracy, Conflict Prevention and Humanitarian Assistance, and Global Health. USAID has offices in many countries, especially poorer countries in Africa, Asia, and Latin America.

USAID's Bureau for Global Health aims to improve health services and enhance the health status of poor and disadvantaged people, particularly in poorer countries. USAID focuses its health work on maternal and child health, HIV/AIDS, other communicable diseases, family planning and reproductive health, nutrition, and health systems. For these purposes, USAID provides grants and technical expertise to other governments, NGOs, and the private sector. In supporting the development of health in other countries, USAID collaborates with other development assistance agencies.[27]

In the 1970s and 1980s, USAID helped support research to develop a number of interventions that are key to saving the lives of poor children in the poorer countries, including oral rehydration therapy, vitamin A supplementation, and immunizations. USAID has also been very supportive of efforts to address malaria, TB, and, most recently, HIV/AIDS. Traditionally, USAID has also been very involved in supporting family planning.

Foundations

Global health has been an area in which foundations have been involved for more than a century. The Rockefeller Foundation[28] and the Ford Foundation[29] have been among the most involved in this field. More recently, the Soros Foundation became involved in health activities in the former Soviet Union. The Soros Foundation[30] focuses largely on the promotion of democracy but became involved in health when it realized the threat that HIV, TB, and drug-resistant TB posed to political and economic stability in this region. Most recently, the Bill & Melinda Gates Foundation has emerged as an extremely important actor in the field of global health. The section below examines the role in global health played by the Rockefeller Foundation, which has historically been the most important foundation involved in health, and the Gates Foundation, which has recently taken the lead in a number of global health areas.

The Rockefeller Foundation

The Rockefeller Foundation is based in New York City and has regional offices in San Francisco, California, Bangkok, Thailand, and Nairobi, Kenya. The foundation aims to "enrich and sustain the lives and livelihoods of poor and excluded people throughout the world."[24] In the health field, the foundation seeks to "reduce avoidable unfair differences in the health status of populations."[28]

The Rockefeller Foundation has focused considerable attention on the development of knowledge and technology that can be applied to addressing the conditions that most affect the health of the poor globally. The Rockefeller Foundation was instrumental in establishing the first schools of public health in the United States and was also deeply involved in the development of a vaccine against yellow fever. The Rockefeller Foundation does finance a small amount of activities in health every year. However, its strength as an organization is the way in which it uses a relatively small amount of money to invest in the generation of knowledge that can make an important difference to the health of the poor globally.

More recently, the Rockefeller Foundation has focused it attention in the health field in three areas. First, the foundation established the framework for developing partnerships between the public and private sector to meet key health needs that had been neglected. In line with this work, the foundation was instrumental in establishing the first and then a number of additional public-private partnerships for health, including the International AIDS Vaccine Initiative, the International Partnership on Microbicides, and the Global Alliance for TB Drug Development. Second, it has tried to help better understand the problems that HIV/AIDS inflicts on families and how they might deal with those problems. Third, the foundation has helped to "strengthen the production, deployment, and empowerment" of key human resources needed for delivering health services in poor countries.[28]

The Bill & Melinda Gates Foundation

The most substantial change in many years in the key actors involved in global health has been the advent of the Bill & Melinda Gates Foundation. The Gates Foundation is based in the United States in Seattle, Washington. The main aims of the foundation in the health field are to help spread known technologies for improving health, such as immunization, to the places where they are most in need. At the same time, the foundation seeks to encourage the development of new technologies that can meet the major health needs of the poor globally. The foundation hopes to meet these aims by "supporting discoveries and inventions essential to solving major global health problems, supporting the development and testing of specific tools and technologies, and helping to ensure that new health interventions and technologies are adopted in the developing world."[31] The foundation has become one of the major financiers of global health efforts. The foundation has an endowment of over $30 billion and it will grow to almost $60 billion with pledged gifts from an American financier.[32] From its establishment in 2002 to 2005, the foundation had provided almost $3.6 billion in grants for health activities.[31]

To a large extent, the foundation has focused its grants in four areas. First, it has paid particular attention to communicable diseases, since they are such an important cause of death for the poor globally. In these areas, it has been particularly involved in financing efforts in AIDS, TB, and malaria. It has supported with major grants, for example, the establishment of AIDS initiatives in Africa and in India, the Global Fund to Fight Against AIDS, TB, and Malaria, the International AIDS Vaccine Initiative, and the International Partnership on Microbicides. Another important area for the foundation is reproductive health, for which it granted $60 million to the Johns Hopkins University to improve reproductive health programs globally.[33] The foundation has also been a major financier of a variety of partnerships and initiatives aimed at key global health problems, including the Vaccine Fund and GAVI to support immunizations, the Global Alliance for Improved Nutrition (GAIN), and an initiative to save the lives of very young children called "Saving Newborn Lives." The foundation gave $750 million to the Vaccine Fund alone. Finally, the foundation has placed major emphasis on encouraging scientific discoveries and their application to the health problems of the poor globally through its program on the "Grand Challenges in Global Health," for which it has provided more than $400 million.[32]

NON-GOVERNMENTAL ORGANIZATIONS

There are thousands of NGOs in the world today that have as one of their primary aims the improvement of the health of poor people in developing countries. Most of these organizations raise money from private sources or receive grants from governments or global health partnerships which they help to invest in activities that address important health issues, such as improving the availability of clean water, strengthening nutrition and immunization programs, or enhancing programs for the treatment of TB and HIV. Some of the organizations are small and focus their attention only on a limited number of activities. Other organizations are very large, comprehensive in the topics they cover, and global in their reach. Some NGOs will be completely secular, while others will be faith-based. Some of the most important NGOs that operate internationally on health are listed in Table 11-5.

Some additional comments are noted later on Save the Children and Doctors Without Borders, which are two of the most important NGOs that work on health globally. These are just two examples of the hundreds of large NGOs and thousands of small NGOs that are involved in health efforts in low- and middle-income countries.

TABLE 11-5 Selected Non-Governmental Organizations Involved in Global Health

CARE
Catholic Relief Services
Christian Children's Fund
Doctors Without Borders
OXFAM
Partners in Health
Save the Children
World Vision

Source: The Author

Save the Children

Save the Children was established in 1932 in New York City by a group of people who wanted to help meet the needs of poor people in the Appalachian region of the United States who had been hurt by an economic depression. Today, it is part of an international alliance of related organizations and it one of the largest NGOs in the world. One affiliate of Save the Children is based in the United States in Westport, Connecticut. It is actively involved in relief and development work in a number of areas in health. Save the Children focuses its attention on working with poor families and communities to identify their most important health and development needs. It then addresses these needs in ways that seek to contribute to individual and community self-sufficiency.[34]

Save the Children (U.S.) is involved in efforts to improve health in more than 30 countries, focusing on community-based efforts for poor and disadvantaged people. The health work of Save the Children also pays particular attention to the survival and well being of newborns and children, reproductive health, and HIV/AIDS. "Saving Newborn Lives," as noted earlier, is an initiative of Save the Children that is financed with the assistance of the Bill & Melinda Gates Foundation. This effort tries to identify and disseminate simple approaches to preventing deaths among newborn children.[35] Save the Children is also deeply involved in nutrition through food relief, enhancing agricultural production, and specific investments in nutrition education and food and micronutrient supplementation.

Doctors Without Borders

Doctors Without Borders was founded in 1971 and is based in Brussels, Belgium. It is an umbrella organization made up of affiliated groups in 18 countries.[36] The groups located in Belgium, France, Holland, Spain, and Switzerland carry out health work in more than 80 countries. Doctors Without Borders, usually referred to by its French name, Medicins Sans Frontieres, or by the abbreviation of that name MSF, is best known for its work in humanitarian crises. It has often been involved in the provision of health services following natural disasters, such as earthquakes and hurricanes, or those humanitarian emergencies related to war and famine.[37] MSF, for example, assisted Nicaragua after an earthquake, Ethiopia during a famine, and Somalia after a war. MSF has also been engaged intensively in health services for refugees and displaced people. In addition, when health services have been severely weakened due to war or conflict, MSF often helps to provide health services temporarily, while trying to help rebuild health system capacity. One example of this was in Liberia after its civil war.

MSF is also well known for its commitment to political independence, medical ethics, and human rights. Related to this, MSF has increasingly sought to become a voice in international health policy arenas for the disenfranchised. More recently, MSF has also become very involved with prevention, care, and treatment for HIV/AIDS. In this work, MSF has helped to mobilize international support for antiretroviral therapy in poor countries and has become a leader in trying to lower the price of those drugs.[37]

PARTNERSHIPS RELATED TO WHO

Some global health problems affect an exceptional number of people in a large number of countries. The costs of addressing these problems are great and the skills needed to combat them are substantial. Most of the resource poor countries can not tackle these problems without aid and no individual development partner can provide enough assistance to help deal effectively with the scale of these problems. Therefore, a number of organizations have decided to work together to help address some of the most important burdens of disease. Some of the partnerships that have ensued are closely related to WHO, as noted in Table 11-6. Two of the most important such partnerships are Stop TB and Roll Back Malaria.

TABLE 11-6 Selected WHO-Related Partnerships for Global Health

Global Alliance for the Elimination of Leprosy
Global Polio Eradication Campaign
Lymphatic Filariasis Control Program
Roll Back Malaria
Stop TB
Tropical Disease Research Program

Source: The Author

Stop TB

The Global Partnership to Stop TB was established in 2000. It aims to "eliminate TB as a public health problem, and ultimately, to obtain a world free of TB."[38] Stop TB is comprised of a wide array of partners including countries, development agencies, private sector organizations, and NGOs. WHO plays a prominent role in Stop TB, and the secretariat for the partnership is housed at WHO headquarters in Geneva, Switzerland. The primary goal of Stop TB is to ensure that 70% of the people in the world with TB will be diagnosed, that 85% of them will be cured, and that by 2015 the burden of TB disease will be cut in half. The partnership tries to encourage the wider use of effective TB strategies, such as DOTS, including those for dealing with HIV/TB co-infection and drug-resistant TB. It also works to promote the development of new TB diagnostics, drugs, and vaccines. Stop TB engages in advocacy, technical assistance, and helps to mobilize funding for the fight against TB.[2]

Roll Back Malaria

Roll Back Malaria was founded in 1998 by WHO, UNICEF, and the World Bank to advocate for malaria control, to promote the development of better approaches and technologies for malaria containment, and to help finance and spread appropriate malaria control and treatment.[39] The partnership has expanded since then to include a variety of public and private actors in a number of countries. In these activities, they promote appropriate prevention and treatment of malaria. In addition, Roll Back Malaria has established a Malaria Medicines and Supplies Service. This aims at helping resource poor countries better organize and manage the procurement of supplies and medicines needed to manage effective malaria control.[40]

OTHER PARTNERSHIPS AND SPECIAL PROGRAMS

In the last decade, global partners have expressed considerable concern over a number of health issues that affect the poor. One has been the need to strengthen immunization programs for children and for pregnant women. Related to this has been a growing interest in trying to more quickly increase the use of several "newer vaccines" that have been used for some time in better-off countries but have only rarely been provided in poorer countries. In addition to this, there has been a growing fear that the pace of progress against HIV, TB, and malaria has been insufficient and that urgent and bold measures need to be taken to move more forcefully against these diseases. To address immunization more effectively, the Global Alliance for Vaccines and Immunization (GAVI) was established. The Global Fund to Fight Against AIDS, TB, and Malaria ("The Global Fund") was established to make more rapid progress against HIV, TB, and malaria.

GAVI

GAVI is a partnership among public and private sector organizations that was established in 2000.[4] The founding partners of GAVI include WHO, UNICEF, and the World Bank. GAVI is based in Geneva, Switzerland. The Bill & Melinda Gates Foundation made a major grant to help establish GAVI and provide for its operations. The main aims of GAVI are to improve the ability of health systems to carry out immunization; raise rates of coverage in low-income countries of key vaccines; promote more rapid uptake of underused vaccines, such as hepatitis B, Haemophilus influenzae type B, and yellow fever; speed up the development of other vaccines of importance; and help countries ensure that vaccines are given safely.[41] GAVI has tried to improve global health work through two innovative approaches. The first is to tie its financing to the achievement of goals that are agreed to by the countries that are being helped. The second is to work closely with countries to develop plans to sustain the investments that are being supported. GAVI is an organization that advocates for the importance of immunization, provides technical assistance to countries to enhance their immunization efforts, and finances those efforts.

The Global Fund

The Global Fund to Fight Against AIDS, TB, and Malaria was also established in 2002 and is based in Geneva, Switzerland.[42] The driving force behind the establishment of the Fund was increasing global concern about HIV and a growing recognition among development partners that measures to address the AIDS epidemic had been insufficient. Interest in establishing the Fund was also heightened by the growing attention to global health discussed hereafter, and a special concern for the exceptional burden of HIV, TB, and malaria, especially in Africa.[43]

The Global Fund is a partnership of the public and private sectors and WHO, UNAIDS, and the World Bank are also key partners. The Fund is governed by a Board of Directors that represents governments, international organizations, civil society, and communities affected by AIDS, TB, and malaria. The fund is financed by grants that come largely from developed country governments, but which also come from the private and foundation sector, including the Bill & Melinda Gates Foundation.

The Global Fund is primarily a financing agency but it also engages in advocacy for global health and the three diseases on which it focuses. The main aim of the Fund is to finance proposed investments in these diseases, with an emphasis on AIDS and Africa. It has a particular interest in helping to scale up programs for anti-retroviral therapy against HIV. The Fund has taken innovative approaches to a number of aspects of development assistance for health, including the following:

- It is strictly a financing mechanism and not a technical or implementing agency.
- It seeks to raise funds for investments that will be additional to other funding already available.
- It tries to work on the basis of a national plan that is developed by a group representing diverse national interests, for the use of Global Fund financing.
- It evaluates proposals through an independent review process.
- It tries to operate in a performance-based manner by supporting investments that are meeting their targets and reducing or eliminating support for programs that are not meeting their aims.[42]

In its first two rounds of funding, the Global Fund committed about $1.5 billion to support 154 programs in 93 countries.[44]

Public–Private Partnerships

As interest in global health rose in the mid-1990s, many of the actors in this field increasingly believed that the mechanisms for developing, manufacturing, and distributing new vaccines, drugs, diagnostics, and medical devices needed to alleviate key global health problems were not sufficient. They noted with growing concern, for example, that the vaccine for TB was over 100 years old and that no new TB drugs had been developed for decades. They saw insufficient attention to the development of vaccines against HIV and malaria in both the public and the private sector and fewer firms willing to engage in vaccine development. They also understood that private pharmaceutical firms did not see a profitable market in the development of low-cost diagnostics, vaccines, drugs, or medical devices that could address the major killers of the poor globally. They knew that without changes in the way the market for these products worked that private sector firms would remain on the sidelines.

In the face of these issues, the Rockefeller Foundation encouraged key global health actors to think creatively about how they could spur the more rapid development of products that could attack global health problems in a low cost but effective way. One idea that emerged from this was the notion of organizations that would combine the strengths of public and private organizations in a common quest for better health. They would also seek broader sources of financing for these health ventures; try to tackle intellectual property issues that constrained the availability of affordable diagnostics, drugs, medical devices, and vaccines in poor countries; and see how they could encourage more private sector involvement in the search for these products. In some respects, they were conceived of as venture capital firms that would have a social goal, rather than a goal that was mostly aimed at maximizing profit. Today, there is a wide array of "public–private partnerships for health," or "PPPs," as they are called. The aim of many of these is to develop new products and these are often called Product Development

Partnerships. Some of the most important of such partnerships are noted in Table 11-7.

IAVI

Two of the more interesting public-private partnerships for health are the International AIDS Vaccine Initiative (IAVI) and the Institute for One World Health. IAVI was established as a not-for-profit corporation in 1996. It is based in New York City but operates globally and has activities in more than 20 countries. IAVI has three main objectives: to advocate for AIDS vaccines, to help develop programs and policies that would encourage the use of an AIDS vaccine if one were developed, and to engage in research and development of candidate AIDS vaccines.[45] IAVI works with a number of scientific partners under agreements to ensure that if any of the partners does develop an AIDS vaccine with IAVI support, the vaccine "would be made available in developing countries at reasonable prices, would be available in sufficient quantities, and would be made available as soon as it is licensed as safe and effective."[46] IAVI has received financial support from a number of governments; from some private companies, such as Becton Dickinson and Co. (BD); the Rockefeller Foundation; the World Bank; and the Bill & Melinda Gates Foundation.

Institute for One World Health

The Institute for One World Health was founded in the United States in San Francisco, California, in 2000 and is similar in many ways to IAVI.[47] The main aims of this not-for-profit pharmaceutical company are to identify "promising drug development opportunities; take responsibility for shepherding those leads through the complex development process; and, enable the development of drugs that can help to address the diseases that disproportionately affect developing countries."[48] The Institute works in collaboration with a number of universities, hospitals, industry, government, and NGOs. The Institute has received funding from a number of foundations, including the Bill & Melinda Gates Foundation. "By partnering and collaborating with industry and researchers, by securing donated intellectual property, and by utilizing the scientific and intellectual capacity of the developing world," One World Health hopes to deliver "affordable, effective, and appropriate new medicines where they are needed most."[48] The Institute has focused primarily on visceral leishmaniasis, diarrheal disease, malaria, and Chagas disease.[48]

Pharmaceutical Firms

In the last decade, international pharmaceutical firms have also engaged in partnerships to try to improve global health at low cost. This has generally been done in one of three ways. First, some firms donate drugs to global health programs. Novartis, for example, donates leprosy drugs to the Global Alliance to Eliminate leprosy, and today no country needs to purchase such drugs.[49] Pfizer and the Edna McConnell Clark Foundation work with the International Trachoma Initiative by donating an antibiotic, azithromycin, to its efforts to reduce trachoma related blindness.[50] Merck donates Ivermectin to the Onchocerciasis Control Program that has been successful in reducing river blindness in Africa.[51] These are only some of the many donation efforts now underway.

In addition, a number of drug companies, including Abbott, Boehringer Ingelheim, Bristol Myers Squibb, Gilead, GSK, and Merck, have agreed to sell anti-retroviral drugs for HIV at greatly discounted prices to developing countries affected by the AIDS epidemic. Some of the drug companies also sponsor programs to address diseases such as HIV in particular countries, such as Merck's support for the national HIV/AIDS control program in Botswana.[52]

The role of the major drug companies in global health is a subject of considerable controversy. There is a serious concern in some members of the global health community, for example, that the approach of the branded drug manufacturers to patents raises the price of drugs beyond what people in low-income countries can afford. Some people also believe that the major manufacturers should be far more generous than they have been in offering their drugs at reduced prices in low- and middle-income countries. Others have expressed concern that these manufacturers have not been open enough in licensing their products to other companies in a way that would reduce their prices in the developing world. The role of pharmaceutical firms in global health is very important, complicated, and controversial and goes considerably beyond the scope of this book.

TABLE 11-7 Selected Public-Private Partnerships for Public Health

Global Alliance for TB Drug Development
International AIDS Vaccine Initiative
International Partnership on Microbicides
Malaria Vaccine Initiative
Medicines for Malaria Venture

Source: The Author

TRENDS IN GLOBAL HEALTH EFFORTS

The notion of cooperating to improve health globally is not a new one. Rather, different countries have realized for more than 100 years that many health problems could not be solved by individual countries and had to be addressed through collective action across countries.

In the ensuing period, in fact, many actors have cooperated in a variety of health activities. This section examines how the themes of those efforts varied over time. The threat of cholera, for example, led to the first international conference on health in 1851.[53] Numerous international conferences on health followed that and by 1903, the world created The International Commission on Epidemics.[54] In 1909, the International Office of Public Hygiene was set up in Paris and this was followed by the establishment of the League of Nations Health Office in 1920 in Geneva, Switzerland. The International Sanitary Bureau was set up in 1924. The Rockefeller Foundation assisted in financing and providing technical support to the League of Nations Health Office. The early international organizations for health focused their efforts on the surveillance of disease, the provision of global standards for drugs and vaccines, and selected technical advice to countries on key health matters, including medical education.[55]

International efforts in health took a substantial leap forward with the establishment of the United Nations agencies after World War II, including WHO and UNICEF. In the 40 years since then there have been a number of areas of focus for international cooperation on health, as noted hereafter.[15,56,57] Following the establishment of WHO, efforts at international cooperation in health shifted to focus on helping to build capacity for global public health efforts, for health systems development in countries that were newly independent, and in working together to fight disease. Perhaps the greatest single effort at global cooperation in health began in 1966 with the start of the global program to eradicate smallpox. During this period of intensive attention to specific diseases, WHO also led work to combat malaria and other communicable diseases that most affected the poor, such as leprosy,[58] lymphatic filariasis,[59] and onchocerciasis.[60,61]

Historically, another important area of focus for global cooperation has been family planning. Much of the early work on family planning was led by the United States. Over time, the focus on family planning shifted from one that was centered almost exclusively on limiting family size to an approach that centered much more on reproductive health. This shift was encouraged by and reflected in a series of global conferences on family planning, safe motherhood, reproductive health, and women starting in 1974 in Bucharest, Romania.[62] The 1987 conference on women in Nairobi, Kenya, for example, was used to launch the Safe Motherhood Initiative.[57]

In 1978, the world launched a major effort when it enacted the Alma Ata declaration on primary health care, as mentioned earlier. This declaration noted that health was a fundamental human right and that countries had the obligation to ensure that all people had access to appropriate primary health care. The Alma Ata declaration heralded a new global focus on primary health care and on the health needs of the poor. It also led to much greater attention to the needs for health systems that could deliver primary care and to the importance of taking a community-based approach to the health needs of poor people. The Alma Ata Declaration was linked to the world's efforts to achieve what was called globally "Health for all by the Year 2000."[63]

An immense amount of attention has also been paid to "Child Survival." These efforts focused on what were called the GOBI interventions: growth monitoring, oral rehydration, breast feeding, and immunization. UNICEF was the leader of this effort. USAID was also instrumentally involved in child survival activities, which ultimately became an important focus of attention for the World Bank, WHO, and a variety of bilateral organizations.[64]

As the world moved into the late 1980s and early 1990s, considerable concern arose that despite more than 30 years of global efforts to improve the health of the poor, the unfinished agenda remained very large. Many of those working on health believed that some of the weaknesses stemmed from an approach to health that was too disjointed and that needed to be better grounded in a more systemic view of health that would focus on trying to improve health services more broadly. This led to considerable work being done on "health sector reform." At the same time, the *1993 World Development Report* of the World Bank articulated the need to take an approach to decision making on health investments that would be grounded in cost-effectiveness analysis.[65] This framework for analysis soon became the foundation for actions of a number of key actors in global health.

At about the same time, much greater attention began to be paid, even in low-income countries, to the role of the private sector in health. Development partners also created around this time new ways of working together cooperatively within individual countries. Increasingly, for example, development partners would cooperate and jointly help countries to develop and finance investments in health. In much of the work done prior to this period, many development partners worked individually with a country, often leading to a lack of coordination across that country's health sector efforts.

Toward the mid-1990s, the global health community began to pay considerably more attention to HIV, as well as to other major killers of the poor in resource poor countries, including malaria and TB. Particular attention has been paid to reducing the cost of AIDS drugs and getting more people treated, raising case finding and cure rates for TB by expanding coverage with DOTS, and strengthening malaria control programs through the use of insecticide-treated bed nets, intermittent treatment of pregnant women, and greater use of artemisinin-based combination therapy. There has also been an enormous increase in cooperation through the many health partnerships that have been formed, as noted earlier in the chapter.

SETTING THE GLOBAL HEALTH AGENDA

As we think about how different actors cooperate in global health activities and the themes on which they focus, it is important to consider how global health policies get established. The next section comments briefly on how the overall global health agenda and the agenda for particular global health topics are set. This is another topic that is quite complicated and often the subject of controversy that readers may wish to explore further.

One important activity in setting global health priorities is the World Health Assembly of the World Health Organization.[66] Once each year, ministers of health of WHO member countries meet in Geneva, Switzerland, to consider important global health matters and resolutions proclaiming their interest in and commitment to addressing key health issues. The World Health Assembly has been the foundation for some of the most important global health efforts undertaken, such as the smallpox eradication campaign.

Some important developments in global health have been encouraged by writings, advocacy efforts, and program activities of WHO, multilateral or bilateral development assistance agencies, and some of the important NGOs involved in health. The *1993 World Development Report* of the World Bank focused on health and was widely read and debated around the world. This document set the basis for the next generation of World Bank-assisted health projects in many countries and for important work done by other development organizations and countries in health, as well. Given the importance of World Bank assistance for health to so many countries, the approaches suggested in the *1993 World Development Report* had a major impact on the world's thinking about health in developing countries.

Movement in the policy agenda for global health can also follow significant investments by development partners. This has clearly been the case, for example, as a result of the substantial funds that the Bill & Melinda Gates Foundation has provided to selected global health activities. As noted earlier, the Gates Foundation has focused considerable attention on improving and disseminating technology for improving the health of the poor, as well as selected investments in key health problems, such as HIV. The investments the Gates Foundation has made, for example, in immunization and in the development of AIDS vaccines has considerably raised the world's attention to these matters and placed them more firmly on the global health agenda.

Popular action, often led by NGOs or other advocates for health, can also influence the setting of the global health agenda. In the late 1990s, for example, Professor Jeff Sachs, then of Harvard University, began to be actively involved in speaking and writing about the importance of health to economic and social development. His work attracted attention to health issues and led to considerable international engagement and action on the health of poor people globally. At about the same time, some important NGOs, such as Doctors Without Borders, became major advocates for AIDS treatment and the reduction of the prices of AIDS drugs. Through their advocacy work and efforts to treat people with anti-retroviral drugs, they attracted considerable attention to these topics and had a major impact on the way the world approached them.

Another good example of how an NGO affected the global health agenda is the impact of Partners in Health, an NGO based in the city of Boston in the United States, on the global agenda for TB and for HIV. Largely led by the work of Dr. Paul Farmer and Dr. Jim Kim of Harvard University, Partners in Health tried to develop in Peru and Haiti a model of how one could treat drug-resistant TB and then HIV at an acceptable cost and in a sustainable way. At the time, the prevailing opinion globally was that drugs for these conditions were so expensive that they could not be treated in resource poor settings. The work of Partners in Health helped to shift global efforts toward finding ways to make treatment affordable for all people.[67]

In other respects, one can think of efforts to set the global health agenda as a kind of ongoing meeting around a negotiating table at which important actors in global health are sitting. The organizations most involved in such discussions will generally be WHO, UNICEF, and the World Bank. Selected bilateral development agencies will also participate, such as USAID, the Department for International Development of the UK, and often the Canadian International Development Agency and the Dutch Development Agency, while AUSAID plays a unique role in some of Asia in the Pacific. Given the importance of AIDS in many ways, UNAIDS is also often involved. The Gates Foundation, the Rockefeller Foundation, and selected NGOs might also be involved. Some other NGOs, such as MSF, may not be present, but through advocacy they do bring their interests to the policy-setting group.

The way in which the agenda is set for specific health topics will be similar to those mentioned previously, but will usually also include actors who have particular interests in the topic at hand. WHO and the World Bank will almost always be involved. The key bilateral agencies will also participate. In addition, the agencies working with the topic under discussion and groups representing people affected by particular conditions increasingly also have inputs to these discussions. If TB is being discussed, for example, then the key NGOs working globally with TB will be involved, as will the TB programs from representative countries. If leprosy is being discussed, then the leprosy programs of some countries will be involved, NGOs working in leprosy will be involved, and groups of people affected by leprosy will also be involved.

FUTURE CHALLENGES

There are a number of challenges to effective collaborative action in global health. First, the types of health conditions that the world faces may change and new conditions might develop. Smallpox was once a disease of considerable importance, as was polio. Smallpox was eradicated, and there are very few cases of polio in the world today. In recent years, however, there have been outbreaks of new and emerging diseases, such as Ebola, the avian flu, and SARS. It is possible that there will be a major epidemic of influenza and that other new and emerging diseases will appear in the future. The world will have to be ready, through collaborative efforts, to carry out surveillance, prevention, and treatment of those diseases.

Second, it will be very important for development partners to work together to help countries strengthen their health systems, as well as to try to combat individual diseases. If countries are to be able to meet their most important health needs in a sustainable manner in the future, then they must have health systems that work. In most low-income countries, this will require better management, more appropriate forms of organization, sounder systems for key public health functions, better trained staff at all levels, and a consistent manner of providing financing for health system needs, while helping to cover the costs of health care for the truly poor. Achieving these aims is not as attractive politically as fighting a specific disease or health problem. Yet, in the long run, a systems approach must be taken to developing health services and different global health actors will have to work together to achieve this, since they are usually only involved in working with a part of the health system of any country.

Another set of future challenges concerns the need to ensure that actors in global health work together to address the knowledge gaps that prevent sufficient progress against health conditions that cause people to be sick too often and to die prematurely, especially poor people in low-income countries. There will continue to be an important need, for example, for increasing our knowledge of the basic science concerning many diseases, including AIDS, TB, and malaria. It will not be possible to develop preventive vaccines for these diseases or better treatment for them, without significant improvements in scientific knowledge. There will also be a need for operational research in global health so that we can learn more about what approaches are effective and efficient. What is the best way, for example, to ensure that people take all of their drugs for HIV or TB? How should a health system in a developing country be organized to ensure that it can operate in a cost-efficient way, while paying sufficient attention to the poor? These questions can only be answered through the generation and sharing of knowledge and experience globally, a process dependent upon cooperation and coordination.

The factors that have encouraged the development of public-private partnerships for health will also continue to challenge the global health community. There are many such partnerships now and it will be very important to learn as quickly as possible which aspects of these partnerships encourage product development in effective and efficient ways and which ones do not. It is also necessary to continue to encourage the development of new and innovative approaches to enabling the development of new diagnostics, vaccines, and therapies that can be affordable in low- and middle-income countries. If any of the public-private partnerships are successful in developing new products, then it will be essential that efforts turn to ensuring that they are used quickly where they are most needed.

The financial needs for addressing global health concerns are very considerable and will continue to have a prominent place on the global health agenda. The multilateral development banks, the bilateral aid agencies, and special programs such as The Global Fund need continuous financing. In addition, some of the important initiatives that have been started, such as the considerable push for treatment against HIV, can not be sustained without many years of additional financing by rich countries, foundations, the private sector, and their partners. The amount of money that is spent on global health is much less than is spent on defense globally. Yet, there are still many risks that donors will develop "aid fatigue" and not have the political will necessary to continue financing global health efforts at the level needed.

It will be important that any development financing for health be as effective as possible. Although the topic of development effectiveness is considerably beyond the scope of this book, Table 11-8 summarizes some of the factors most closely associated with the success of development assistance in health.

There are also a number of important challenges to the way that actors in global health cooperate to assist countries in investing in the health sector. In recent years, development assistance agencies have increasingly tried to cooperate closely in their aid work on specific countries. However, there are always tendencies in development agencies to act independently rather than in coordination with other agencies. Although we should expect these tensions to continue, it is important if development assistance in health is to be effective that agencies work increasingly in a cooperative fashion.

Finally, it will be very important that good leadership in the global health field continues. Different agencies will need to work together in ways that address the challenges noted earlier. New groups and organizations need to join the community of global health actors to continue to inspire innovative and efficient methods of addressing and financing global health needs.

TABLE 11-8 Factors Associated with Positive Outcomes in Development Assistance

- Strong leadership in the host government and in the development partner agencies
- Close collaboration among governments, donors, and non-governmental organizations in the design and implementation of the program
- Household and community participation in the design, implementation, and monitoring of programs
- Simple and flexible technologies and approaches that can be adapted to local conditions and do not require complex skills to operate and maintain
- Approaches that help to strengthen health systems, especially human resources for health
- Consistent, predictable funding

Source: Adapted with permission from The World Bank. Hecht RM, Shah R. Recent trends and innovations in development assistance in health. In: Jamison DT, Breman JG, Measham AR, et al., eds. *Disease Control Priorities in Developing Countries.* 2nd ed. New York: Oxford University Press 2006:246.

CASE STUDY

It is fitting that one of the last chapters of the book should include a case study of the successful effort to eliminate onchocerciasis in Africa. This case study complements a discussion of the integrated provision of drugs to treat onchocerciasis and vitamin A. More detailed information on this case is available in *Case Studies in Global Health: Millions Saved.*

Background

Onchocerciasis, or river blindness, is a pernicious disease afflicting approximately 18 million people worldwide. More than 99% of its victims are in Sub-Saharan Africa. In the most endemic areas, over a third of the adult population is blind, and infection often approaches 90%.[68] In 11 West African countries in 1974, nearly 2.5 million of the area's 30 million inhabitants were infected with onchocerciasis, and approximately 100,000 were blind. The remaining 19 endemic countries in central and east Africa were home to 60 million people at risk of the disease.

The Intervention

Onchocerciasis is caused by a worm called *Onchocerca volvulus* which enters its human victim through the bite of an infected blackfly. The flies breed in fast-moving waters in fertile riverside regions. Once inside a human, the tiny worm grows to a length of one to two feet and produces millions of microscopic offspring called microfilarie. The constant movement of the microfilarie through the infected person's skin causes torturous itching, lesions, muscle pain, and, in severe cases, blindness. Fertile land is often abandoned for fear of the disease.

Early efforts to control the disease proved ineffective because blackflies cover long distances and cross national borders, rendering unilateral efforts ineffective. An international conference in Tunisia in 1968 concluded that onchocerciasis could not be controlled without regional collaboration and long-term funding of at least 20 years to break the life cycle of the worm. World Bank President Robert McNamara's tour of drought-stricken West Africa in 1972 served as a catalyst to progress. Moved by seeing communities where nearly all the adults were blind and were led by children, McNamara decided to spearhead an international effort against onchocerciasis.[68]

The Onchocerciasis Control Program (OCP), the World Bank's first large-scale health program, was launched in 1974 in conjunction with the WHO, the UN Food and Agriculture Organization (FAO), and UNDP. The program included a significant research budget and set out to eliminate onchocerciasis in 7, and eventually in 11, West African countries.[69] Breeding grounds of blackflies were sprayed with larvicide, and the spraying program was able to persist even through regional conflicts and coups. In the 1980s, a Merck drug called Ivermectin was included as a powerful new weapon against the disease, a single dose of which could effectively paralyze the tiny worms for up to a full year.[70] The drug proved popular because it quickly reduced uncomfortable symptoms and provided protection against other parasites. Merck donated Ivermectin and Dr. William Foege of the Carter Center managed its distribution.

The African Programme for Onchocerciasis Control (APOC) was established in 1995 as a broad international partnership to control the disease throughout Africa and to carry onchocerciasis control to 19 countries in East and Central Africa. These were countries in which long distances and thick forests made spraying difficult. APOC pioneered a system of Community-Directed Treatment with Ivermectin (ComDT) to ensure local participation, reach remote villages, and maintain distribution of the drug after donor funding expires in 2010.[71] ComDT workers are often the only health personnel to reach distant villages, and their access could be used for other health interventions in the future.

The Impact

By 2002, OCP halted transmission of onchocerciasis in 11 West African countries, preventing 600,000 cases of blindness, and protecting 18 million children born in the OCP area from the risk of the disease. About 25 million hectares of arable land—enough to feed an additional 17 million people—is now safe for resettlement.[72] APOC is expanding this success to central and east Africa, where 40,000 cases of blindness are expected to be prevented each year.

Costs and Benefits

OCP operated with an annual cost of less than $1 per protected person. Total commitments from 22 donors amounted to $560 million. The annual return on investment, due mainly to increased agricultural output, was 20%, and it is estimated that $3.7 billion will be generated from improved labor and agricultural productivity.[73] APOC coverage cost even less, at just 11 cents per person. The economic rate of return for the program is 17% for the years 1996 to 2017, and it is estimated that 27 healthy life days will be added per dollar invested.[74]

Lessons Learned

Success in controlling onchocerciasis could not have been attained without a genuinely shared vision among all partners in the program. Commitment among the African governments was critical to coordinating a regional effort across national borders. Long-term commitments from donors, along with Merck's decision to donate Ivermectin indefinitely, were essential elements for the program's sustainability. The participation of a wide range of organizations, such as multilateral institutions, private companies, and local NGOs, allowed for a cost-effective and efficient intervention. The ComDT framework, by emphasizing local ownership and participation, proved a cost-effective and self-sustaining means of delivering drugs to remote populations. The onchocerciasis program proved that effective aid programs, implemented with transparency and accountability, can deliver lasting results.

MAIN MESSAGES

It is very important that key actors work together to address global health problems because they may have effects that go beyond one country, they may be expensive to deal with, and they may require technical and managerial resources larger than some poorer countries can bring to bear on their own. In addition, it is very important that there be global standards in some health fields and these standards need to be broadly developed and widely accepted. Good examples of areas in which it is imperative that different actors work together globally would include efforts to carry out disease surveillance, the global fight for polio eradication, and the standards for some disease control programs, such as TB.

There are many actors in global health and among the most actively involved are WHO, UNICEF, UNAIDS, and the World Bank. Most high-income countries have development assistance organizations and they often play important roles in global health, such as USAID, AUSAID, and DFID. A number of foundations are also deeply involved in global health work and the Bill & Melinda Gates Foundation has become a major actor in global health since the late 1990s. Many NGOs are also very involved in global health efforts and Doctors Without Borders is among the best known of these. These organizations play one of several roles, singly or all together, including advocacy, knowledge generation, technical assistance, or financing.

A relatively new form of organization was created specifically to deal with difficult global health problems, called public-private partnerships for health. These organizations include, among others, the International AIDS Vaccine Initiative and the International Partnership on Microbicides. Essentially, they try to combine the skills and financing of public and private sector organizations, in order to advocate for specific health issues, develop new vaccines, diagnostics, or drugs, and ensure that what they develop will be appropriate to the health needs of poor countries and affordable to them, as well. Some other new organizations, such as GAVI and the Global Fund were established to try to dramatically increase the pace of immunizing children and combating AIDS, TB, and malaria.

The global health community is likely to face many challenges that will continue to require collective action by global health actors. Some of the key challenges will include filling key gaps in knowledge and encouraging public and private sector organizations to develop the diagnostics, vaccines, and drugs needed to address the most important global health issues. They will also include the need for organizations to work together to strengthen health systems, to combat individual diseases, and to try to ensure that critical global health needs have adequate financing.

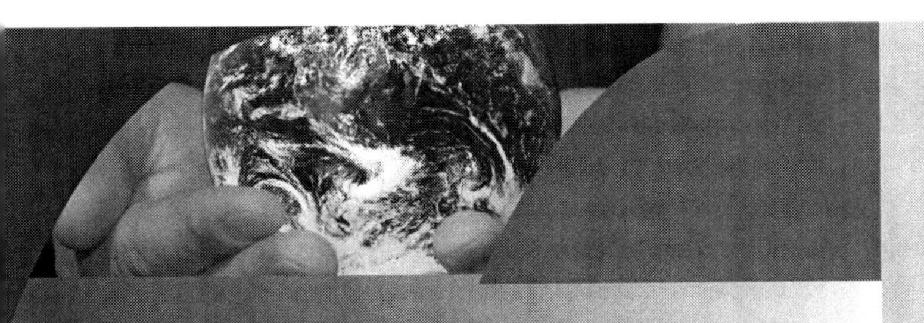

Discussion Questions

1. What are the most important organizations that work on global health issues?
2. What functions do these organizations play?
3. Why is it important that different actors cooperate to address global health concerns?
4. Name some of the most important successes of cooperative action on global health.
5. What were some of the key factors that led to those successes?
6. What are the lessons of these successes for future global health efforts?
7. What are some of the future challenges that demand continued or strengthened collaboration in global public health?
8. What is a public-private partnership for health and why might they be valuable?
9. Why is cooperative action needed to address problems like onchocerciasis and Guinea worm?
10. How might the world raise the money needed to further address problems like HIV and the need for drug treatment against AIDS?

REFERENCES

1. UNICEF. Polio experts warn of largest epidemic in recent years, as polio hits Darfur: Epidemiologists "alarmed" by continuing spread of virus —warn thousands of children could be paralyzed across west and central Africa. *Joint Press Release.* Available at: http://www.unicef.org/media/media_21872.html. Accessed July 12, 2006.

2. World Health Organization. Tuberculosis: Fact sheet No 104. Available at: http://www.who.int/mediacentre/factsheets/fs104/en/. Accessed July 12, 2006.

3. Global Alliance for TB Drug Development. No R&D in 30 Years. Available at: http://www.tballiance.org/2_3_C_NoRandDin30Years.asp. Accessed July 12, 2006.

4. The GAVI Alliance. GAVI Alliance for Vaccines and Immunization. Available at: http://www.gavialliance.org/. Accessed July 5, 2006.

5. The GAVI Alliance. General Principles for Use of GAVI/Vaccine Fund Resources. Available at: http://www.gavialliance.org/General_Information/About_alliance/GAVI/Principles.php. Accessed July 12, 2006.

6. Merson MH, Black RE, Mills AJ. *International Public Health: Diseases, Programs, Systems, and Policies.* Gaithersburg, MD: Aspen Publishers; 2001.

7. Lele U, Ridker R, Upadhyay J. Health System Capacities in Developing Countries and Global Health Initiatives on Communicable Diseases. Available at: http://www.umalele.org/content/view/85/109/. Accessed July 12, 2006.

8. Heymann DL, Rodier G. Global surveillance, national surveillance, and SARS. *Emerg Infect Dis.* Feb 2004;10(2):173–175.

9. Walt G. Global Cooperation in International Public Health. In: Merson MH, Black RE, Mills AJ, eds. *International Public Health.* Gaithersburg, Maryland: Aspen Publishers; 2001:667–669.

10. Basch P. *Textbook of International Health.* 2nd ed. New York: Oxford University Press; 2001:486–509.

11. Basch P. *Textbook of International Health.* 2nd ed. New York: Oxford University Press; 2001:42–72.

12. Kickbusch I, Buse K. Global influences and global responses: international health at the turn of the twenty-first centery. In: Merson MH, Black RE, Mills AJ, eds. *International Public Health.* Gaithersburg, MD: Aspen Publishers; 2001:701–733.

13. World Health Organization. About WHO. Available at: http://www.who.int/about/en/. Accessed July 12, 2006.

14. World Health Organization. Declaration on Occupational Health for All. Available at: http://www.who.int/occupational_health/publications/declaration/en/index.html. Accessed July 12, 2006.

15. Merson MH, Black RE, Mills AJ. *International Public Health: Diseases, Programs, Systems, and Policies.* Gaithersburg, MD: Aspen Publishers; 2000:667–669.

16. Merson MH, Black RE, Mills AJ. *International Public Health: Diseases, Programs, Systems, and Policies.* Gaithersburg, MD: Aspen Publishers; 2000:701–733.

17. UNICEF. The Structure of UNICEF. Available at: http://www.unicef.org/about/structure/index.html. Accessed July 12, 2006.

18. UNICEF. What We Do. Available at: http://www.unicef.org/whatwedo/index.html. Accessed July 12, 2006.

19. UNICEF. Support UNICEF. Available at: http://www.unicef.org/support/14884.html. Accessed July 12, 2006.

20. Joint United Nations Programme on HIV/AIDS. Cosponsors. Available at: http://www.unaids.org/en/Cosponsors/default.asp. Accessed July 12, 2006.

21. Joint United Nations Programme on HIV/AIDS. Focus Areas. Available at: http://www.unaids.org/en/Coordination/FocusAreas/default.asp. Accessed July 12, 2006.

22. UNAIDS. United Nations Joint Programme on HIV/AIDS. Available at: http://www.unaids.org/en/. Accessed July 5, 2006.

23. The World Bank. *World Bank Annual Report 2002.* Washington, DC: The World Bank; 2002.

24. Health, Nutrition, & Population. Available at: http://www.worldbank.org/html/extdr/hnp/hnp.htm. Accessed July 6, 2006.

25. World Bank. Working for a World Free of Poverty. Available at: http://siteresources.worldbank.org/EXTABOUTUS/Resources/wbgroupbrochure-en.pdf. Accessed July 12, 2006.

26. The World Bank. The World Bank Lending by Theme and Sector. *The World Bank Annual Report 2005.* Washington, DC: The World Bank; 2005.

27. USAID. Health: Overview. Available at: http://www.usaid.gov/our_work/global_health/. Accessed July 12, 2006.

28. The Rockefeller Foundation. Available at: http://www.rockfound.org/. Accessed July 6, 2006.

29. Ford Foundation. Available at: http://www.fordfound.org/. Accessed July 6, 2006.

30. The Soros Foundation. Available at: http://www.soros.org/. Accessed July 6, 2006.

31. Bill & Melinda Gates Foundation. Available at: http://www.gatesfoundation.org/default.htm. Accessed June 9, 2006.

32. Bill & Melinda Gates Foundation. About Us. Available at: http://www.gatesfoundation.org/AboutUs/. Accessed June 9, 2006.

33. Bill & Melinda Gates Foundation. Global Health Program Fact Sheet. Available at: http://www.gatesfoundation.org/GlobalHealth/RelatedInfo/GlobalHealthFactSheet-021201.htm. Accessed July 12, 2006.

34. Save the Children. Mission and Strategy. Available at: http://www.savethechildren.org/mission/index.asp. Accessed July 12, 2006.

35. Save the Children. Save the Children Receives $60 Million Grant from the Bill & Melinda Gates Foundation to Save Newborn Lives Globally. Available at: http://www.savethechildren.org/news/releases/release_120205.asp. Accessed July 12, 2006.

36. Doctors Without Borders. Available at: http://www.doctorswithoutborders.org/. Accessed July 15, 2006.

37. Doctors Without Borders. About Us. Available at: http://www.doctorswithoutborders.org/aboutus/index.cfm. Accessed July 12, 2006.

38. World Health Organization. The Stop TB Department. Available at: http://www.who.int/tb/about/en/. Accessed July 12, 2006.

39. Roll Back Malaria Global Partnership. Available at: http://rbm.who.int/. Accessed July 15, 2006.

40. Roll Back Malaria Global Partnership. What is MMSS? Available at: http://rbm.who.int/mmss/. Accessed July 13, 2006.

41. The GAVI Alliance. Progress and Challenges 2004. Available at: http://www.gavialliance.org/General_Information/About_alliance/pandc2004_index.php. Accessed July 12, 2006.

42. The Global Fund. The Global Fund to Fight AIDS, Tuberculosis, and Malaria. Available at: http://www.theglobalfund.org/en/. Accessed July 6, 2006.

43. The Global Fund. The Global Fund to Fight AIDS, Tuberculosis, and Malaria. History of the Fund in Detail. Available at: http://www.theglobalfund.org/en/about/road/history/default.asp. Accessed July 6, 2006.

44. The Global Fund. The Global Fund to Fight AIDS, Tuberculosis, and Malaria. How the Fund Works. Available at: http://www.theglobalfund.org/en/about/how/. Accessed July 6, 2006.

45. International AIDS Vaccine Initiative. About IAVI. Available at: http://www.iavi.org/viewpage.cfm?aid=24. Accessed July 12, 2006.

46. International AIDS Vaccine Initiative. IAVI's Intellectual Property Agreements for AIDS Vaccine Development. Available at: http://www.iavi.org/viewpage.cfm?aid=40. Accessed July 12, 2006.

47. Institute for One World Health. History: A nonprofit pharmaceutical company is born. Available at: http://www.oneworldhealth.org/about/history.php. Accessed

48. Institute for One World Health. Extraordinary Opportunities, Inspired Solutions. Available at: http://oneworldhealth.org/business/index.php. Accessed July 12, 2006.

49. International Federation of Pharmceutical Manufacturers & Associations. Global Alliance to Eliminate Leprosy. Available at: http://www.ifpma.org/Health/other_infect/health_lep.aspx. Accessed July 12, 2006.

50. National Institutes of Health. A Leading Cause of Blindness May Be Controlled by Simple Course of Oral Antibiotic. Available at: http://www3.niaid.nih.gov/news/newsreleases/1999/trachoma.htm. Accessed July 12, 2006.

51. Benton B. The Onchocerciasis (Riverblindness) Programs: Visionary Partnerships. Available at: http://www.worldbank.org/afr/findings/english/find174.htm. Accessed July 12, 2006.

52. African Comprehensive HIV/AIDS Partnerships. Available at: http://www.achap.org/. Accessed July 12, 2006.

53. Basch P. *Textbook of International Health.* 2nd ed. New York: Oxford University Press; 2001:38–39.

54. Basch P. *Textbook of International Health.* 2nd ed. New York: Oxford University Press; 2001:43.

55. Basch P. *Textbook of International Health.* 2nd ed. New York: Oxford University Press; 2001:45.

56. Basch P. *Textbook of International Health.* 2nd ed. New York: Oxford University Press; 2001:47–70.

57. Whaley RF, Hashim TJ. *A Textbook of World Health: A Practical Guide to Global Health Care.* New York: Parthenon Pub. Group; 1994:187–199.

58. World Health Organization. Fact Sheet No 101: Leprosy. Available at: http://www.who.int/mediacentre/factsheets/fs101/en/. Accessed July 7, 2006.

59. World Health Organization. Fact Sheet No 102: Lymphatic Filariasis. Available at: http://www.who.int/mediacentre/factsheets/fs102/en/. Accessed July 7, 2006.

60. World Health Organization. Onchocerciasis. Available at: http://www.who.int/topics/onchocerciasis/en/. Accessed July 7, 2006.

61. Whaley RF, Hashim TJ. *A Textbook of World Health: A Practical Guide to Global Health Care.* New York: Parthenon Pub. Group; 1994:197.

62. Bruce FC. Highlights From the National Summit on Safe Motherhood: Investing in the Health of Women. *Maternal Child Health J.* 2002 2002;6(1):67–69.

63. WHO. Declaration of Alma-Ata. *International Conference on Primary Health Care.* Alma-Ata, USSR: WHO; 1978.

64. Merson MH, Black RE, Mills AJ. *International Public Health: Diseases, Programs, Systems, and Policies.* Gaithersburg, MD: Aspen Publishers; 2000:682.

65. The World Bank. *World Development Report 1993.* New York: The World Bank, Oxford University Press; 1993:25–29.

66. World Health Organization. Fifty-eighth World Health Assembly. Available at: http://www.who.int/mediacentre/events/2005/wha58/en/. Accessed July 7, 2006.

67. Kidder T. *Mountains Beyond Mountains.* New York: Random House; 2003.

68. Benton B, Bump J, Seketeli A, Liese B. Partnership and promise: evolution of the african river blindness campaigns. *Ann Trop Med Parasitol.* 2002;96(suppl 1):S5–S14.

69. Laolu A. Victory over river blindness. *Africa Recovery.* 2003;17(1):6.

70. The Story of Mectizan®. Available at: http://www.merck.com/about/cr/mectizan/ Accessed August 6, 2004.

71. Amazigo U, Brieger W, Katabarwa M, et al. The challenges of community-directed treatment with Ivermectin (CDTI) within the African Programme for Onchocerciasis Control (APOC). *Ann Trop Med Parasitol.* 2002;96(1):S41–S58.

72. The World Bank. Defeating Onchocerciasis in Africa. Available at: http://www.worldbank.org/operations/licus/defeatingoncho.pdf. Accessed October 1, 2003.

73. Hopkins D, Richards F. Visionary campaign: eliminating river blindness. *Med Health Ann.* 1997:8–23.

74. Benton B. Economic impact of onchocerciasis control through the African Programme for Onchocerciasis Control: an overview. *Ann Trop Med Parasitol.* 1998;92(supplement 1):S33–S39.

CHAPTER 12

Culture and Health

Learning Objectives

By the end of this chapter the reader will be able to:

- Define *culture*
- Describe the most important relationships between culture and health
- Outline some of the theories of how behavior change occurs in health
- Describe some key measures to promote behavior change for better health
- Discuss the importance of social assessments

VIGNETTES

Joshua was just older than 1 year of age and lived in eastern Zimbabwe. His mother could tell that he had a fever. She wondered what had caused it. Was it the food that he ate? Was it the mixing of the "hot" foods and the "cold" foods? Or was it possible that they had done something to offend local custom? If the fever did not get better tomorrow, then she would take Joshua to the local healer.

Siu-Hong was 80 years old and lived in Hong Kong. He had a severe toothache for more than a week. His children repeatedly encouraged him to go to the dentist, but he would not go. He did not like dentists or "western medicine." In addition, he would have to wait in line to be seen at the dentist's office and would miss work at the clothes market. His children finally convinced him to go to the dentist by giving him a "present" of $25 and offering to take him to "dim sum," the traditional South Chinese "brunch."

Dorji lived in Bhutan, just outside the capital city of Thimpu. He felt tired, weak, and dizzy for some time but had no fever. After another week of feeling this way, Dorji went to visit his local health clinic. Each clinic in Bhutan had two medical practitioners, one who practiced the indigenous system of medicine and the other who practiced "Western biomedical medicine."[1] In light of Dorji's symptoms, he visited the indigenous practitioner inside the clinic. The "doctor" gave him some herbs that he thought would help his condition. However, he also thought Dorji had an underlying infection and took him across the hall to the "other doctor" who prescribed antibiotics for him.

Arathi was a young mother in southeast India. She and the other women in her village were participating in the Tamil Nadu Nutrition Project. They were all young mothers, many of whose babies were underweight for age. Arathi nursed her baby as she had learned from her mother to do. She also gave the baby some other foods as she had learned from her mother and grandmother. Despite this, her baby was quite small for her age. As part of the project, the community nutrition workers taught all the women and children in the village songs about proper feeding and about the vitamins the children needed. They also sponsored weekly weighing parties, in which all of the babies of the village were weighed and the mothers together decided if the baby was growing properly and what could be done to make the baby healthier. They also helped the mothers to make a food supplement for the babies who were "too small."

THE IMPORTANCE OF CULTURE TO HEALTH

Culture is an important determinant of health in a number of ways. First, culture is related to health behaviors. People's attitudes toward foods and what they eat, for example, are closely related to culture. The food that pregnant women eat, birthing practices, and how long women breastfeed are also linked to their cultural backgrounds. Hygiene practices are closely tied to culture, as well. Second, culture is an important determinant of people's perceptions of illness. Different culture groups may have different beliefs about what constitutes good health and what constitutes illness. Third, the extent to which people use health services is also very closely linked with culture. Some groups may use health services as soon as they feel ill. Others, however, may visit health practitioners only when they are very sick. Fourth, different cultures have different practices concerning health and medical treatment. Chinese and Indian cultures have well defined systems of medicine. There is a long history in many other societies, as well, of local systems of medicine that include notions of illness, various types of practitioners of medicine, and different kinds of medicines.

The purpose of this chapter is to introduce you to the most important links between health and culture, particularly as they relate to global health and people in low- and middle-income countries. The chapter begins by introducing you to the concept of "culture." It then examines how views of health, illness, the use of health services, and the role of different health providers vary by culture. The chapter also reviews some of the theories of behavior change that relate to enhancing people's health. The chapter concludes with comments about how one can ensure that investments take appropriate account of health and related cultural issues.

As you review this chapter, it is important to note that some cultural values enhance health. A culture, for example, that puts a strong emphasis on monogamy in marriage should have lower rates of HIV/AIDS than cultures in which having multiple sexual partners is more tolerated. However, some cultural values may not enhance health. A cultural emphasis on heaviness in people, for example, as a sign of prosperity or wealth, may be harmful to health, because it would encourage cardiovascular disease and diabetes. Some cultures have food taboos that prevent pregnant women from getting all of the nutrients they need in pregnancy. This chapter aims to help you to understand the relationship between culture and health, identify practices helpful and hurtful to good health, and learn about approaches to promoting healthier behaviors.

THE CONCEPT OF CULTURE

The concept of **culture** was developed at the end of the 19th century by anthropologists. There have been many definitions of culture. An early definition suggested that culture was:

> that complex whole which includes knowledge, beliefs, art, law, morals, custom and any other capabilities and habits acquired by man as a member of society."

A relatively modern definition states that culture is "a set of rules or standards shared by members of a society, which when acted upon by the members, produce behavior that falls within a range of variation the members consider proper and acceptable."[3] In the simplest terms, one may call culture "behavior and beliefs that are learned and shared."[4]

Cultures operate in a variety of domains, including:

- The family
- Social groups beyond the actor's family
- Individual growth and development
- Communication
- Religion
- Art
- Music
- Politics and law
- The economy[4]

As one thinks about the links between culture and health, it is also important to understand the term **society**, which refers to "a group of people who occupy a specific locality and share the same cultural traditions."[3] Societies have social structures that are the "relationships of groups within society that hold it together."[5] In addition, we must note that there is heterogeneity within all cultures. Sometimes this is reflected in what people call subcultures. There are many shared aspects, for example, of Chinese culture. However, China is a very large country and even among the Han Chinese, there are important variations as one moves across China in language, food, wedding customs, and music, among other things. The same would be true of North India. People across North India have much in common. Yet, there are many variations of North Indian culture in different places, such as in the state of West Bengal, on the one hand, and Rajasthan, on the other. This can be seen, again, in language, music, art, and food.

When thinking about the links between culture and health, one also needs to consider that some cultural practices may be well adapted to some settings but poorly adapted to others. Alternatively, they may be well adapted to the way people have been living, but less well adapted to the way people live after important changes or developments in their communities.[6] The culture of nomadic people, for example, may be well suited to their nomadic lifestyle. However, their culture may be very ill equipped to deal with a life style after societal change that would cause them to be more sedentary.

As we consider the relationship between culture and health, we should be aware of the ways in which a culture is viewed by people from outside that culture group. First, we should distinguish between the views of outsiders to a culture and insiders to a culture. This helps us to understand when we are looking at something from our perspective, compared to looking at it from the perspective of those who live within that culture.

Especially in the early days of anthropology, those who studied cultures other than their own often viewed them solely through the prism of their own society and judged much of what they saw to be lacking. This view is called ethnocentrism. Contrary to this view is "cultural relativism," or the idea that "because cultures are unique, they can be evaluated only according to their own standards and values."[7]

The approach that will guide the rest of this chapter and, indeed, the book as a whole, is the question: "How well does a given culture satisfy the physical and psychological needs of those whose behavior it guides?"[7] For example, is female circumcision, also called female genital mutilation, a health-enhancing procedure or a harmful procedure? Is it good or bad for the health of a newborn to be given sugar water? How should one see cultural practices that discriminate against women and cause them to eat less well than men or that might lead to the disproportionate abortion of female fetuses, as in India and China? On the other hand, what about cultures that do encourage exclusive breastfeeding for six months? What about male circumcision, which is associated with reduced transmission of HIV?

You will realize as you make your way through the book that those responsible for guiding health policies and programs in different countries must have a good understanding of the cultures with which they are working if they are to be helpful in enhancing health for the members of those societies. This is also true of outsiders, including development assistance agencies. They must be very sensitive to local cultures, while simultaneously considering with their government partners and in conjunction with insiders to the culture, what behavior changes may be needed to enhance individual and population health in a particular setting.[8]

HEALTH BELIEFS AND PRACTICES

Different cultures vary in their perceptions of their bodies and their views of what is illness, what causes illness, and what should be done about it. They have different views on how to prevent health problems, what health care they should seek, and the types of remedies that health providers might offer.[4] The next section will highlight selected aspects of belief systems about health that one would see most in low- and middle-income countries and in immigrant populations in developed countries.

Perceptions of Illness

Perceptions of illness vary considerably across culture groups. What one culture may view as entirely normal, for example, another culture may see as an affliction. Worms are so common among children in some cultures that people do not see infection with worms as an illness. Malaria is so common in much of Sub-Saharan Africa that many families see it as normal. In much of South Asia, back pain among women is very common and is also seen by women as just a normal part of being a woman.[9] Schistosomiasis is very common in Egypt. It causes blood in the urine, which is referred to in Egypt as "male menstruation" and seen as normal because it is so common.[10]

Perceptions of Disease

Medical anthropologists, among others, define disease as the "malfunctioning or maladaptation of biologic and psychophysiologic processes in the individual."[11] Pneumonia is a disease. HIV/AIDS is a disease. Polio is a disease. Illness, however, is different from disease. "Illness represents personal, interpersonal, and cultural reactions to disease or discomfort."[11] People may feel like they have an illness. They can describe it and its symptoms. They may have a name in their culture for this problem. However, they may not have a "disease," which is a physiological condition. This is a very important point, because different cultures may have very different perceptions of the causes of illness.

Most people in the developed countries follow the "Western medical paradigm" in explaining the causes of disease. This will be familiar to you. You get influenza and colds from viruses. You get diabetes as an adult from an inability to control your blood sugar, although there may be a genetic component to this. You get heart disease from smoking, from being obese, or from having cholesterol that is too high.

On the other hand, many people, especially those in or from the developing world and more "traditional societies" often see illness as being caused by factors other than disease, as defined in the biomedical model. There are many cultures, for example, that believe that illness is brought on by the body being "out of balance." Among the most common of these concepts is the notion of "hot" and "cold." In this case, the body may get out of balance if one engages in certain unhealthy practices. In Chinese culture, for example, one should not drink cold liquids while eating hot food. In some cultures, some foods are regarded as "hot" and some foods are regarded as "cold" and people have to eat them in certain appropriate proportions or only at certain times to avoid illness.

Many people also believe that illness has supernatural causes. A study done among Americans of Caribbean and African descent living in the southern United States showed that many people believed that the symptoms of illness stem from supernatural causes.[12] There are many cultures in which people believe that illness comes from being affected by "the evil eye," being bewitched or possessed, losing their soul, or offending gods.[13] Some indigenous Canadians have a belief that "illness is not necessarily a bad thing, but instead a sign sent by the Creator to help people re-evaluate their lives."[14] A study of the cultural perceptions of illness among Yoruba people in Nigeria found that illness could be "traced to enemies, including witchcraft, sorcery, gods, ancestors, natural illnesses, or hereditary illness."[15]

Emotional stresses are also seen in different cultures as causes of illness. This could come about as a result of being stressed or extremely frightened. Being too envious is also viewed as a cause of illness.[13] Sexual matters are seen as causes of illness in some cultures, as well. In several cultures, for example, frequent sexual relations is believed to weaken men, by taking away their blood.[13] These beliefs are quite common in parts of India.

Folk Illness

Many cultures also have what are called "folk illnesses." These are local cultural interpretations of physical states that people perceive to be illness, but that do not have a physiologic cause. "Empacho" is an illness that is commonly described in a number of Latin American cultures. This is often discussed as a condition caused by food that "gets stuck to the walls of the stomach or intestines, causing an obstruction."[16] It is said to be caused by any of a variety of inappropriate food practices, and in children it is said to produce a number of gastrointestinal symptoms, including bloating, diarrhea, and a stomachache.

To cure empacho, families may limit some foods, give abdominal massages with warm oil, or pop the skin on the small of the back. They will also often consult a local healer, such as the *santiguadora* in the Puerto Rican community and *sobadora* in the Mexican community. Some Mexican communities in both the United States and Mexico also treat this "illness" with some powders.

To understand health problems in low- and middle-income countries, it is very important to understand the existence of folk illnesses such as empacho. It may be that the condition described by communities as empacho has no known or real biomedical basis. However, even if this condition has no biomedical basis, people believe this is an important illness and any efforts to improve the health of the community will have to consider such beliefs.[16] Table 12-1 lists some of the culturally defined causes of illness.

The Prevention of Illness

Given the wide range of views of what causes illness, it is not surprising that there are many different cultural practices that concern avoiding illness. Many cultures, for example, have taboos, or things that they forbid people to do if they are to stay healthy. A large number of taboos concern what not to eat during pregnancy, as was suggested in a study of traditional beliefs in Western Malaysia, which indicated that pregnant women should avoid certain important sources of protein.[17] A study in southern Nigeria about traditional beliefs concerning eating in pregnancy found widespread belief that pregnant women must avoid:

- sweet foods, so the baby would not be weak
- eggs, so the baby would not grow up to be a thief
- snails, so the baby would not be dull, salivate excessively, or not develop speech properly.[18]

A study in Brazil suggested that women should not eat game meat and fish during pregnancy, although both could be good sources of protein.[19] A study of poor women in South India showed that "taboos affected the intake of fruits and legumes" and legumes are among the most important sources of protein for many Indian women.[20]

There is also a wide array of ritual practices that people undergo to avoid illness. Related to this, there are traditions in some cultures to get rid of bad spirits or evil forces to ensure that one does not fall ill. There are beliefs among the Yoruba people in Nigeria, for example, that charms, amulets, scarification, or some oral potions can prevent illness that is caused by one's enemies.[15] Some tribal groups in Rajasthan, India, put charms at certain crossings to inflict harm on others, to avoid harm to themselves, to appease an evil spirit, or to leave their affliction there with the spirit.[21] In rural Senegal, a special ritual is performed for women who have lost two children, or had two miscarriages, or appear to be infertile. The ritual is intended to prevent the causes of child death and infertility.[22]

The Diagnosis and Treatment of Illness and the Use of Health Services

In many cultures, when people are ill, it is common that they first try to care for the illness themselves with home remedies.

This is often followed by a visit to some type of local healer and the use of indigenous medicines from that healer. Only if the illness does not resolve after that will families seek the help of a "western doctor." Even then, it is quite common for people to use modern medicines and indigenous medicines at the same time.

Studies that were done of the treatment of diarrheal disease in Central America showed very clearly, for example, that people tried a variety of mechanisms for diagnosing and treating their illnesses.

The manner in which people and families care for illnesses is called "patterns of resort." People seek help from different healthcare providers at different times for a number of reasons.[23] One important concern is the cost of services, both direct, such as fees, and indirect, such as the cost of transportation, time en route, or waiting. Another concern is the means of payment. People with little cash may prefer to visit a healer or doctor who takes payment in kind, rather than in cash. This could be in small gifts or payment in farm products such as fruits, vegetables, or poultry. People are also driven by the reputation of the provider. They will go to a provider that is reputed in their community to have good results over a provider who does not enjoy this type of reputation.

The manner in which the provider treats them socially is also an important determinant of the use of services. People generally prefer to go to a provider who is from their community, speaks their language, is known to them, and treats them with respect, rather than an outsider who may be disrespectful. It is interesting to note that people tend to treat folk illnesses at home and then go to a local healer. As a last resort, they may go to a physician, even if they understand that the physician "does not treat empacho."[16]

It is also very important to understand the extent to which a large share of the treatment of illness in most cultures takes place first at home. People in developed countries may take some aspirin, drink plenty of water, eat a certain soup, and try to rest when they first develop symptoms. They may also take a variety of different types of herbal products or vitamins. Only if people do not feel better by a certain time will they try to see a health provider. People in more traditional societies have analogous patterns of behavior when they believe themselves to be ill. Understanding these patterns, of course, is central to any efforts to enhance their health through efforts such as maternal care, vaccination programs, or treatment of infectious diseases, such as AIDS, TB, or malaria.

Health Providers

There are many different types of health service providers. Some of these are shown in Table 12-2. As you can see in the table, some of the providers are practitioners of indigenous systems of medicine, such as ayurvedic practitioners in India and practitioners of Chinese systems of medicine, such as herbalists and acupuncturists. Other practitioners will be part of a wide array of local health providers. These include, for example, traditional birth attendants, priests, herbalists, and bonesetters. The types of practitioners of western medicine will depend on the size and location of the place in which they work and could include, for example, community health workers, nurses, midwives, nurse-midwives, physicians, and dentists. You should also be aware that in many low- and middle-income countries, pharmacists, or stores that sell drugs, also frequently dispense both drugs and medical advice. Although prescriptions for drugs may be legally required, many low- and middle-income countries are unable or unwilling to enforce this requirement. It is also important to note that many health providers will combine indigenous health practices with western medicine.[24]

TABLE 12-1 Selected Examples of Cultural Explanations of Disease

Body Balances	Emotional	Supernatural	Sexual
Temperature	Fright	Bewitching	Sex with forbidden person
Energy	Sorrow	Demons	Overindulgence in sex
Blood	Envy	Spirit possession	
Dislocation	Stress	Evil eye	
Problems with organs		Offending god or gods	
Incompatibility of horoscopes		Soul loss	

Source: Adapted with permission from Scrimshaw SC. Culture, behavior, and health. In: Merson MH, Black RE, Mills A, eds. *International Public Health: Diseases, Programs, Systems, and Policies.* Sudbury, MA: Jones and Bartlett; 2006:53–78.

TABLE 12-2 Selected Examples of Health Service Providers

Indigenous	Western Biomedical	Other Medical Systems
Midwives	Pharmacists	Chinese medical system
Shamans	Nurse-midwives	• practitioners
Curers	Nurses	• chemists/herbalists
Spirtualists	Nurse-practitioners	• acupuncturists
Witches	Physicians	Ayurvedic practitioners
Sorcerers	Dentists	
Priests		
Diviners		
Herbalists		
Bonesetters		

Source: Adapted with permission from Scrimshaw SC. Culture, behavior, and health. In: Merson MH, Black RE, Mills A, eds. *International Public Health: Diseases, Programs, Systems, and Policies.* Sudbury, MA: Jones and Bartlett; 2006:53–78.

HEALTH BEHAVIORS AND BEHAVIOR CHANGE

The leading causes of death in low- and middle-income countries are ischemic heart disease, cerebrovascular disease, HIV, and pneumonia. Malaria, TB, and diarrhea are also among the top 10 causes of death in these countries.[25] The risk factors for these diseases and conditions include nutrition (both undernutrition and overnutrition), tobacco use, unsafe sex, and unsafe water and sanitation.[26] There are many behaviors that *are* conducive to good health. However, what is the extent to which behavior is a contributing factor to the leading risk factors for illness and premature death in the developing world? A number of examples are discussed next.

An infant's being underweight for age is the most important risk factor for premature death in the developing world. Although income and education are closely linked with nutritional status of both mother and child, cultural variables are also important determinants of their nutrition. As noted earlier, there are many cultures that have food taboos for pregnant women that are not helpful to birth outcomes, and other cultures encourage pregnant women to eat less rather than more. In addition, the extent to which women breastfeed their babies is closely linked with culture, as is the timing for the introduction of complementary foods. Undernutrition also stems from other eating practices that are also closely tied to culture. Can behaviors be changed so that pregnant women will eat the most nutritious foods they can, given their level of income, and exclusively breastfeed their babies for six months?

Unsafe sex is the major risk factor for HIV/AIDS in low- and middle-income countries. Some people, such as commercial sex workers, may not have the bargaining power with their clients to negotiate sex with a condom. The same will often be true of women who are forced into unsafe sex by their husbands and boyfriends or because of their own economic position. However, many people who engage in unsafe sex do have control over whether or not to use a condom. What would it take to ensure that they do so?

Hygiene is another area that closely relates to health behaviors and the lack of safe water and sanitation is a risk factor of importance for diarrheal disease. In many low- and middle-income countries hygiene may be low, and families need to learn to use water safely, dispose of human waste in sanitary ways, and wash their hands with soap after defecating. Behaviors regarding hygiene, of course, are intimately linked with culture. How can they be changed?

As you will read about later, indoor air pollution is a major risk factor for respiratory infections. This relates largely to the fact that families in many cultures cook indoors without appropriate ventilation. Some families may not be able to afford an improved stove. However, other families cook as they do because of tradition and the lack of knowledge of the health impacts of indoor air pollution. How could one change such fundamental matters as the way that people cook?

Cigarettes are the leading risk factor for cardiovascular disease and cancer. Most people who smoke cigarettes start smoking as adolescents. Are there measures that can be taken to change these behaviors? How would the efforts to change behavior have to differ if one tried to stop adolescents from taking up smoking, compared to helping adult smokers to quit?

Of course, behaviors are closely linked with culture and health not only in developing countries, but in developed countries, as well. Moreover, in developed, as well as in developing countries, there is a wide array of behaviors that do not promote good health. In the developed countries, for example, an increasing number of people are obese and have diabetes, associated with poor diet and a sedentary lifestyle. Many people also continue to smoke, even though smoking is the single largest risk factor for both cardiovascular disease and cancers. Despite the widespread availability of seat belts in cars, some people still do not use them. What needs to be done to get people to change these behaviors to ones that are healthier?

Improving Health Behaviors

There are a number of models or theories that explain why people engage in certain health behaviors and what can be done to encourage changes in those behaviors. Those interested in greater detail in how to change health behaviors can review *The Essentials of Health Behavior*, another book in this series.[27] Some of the most important concepts about health behavior and models about behavior change, however, are examined very briefly here.

The Ecological Perspective

As one considers the factors that influence behaviors that relate to health, it is important to take what is called an ecological perspective. This is a concept that suggests that the factors influencing health behaviors occur at several levels. These are noted in Table 12-3.

The basic precepts concerning the ecological approach are:

- "health related behaviors are affected by, and affect, multiple levels of influence: intrapersonal or individual factors, interpersonal factors, institutional factors and public policy factors."
- "behavior both influences and is influenced by the social environments in which it occurs."[28]

You can try to imagine, for example, whether or not an adolescent male will take up smoking. This will depend on how he feels about smoking, what he thinks others think of his smoking, the setting in which he operates, how expensive it is to buy cigarettes, and how easy it is to buy them. Of course, if he does start smoking, some of his own peer group may follow.

TABLE 12-3 The Ecological Perspective

Factors	Definition
Individual	Individual characteristics that influence behavior such as knowledge, attitudes, beliefs, and personality traits
Interpersonal	Interpersonal processes, and primary groups including family, friends, and peers
Institutional	Rules, regulations, policies, and informal structures
Community	Social networks and norms or standards that exist formally or informally among individuals, groups, and organizations
Public policy	Local, state, and federal policies and laws that regulate or support healthy actions and practices for disease prevention, early detection, control, and management

Source: Adapted with permission from Murphy E. *Promoting Healthy Behavior, Health Bulletin 2.* Washington, DC: Population Reference Bureau; 2005.

The Health Belief Model

The Health Belief model was the first effort to articulate a coherent understanding of the factors that enter into health behaviors. It was developed by the U.S. Public Health Services as they tried to understand why people did or did not avail themselves of the opportunity to get chest X-rays for tuberculosis.[29] The premises of this model are that people's health behaviors depend on their perceptions of:

- Their likelihood of getting the illness
- The severity of the illness if they get it
- The benefits of engaging in behavior that will prevent the illness
- The barriers to engaging in preventive behavior

In this model, people's health behavior also depends on whether or not people feel that they could actually carry out the appropriate behavior if they tried, which is called "self-efficacy."[30]

One could think about how this model pertains to engaging in safe sex. The extent to which a young man uses a condom will be influenced by his fear of getting HIV/AIDS, how serious a disease he believes it to be, the extent to which a condom can prevent HIV/AIDS, and how easy it is to buy a condom and get a partner to agree to use it. The young man must also feel that he will buy the condom and use it.

Stages of Change Model

The Stages of Change model was developed in the 1990s in the United States in conjunction with work on alcohol and drug abuse.[31] The premise behind this model is that change in behavior is a process and that different people are at different stages of readiness for change. The stages of change are outlined in Table 12-4.

It is easy to see how this model might apply to alcohol and drug abuse. You can imagine an excessive drinker who is not aware of his problem or who will not face it and needs help in doing so. Other people, who are aware of their problem and willing to do something about it, may need help to stop. Still others, who have already broken their addictions, need positive reinforcement to maintain their health.[30]

TABLE 12-4 The Stages of Change Model

Stages
Precontemplation
Contemplation
Decision/Determination
Action
Maintenance

Source: Data with permission from Murphy E. *Promoting Healthy Behavior, Health Bulletin 2.* Washington, DC: Population Reference Bureau; 2005.

TABLE 12-5 Diffusions of Health Innovations Model

Stages of Diffusion
Recognition of a problem or need
Conduct of basic and applied research to address the specific problem
The development of strategies and materials that will put the innovative concept into a form that will meet the needs of the target population
Commercialization of the innovation, which will involve prodution, marketing, and distribution efforts
Diffusion and adoption of the innovation
Consequences associated with adoption of the innovation

Source: Adapted with permission from Scrimshaw SC. Culture, behavior, and health. In: Merson MH, Black RE, Mills A, eds. *International Public Health: Diseases, Programs, Systems, and Policies.* Sudbury, MA: Jones and Bartlett; 2006:53–78.

The Diffusions of Innovations Model

The Diffusions of Innovations model had its origins in work that was done on promoting agricultural change in the United States. In this model, "an innovation is an idea, practice, service, or other object that is perceived as new by the individual or group."[32] This model is based on the notion that communication is needed to promote social change and that "diffusion" is the process by which innovations are communicated over time among members of different groups and societies.[33] This model focuses on how people adopt and can be encouraged to adopt "innovations" but does not get involved with how they might maintain what they have adopted.

Table 12-5 outlines the stages that have to be undertaken to try to diffuse a health innovation.

This model also suggests that as the innovation begins to be diffused, people will fall into six groups:

- Innovators
- Early adopters
- Early majority
- Late majority
- Late adopters
- Laggards[32,33]

In addition, the model also indicates that the pace of adoption will be influenced by:

- The gains people think they will get by adopting the innovation
- How much the innovation fits in with their existing culture and values
- How easy it is to try out the innovation
- Whether or not there are role models who are already trying out the innovation
- The extent to which potential adopters see the innovation as cost-efficient and not taking too much of their time, energy, or money[32,33]

One can imagine how the Diffusions of Innovations model may apply to efforts to change diets in developed countries away from certain fats and toward more fruits and vegetables, fewer processed foods, and more whole grains. Some people change their diets relatively quickly. Others in the community make these shifts only as they can overcome some of their long held dietary patterns. Some people shift as they learn more from their friends, some of whom become role models for change. The relatively high costs of some of the organic and other healthy foods may be a constraint to adoption of change by some people. Others may simply not be willing or able to change the way they and their families have always eaten.

UNDERSTANDING AND ENGENDERING BEHAVIOR CHANGE

As you can clearly see, in many instances, improving health requires that the behaviors of individuals, families, and communities be changed. You also see, however, that behaviors are intimately connected to culture, which is inherently not easy to change. Under these circumstances, what can be done, first to understand what behaviors need to be changed and, second, to change them? These questions are answered briefly here.

Understanding Behaviors

A first step in trying to promote behavior change must be to gain a good understanding of the behaviors that are taking place. This requires a careful assessment of:

- The behaviors that are taking place
- The extent to which they are helpful or harmful to health
- The underlying motivation for these behaviors
- The likely responses to different approaches to changing the unhealthy behaviors

By taking a look at breastfeeding, for example, we can get a sense of how one would carry out such an assessment. One can consider how infant deaths might be reduced. As part of this effort, it is important to get a better sense of the extent to which any nutritional issues are harmful to infant health and how they might be improved. One important part of this effort would be to examine breastfeeding practices. In doing so, we would try to answer the following questions, among others:

- When do women start breastfeeding?
- Do they feed on schedule or on demand?
- Do they feed male and female children the same way?
- For how long do they breastfeed exclusively?
- At what age do they introduce complementary foods?
- Until what age do they continue to breastfeed, even while the children are getting complementary foods?
- Why do they engage in these practices?
- Why do some women not breastfeed?
- Who breastfeeds and who does not?
- Who has influence over their breastfeeding practices?

The answers to these questions, of course, will vary by culture group; however, once we get answers to them, we can begin to formulate a plan for behavior change that is built on the cultural values and approaches of the people. Without understanding current practices, the rationale for them, and who has influence over them, it will be impossible to promote behavior change in the appropriate directions. When we do have a sense of the existing practices and why they take place, what can be done to change behaviors?

Changing Health Behaviors

There are many different approaches to changing health behaviors. Some operate at the level of the individual, some at the level of the community, and some at the level of society as a whole. Generally, they include some combination of communication through the mass media and more personal communication. Several approaches to behavior change are discussed briefly here.

Community Mobilization

One very important way to encourage change in health behaviors is to engage in community mobilization. In this case, the effort focuses on getting an entire community to engage in the effort at promoting more healthy behaviors. This requires considerable efforts aimed at helping people across the community to identify the problems that they face, identify potential solutions to them, and then work together to put those solutions in place. Generally, it also requires that the leaders within the community are themselves mobilized, willing to be "champions" for the needed change, and then promote that change.[34] You will read more later, for example, about the Tamil Nadu Nutrition Project which was noted in one of the vignettes at the opening of this chapter and the manner in which the affected communities were involved in promoting a variety of innovations, including weighing babies together, identifying together the babies who were not thriving, and working together to make supplementary food for their children. In addition, all of the community was involved in learning about appropriate foods and about needed micronutrients. You will also read later about a variety of community-based activities, including efforts to address diarrheal disease through oral rehydration in Egypt and polio campaigns in Latin America.

Mass Media

The mass media are often used to promote change in health behaviors. Most people in developing countries have access to radio, which is often used for this purpose. Increasingly, however, those engaged in promoting better health are using a tool referred to as "entertainment-education." Many of these efforts have focused on soap opera series in which the characters bring out the main messages about healthy behaviors. The British Broadcasting Company has a group, for example, that works with developing countries to produce soap operas on health topics of importance such as

HIV/AIDS. Such a series was done on HIV in India, and one is under production on HIV for Nigeria. The government of Myanmar had a soap opera about leprosy that featured Myanmar's best known actress. The aims of the soap opera were to help people know how to diagnose leprosy, to inform them that it could be treated completely if treated early, and to get people to come forward for treatment at an early stage.

Social Marketing

Social marketing is the application of the tools of commercial marketing to try to promote behavior change and the uptake of important health actions or products. This has been used widely in family planning work. It is also being used in other fields, such as in selling bed nets for malaria control. In social marketing, a local brand of a product is often created, such as a condom, a contraceptive pill, or an insecticide-treated bed net. Mass media and other forms of communication are then used to promote the brand and the behaviors related to the product. Of course, successful marketing depends on very careful market research and a good understanding of the local culture, values, and behaviors. It also depends on what is called "the four Ps" in social marketing:

- Attractive product
- Affordable price
- Convenient places to buy the product
- Persuasive promotion[35,36]

Often the products being marketed through social marketing are sold through commercial channels but their price is subsidized by the government.

Health Education

Health education is something with which every reader of this book will be familiar. It comes in many forms, such as in the classroom, in the news media, on the radio and television, and on the Internet. Successful health education programs that were aimed at sex education have several features in common that hold lessons for other efforts at making health education effective.

- They focused on risky behaviors and were clear about abstinence and consistent condom use
- They provided accurate information
- They addressed how to deal with social pressures
- They selected teachers and peer educators who believed in the program
- They geared the content of the program to the age, sexual experience, and culture of the students[37]

Achieving Success in Health Promotion

The previous section refers to specific types of health promotion that can be used to encourage a change in health behaviors or the adoption of healthy behaviors. There are a number of lessons that have emerged both about these approaches and when looking broadly at what constitutes an effective health promotion effort. These are noted in Table 12-6.

TABLE 12-6 Selected Factors for Success in Health Promotion

Identify specific health problems, related behaviors, and key stakeholders
Know and use sound behavioral theories
Research motivations and constraints to change, considering biologic, environmental, cultural, and other contextual factors
Use participatory assessment tools and include relevant stakeholders in the design, implementation, and evaluation of the intervention
Plan and budget carefully
Identify people who exhibit healthy behaviors that differ from the social norm
Create an environment that enables behavior change through policy dialogue, advocacy, and capacity building
Organize an intervention that addresses both specific behaviors and contextual factors
Work to ensure sustainability
Evaluate from the beginning
Form partnerships to scale up and/or adapt the most successful interventions for implementation in other settings.

Source: Adapted with permission from Murphy E. *Promoting Healthy Behavior, Health Bulletin 2.* Washington, DC: Population Reference Bureau; 2005.

SOCIAL ASSESSMENT

There is one additional area that it is important to cover concerning the links between health and culture. This is "social assessment" or "social impact assessment." A social impact assessment is "a process for assessing the social impacts of planned interventions or events and for developing strategies for the ongoing monitoring and management of those impacts."[38] In more expansive terms, "Social impact assessment includes the processes of analyzing, monitoring, and managing the intended and unintended social consequences, both positive and negative, of planned interventions (policies, programs, plans, projects) and any social change processes invoked by those interventions. Its primary purpose is to bring about a more sustainable and equitable biophysical and human environment."[38]

The social impact assessment looks at a variety of domains that go beyond health. These include impact, among other things, on historical artifacts and buildings, communities, demography, gender, minority groups, culture, and health. The assessment should be carried out in a way that builds on local processes, engages the community fully, and proactively tries to maximize the potential good that can come from the proposed investment. It "promotes community development and empowerment, builds capacity, and develops social capital."[38] The detailed approach of a social impact assessment is outlined in Table 12-7.

Many readers will be familiar with environmental assessment of proposed investment schemes and many countries require such assessments be done before any major physical investment. In some respects, a social assessment is the social analogue to the environmental assessment. In this case, let us suppose that a development agency and a government are going to collaborate to develop a series of health centers in a particular region of a country. If the country carried out the recommended social assessment before it designed the project, then it would aim as it carried out the design to involve the community in this work. The country would also ensure that the design took account of the needs of various groups in the community and was based on their culture and values, and it would keep in mind how programs need to be tailored to address them. The assessment would seek to identify any negative consequences that might emerge from the investment and how those consequences might be mitigated. The plan emerging from the assessment would also have an approach to monitoring and evaluation of the proposed investment to ensure that the social impacts that were foreseen were correct and that the program design really is consistent with local values and the underlying needs of the community.

Some years ago, very little attention was paid in some development assistance agencies and in some governments to social assessment. Little effort was spent on examining the social and cultural issues involved in designing appropriate interventions in health. In addition, little attention was paid to the potential impact on health or on other social areas of investments in sectors outside of health. Although the quality of social assessment may vary both within and across some agencies and governments, it is now a normal practice that social assessments are done for all major development projects.

TABLE 12-7 Selected Focuses of Social Impact Assessment

Identifies interested and affected peoples
Facilitates and coordinates the participation of stakeholders
Analyzes the local setting of the planned intervention to assess likely impacts to it
Collects baseline data to allow for evaluation of the impact of the intervention
Gives a picture of the local cultural context, and develops an understanding of local community values, particularly how they relate to the planned intervention
Identifies and describes the activities that are likely to cause impacts
Predicts likely impacts and how different stakeholders are likely to respond
Assists in evaluating and selecting alternatives
Recommends measures to mitigate any likely negative impacts
Assists in the valuation process and provides suggestions about compensation for affected peoples
Describes potential conflicts between stakeholders and advises on resolution processes
Develops coping strategies for dealing with residual and non-mitigatable impacts
Contributes to skill development and capacity building in the community
Assists in devising and implementing monitoring and management programs

Source: Adapted with permission from Vanclay F. Social Impact Assessment: International Principles. Available at http://www.iaia.org/Members/Publications/Guidelines_Principles/SP2.pdf. Accessed on July 5, 2007.

MAIN MESSAGES

Culture is a set of beliefs and behaviors that are learned and shared. Culture operates, among other areas, in the domains of the family, social groups beyond the family, religion, art, music, and law. Culture is an important determinant of health, in many ways. It relates to people's health behaviors, their perceptions of illness, the extent to which they use health services, and forms of medicine that they have practiced traditionally. This chapter examines the links between culture and health from the perspective of the extent to which a culture satisfies the physical and psychological needs of those who follow it.

Perceptions of illness vary considerably across cultures. What is seen as normal in some societies may be seen as illness in others. Different societies also have differing perceptions of the causes of illness and of disease. In addition to perceptions related to the "western medical paradigm," diseases may be viewed, for example, as due to the body "being out of balance," supernatural causes, offending the gods, emotional stress, or witchcraft. Different cultures also take an array of steps, beyond the western medical paradigm, to prevent illness. Some of these include rituals, the wearing of charms, and the observance of certain food taboos.

When people believe themselves to be ill, they usually resort to trying "home remedies" first. Following that, people in traditional societies often visit some type of traditional healer. It may be some time before they consult a physician practicing "modern medicine," and often only when they are certain they are quite ill and other forms of treatment have not brought relief.

Many forms of traditional behavior are conducive to good health. This might include, for example, traditional practices that provide for the mother to spend some time with her baby before she returns to her normal work and household chores. Male circumcision, as practiced in many cultures, reduces the transmission of HIV/AIDS. Other traditional practices, however, are not health promoting. Feeding sugar water to infants, for example, is not good for the health of the infants, who should be exclusively breastfed for six months. How can healthy behaviors be promoted?

There are a number of "models" of how behaviors can be changed, including: "The Health Belief Model," "The Diffusions of Innovation Model," and the "Stages of Change Model." To encourage behavior change, of course, requires a good understanding of the behaviors that are taking place, how they relate to health, the underlying motivation for them, and the likely response to various approaches to changing them.

When thinking about trying to change behavior on a large scale, such as promoting an immunization program, the use of seat belts, the willingness to seek treatment for leprosy, several approaches are important. One way to engender change is to engage in community mobilization. Promoting messages about desirable and undesirable health behaviors can also be done effectively using the mass media. Social marketing and health education efforts are also important. An effective tool for any efforts at investing in health or trying to change behaviors is to carry out a social assessment, which will identify the social basis of the health issues one is trying to influence, as well as the likely social impacts of the proposed activities.

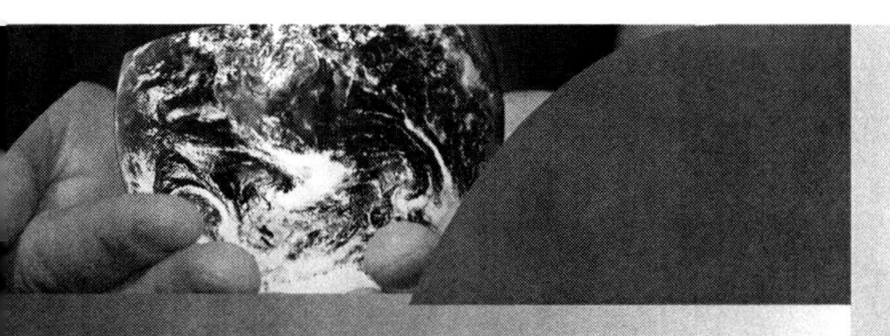

Discussion Questions

1. What is culture? Give some examples of aspects of culture that vary across different societies.
2. Why is it important to assess the relationship between culture and health in specific societies by the extent to which cultural practices promote or discourage good physical and mental health?
3. Name three cultural practices that are health promoting. Name three cultural practices that are harmful to health.
4. How does culture relate to people's perceptions of illness? Why would some cultures regard some illnesses as "normal?"
5. What would low-income people in traditional societies likely see as possible causes of illness?
6. What is the difference between "illness" and "disease?"
7. When an infant is ill in a traditional society in a low-income country, from whom and in what order are the parents likely to seek help?
8. Why would members of the community seek treatment for illness from traditional healers?
9. If you wanted to encourage the large scale adoption of a healthy behavior, such as giving up cigarette smoking, what information would you want to know as you plan your effort?
10. Why are social assessments important? If they are done well, what gains would they produce that might not come if there were no such assessment?

REFERENCES

1. Scrimshaw SC. Culture, Behavior, and Health. In: Merson MH, Black RE, Mills A, eds. *International Public Health: Diseases, Programs, Systems, and Policies.* Gaithersburg, MD: Aspen Publishers; 2001:53–78.

2. Tylor E. *Primitive Culture.* London: J. Murray; 1871.

3. Haviland WA. The Nature of Culture. *Cultural Anthropology.* 6th ed. Fort Worth, TX: Holt, Rinchart & Winston, Inc.; 1990:30.

4. Miller B. Culture and Health: George Washington University; 2004.

5. Haviland WA. The Nature of Culture. *Cultural Anthropology.* 6th ed. Fort Worth, TX: Holt, Rinchart & Winston, Inc.; 1990:31.

6. Haviland WA. The Nature of Culture. *Cultural Anthropology.* 6th ed. Fort Worth, TX: Holt, Rinchart & Winston, Inc.; 1990:46.

7. Haviland WA. The Nature of Culture. *Cultural Anthropology.* 6th ed. Fort Worth, TX: Holt, Rinchart & Winston, Inc.; 1990:51.

8. Scrimshaw SC. Culture, Behavior, and Health. In: Merson MH, Black RE, Mills A, eds. *International Public Health: Diseases, Programs, Systems, and Policies.* Gaithersburg, MD: Aspen Publishers; 2001:56.

9. Murphy EM. Being born female is dangerous for your health. *The American Psychologist.* Mar 2003;58(3):205–210.

10. Scrimshaw SC. Culture, Behavior, and Health. In: Merson MH, Black RE, Mills A, eds. *International Public Health: Diseases, Programs, Systems, and Policies.* Gaithersburg, MD: Aspen Publishers; 2001:57.

11. Kleinman A, Eisenberg L, Good B. Culture, illness, and care: clinical lessons from anthropologic and cross-cultural research. *Ann Intern Med.* Feb 1978;88(2):251–258.

12. Hopper S. The Influence of ethnicity on the healthcare of older women. *Clin Geriatric Med.* 1993;9:231–259.

13. Scrimshaw SC. Culture, Behavior, and Health. In: Merson MH, Black RE, Mills A, eds. *International Public Health: Diseases, Programs, Systems, and Policies.* Gaithersburg, MD: Aspen Publishers; 2001:58.

14. Letendre AD. Aboriginal Traditional Medicine: Where Does It Fit? *Crossing Boundaries - an interdisciplinary journal.* 2002;1(2).

15. Jegede AS. The Yoruba Cultural Construction of Health and Illness. *Nordic Journal of African Studies.* 2002;11(3):322–335.

16. Pachter LM. Culture and clinical care. Folk illness beliefs and behaviors and their implications for health care delivery. *Jama.* Mar 2 1994;271(9):693.

17. Bolton JM. Food taboos among the Orang Asli in West Malaysia: a potential nutritional hazard. *The American Journal of Clinical Nutrition.* August 1972 1972;25:788–799.

18. Chiwuzie J, Okolocha C. Traditional Belief Systems and Maternal Mortality in a Semi-Urban Community in Southern Nigeria. *African Journal of Reproductive Health.* August 2001 2001;5(1):75–82.

19. Trigo M, Roncada MJ, Stewien GT, Pereira IM. [Food taboos in the northern region of Brazil]. *Rev Saude Publica.* Dec 1989;23(6):455–464.

20. Sundararaj R, Pereira SM. Dietary intakes and food taboos of lactating women in a South Indian community. *Trop Geogr Med.* Jun 1975;27(2):189–193.

21. Bhasin V. Sickness and Therapy Among Tribals of Rajasthan. *Stud Tribes Tribals.* 2003;1(1):77–83.

22. Fassin D, Badji I. Ritual buffoonery: as coail preventive measure against childhood mortality in Senegal. *Lancet.* January 1986;18(1):142–143.

23. Scrimshaw SC. Culture, Behavior, and Health. In: Merson MH, Black RE, Mills A, eds. *International Public Health: Diseases, Programs, Systems, and Policies.* Gaithersburg, MD: Aspen Publishers; 2001:62.

24. Scrimshaw SC. Culture, Behavior, and Health. In: Merson MH, Black RE, Mills A, eds. *International Public Health: Diseases, Programs, Systems, and Policies.* Gaithersburg, MD: Aspen Publishers; 2001:63.

25. Lopez AD, Mathers CD, Murray CJL. The Burden of Disease and Mortality by Condition: Data, Methods, and Results for 2001. In: Lopez AD, Mathers CD, Ezzati M, Jamison DT, Murray CJL, eds. *Global burden of disease and risk factors.* New York: Oxford University Press; 2006:70.

26. Lopez AD, Mathers CD, Ezzati M, Jamison DT, Murray CJL. Measuring the Global Burden of Disease and Risk Factors 1990-2001. In: Lopez AD, Mathers CD, Ezzati M, Jamison DT, Murray CJL, eds. *Global burden of disease and risk factors.* New York: Oxford University Press; 2006:10.

27. Edberg M. *Essentials of Health Behavior: An Introduction to Social and Behavioral Therory Applied to Public Health.* Sudbury, MA: Jones & Bartlett Publishers, Inc.; 2007.

28. Murphy E. *Promoting Healthy Behavior, Health Bulletin 2.* Washington, DC: Population Reference Bureau; 2005.

29. Rosenstock IM, Strecher VJ, Becker MH. Social learning theory and the Health Belief Model. *Health Educ Q.* Summer 1988;15(2):175–183.

30. Murphy E. *Promoting Healthy Behavior, Health Bulletin 2.* Washington, DC: Population Reference Bureau; 2005.

31. Murphy E. *Promoting Healthy Behavior, Health Bulletin 2.* Washington, DC: Population Reference Bureau; 2005.

32. Scrimshaw SC. Culture, Behavior, and Health. In: Merson MH, Black RE, Mills A, eds. *International Public Health: Diseases, Programs, Systems, and Policies.* Gaithersburg, MD: Aspen Publishers; 2001:66.

33. Rogers E. *Diffusion of Innovations.* 3rd ed. New York: Free Press; 1983.

34. Murphy E. *Promoting Healthy Behavior, Health Bulletin 2.* Washington, DC: Population Reference Bureau; 2005.

35. Murphy E. *Promoting Healthy Behavior, Health Bulletin 2.* Washington, DC: Population Reference Bureau; 2005.

36. Murphy E. *Promoting Healthy Behavior, Health Bulletin 2.* Washington, DC: Population Reference Bureau; 2005.

37. Murphy E. *Promoting Healthy Behavior, Health Bulletin 2.* Washington, DC: Population Reference Bureau; 2005.

38. Vanclay F. Social Impact Assessment: International Principles. Available at: http://www.iaia.org/Members/Publications/Guidelines_Principles/SP2.pdf. Accessed October 27, 2006.

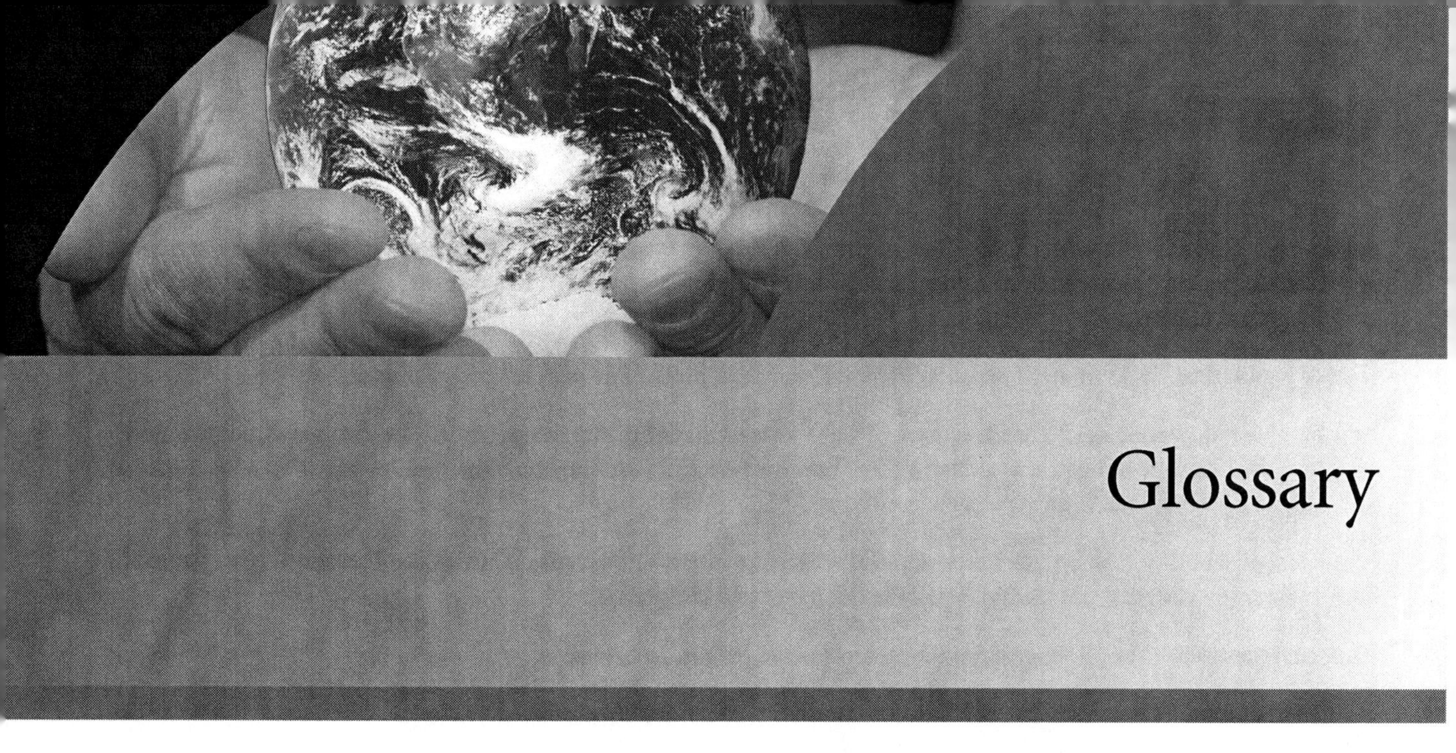

Glossary

TERM DEFINITION (*NOTE: Some definitions are quoted from other sources; refer to text for citations.)

Abortion The premature expulsion or loss of embryo, which may be induced or spontaneous.

Absolute risk The actual chances or probability of developing the disease expressed as a probability such as 0.01 or a percentage such as 1%.

Access The potential for or actual entry of a population into the health system. Entry is dependent on the wants, resources, and needs that individuals bring to the care-seeking process. Ability to obtain wanted or needed services may be influenced by many factors, including travel distance, waiting time, available financial resources, and availability of a regular source of care.

Actual cause of death A primary determinant or risk factor associated with a pathologic or diagnosed cause of death. For example, tobacco use would be the actual cause for deaths from many lung cancers.

Age adjustment Taking into account age-distribution of a population when comparing population or when comparing the same population at two different points in time.

Age distribution The number of people in each age group in a population.

Anemia A low level of hemoglobin in the blood.

Artifactual difference or changes Differences between population or changes in a population over time due to changes in interest in identifying the disease, change in ability to recognize the disease or changes in the definition of the disease.

Assessment One of public health's three core functions. Assessment calls for regularly and systematically collecting, analyzing, and making available information on the health of a community, including statistics on health status, community health needs, and epidemiologic and other studies of health problems.

Assets Resources available to achieve a specific end, such as community resources that can contribute to community health improvement efforts or emergency response resources, including human, to respond to a public health emergency.

Association The relationship between two or more events or variables. Events are said to be associated when they occur more frequently together than one would expect by chance. Association does not necessarily imply a causal relationship.

Assurance One of public health's three core functions. It involves assuring constituents that services necessary to achieve agreed-upon goals are provided by encouraging actions on the part of others, by requiring action through regulation, or by providing services directly.

At-risk population The group of people who have a chance or probability of developing a disease.

Attributable risk percentage The percentage of the disease or disability that can potentially be eliminated, among those with the factor being investigated, assuming a contributory cause and assuming the impact of the "cause" can be immediately and completely eliminated (*Synonym*: percent efficacy).

Biological plausibility An ancillary or supportive criteria for contributory cause in which the disease can be explained by what is currently known about the biology of the risk factor and the disease.

Built environment The physical environment constructed by human beings.

Burden of disease Generically an analysis of the morbidity and mortality produced by disease. Often used to refer to the use of DALYs to estimate the burden of morbidity and mortality.

Capacity The capability to carry out the core functions of public health. Also see *infrastructure.*

Cardiovascular disease (CVD) A disease of the heart or blood vessels.

Case-control studies A study that begins by identifying individuals with a disease and individual without a disease. Those with and without the disease are identified without knowledge of an individual's exposure or non-exposure to the factors being investigated (*Synonym*: retrospective study).

Case fatality rate The proportion of cases of a specified condition which is fatal within a specified period of time.

Casualty Any person suffering physical and/or psychological damage that leads to death, injury, or material loss.

Cataract A clouding of the lens of the eye.

Cause of Death For the purpose of national mortality statistics, every death is attributed to one underlying condition, based on the information reported on the death certificate and utilizing the international rules for selecting the underlying cause of death from the reported conditions.

Centers for Disease Control and Prevention (CDC) The Centers for Disease Control and Prevention, based in Atlanta, Georgia, is the federal agency charged with protecting the nation's public health by providing direction in the prevention and control of communicable and other diseases and responding to public health emergencies. CDC's responsibilities as the nation's prevention agency have expanded over the years and will continue to evolve as the agency addresses contemporary threats to health, such as injury, environmental and occupational hazards, behavioral risks, and chronic diseases; and emerging communicable diseases, such as the Ebola virus.

Cesarean delivery (section) The delivery of a fetus by surgical incision through the abdominal wall and uterus.

Chronic disease A disease that has one or more of the following characteristics: (1) it is permanent, (2) it leaves residual disability, (3) it is caused by a nonreversible pathologic alteration, (4) it requires special training of the patient for rehabilitation, or (5) it may be expected to require a long period of supervision, observation, or care.

Cohort study An investigation that begins by identifying a group that has a factor under investigation and a similar group that does not have the factor. The outcome in each group is then assessed (*Synonym*: prospective study).

Communicable disease Illness that is caused by a particular infectious agent and that spreads directly or indirectly from people to people, from animals to animals, from animals to people, or from people to animals.

Community A group of people who have common characteristics; communities can be defined by location, race, ethnicity, age, occupation, interest in particular problems or outcomes, or other common bonds. Ideally, there should be available assets and resources, as well as collective discussion, decision making, and action.

Community oriented primary care (COPC) A structured six-step process designed to move the delivery of health services from a focus on the individual to an additional focus on the needs of communities.

Community oriented public health (COPH) An effort on the part of governmental health agencies to reach out to the community and to the healthcare delivery system to address specific health issues.

Condition A health condition is a departure from a state of physical or mental well-being. An impairment is a health condition that includes chronic or permanent health defects resulting from disease, injury, or congenital malformations. All health conditions except impairments are coded according to an international classification system. Based on duration, there are two types of conditions—acute and chronic.

Confounding variable A difference in the groups being compared that makes a difference in the outcome being measured.

Consistency A supportive or ancillary criteria implying that the relationship has been observed in a wide range of populations and settings.

Contamination An accidental release of hazardous chemicals or nuclear materials that pollute the environment and place humans at risk.

Contributing factor A risk factor (causative factor) that is associated with the level of a determinant. Direct contributing factors are linked with the level of determinants; indirect contributing factors are linked with the level of direct contributing factors.

Contributory cause A definition of causation that is established when all three of the following have been established: (1) the existence of an association between the "cause" and the "effect" at the individual level; (2) the "cause" precedes the effect in time; and (3) altering the "cause" alters the probability of the "effect."

Control Reduction of disease incidence, prevalence, morbidity, or mortality to a locally acceptable level.

Core functions Three basic roles for public health for assuring conditions in which people can be healthy. As identified in the Institute of Medicine's landmark report, *The Future of Public Health*, these are assessment, policy development, and assurance.

Cost-benefit analysis An economic analysis in which all costs and benefits are converted into monetary (dollar) values, and results are expressed as dollars of benefit per dollars expended.

Cost-effectiveness analysis In health, a tool for comparing the relative cost of two or more investments with the amount of health that can be purchased with those investments.

Crude mortality rate The total number of deaths per unit of population reported during a given time interval, often expressed as the number of deaths per 1,000 or 100,000 persons.

Culture A set of rules or standards shared by members of a society, which when acted upon by the members, produce behavior that falls within a range of variation that members consider proper and acceptable.

Demographic transition The shift from high fertility and high mortality to low fertility and low mortality.

Demographics Characteristic data, such as size, growth, density, distribution, and vital statistics, which are used to study human populations.

Determinant A primary risk factor (causative factor) associated with the level of health problem (i.e., the level of the determinant influences the level of the health problem).

Diabetes Medical illness caused by too little insulin or poor response to insulin.

Diarrhea A condition in which the sufferer has frequent and watery or loose bowel movements.

Disability The temporary or long-term reduction in a person's capacity to function.

Disability adjusted life year (DALY) A composite measure of premature deaths and losses due to illnesses and disabilities in a population.

Disaster Any event, typically occurring suddenly, that causes damage, ecologic disruption, loss of human life, or deterioration of health and health services and which exceeds the capacity of the affected community on a scale sufficient to require outside assistance.

Distribution of disease How a disease is spread out in a population often using factors such as person, place, and time.

Dose-response relationship A relationship which is present if changes in levels of an exposure are associated with changes in frequency of the outcome in a consistent direction.

Drug resistance The extent to which infectious and parasitic agents develop an ability to resist drug treatment

Early case finding and treatment An intervention strategy that seeks to identify disease or illness at an early stage so that prompt treatment will reduce the effects of the process.

Effectiveness The improvement in health outcome that a strategy can produce in typical community-based settings. Also, the degree to which objectives are achieved.

Efficacy The improvement in health outcome effect that a strategy can produce in expert hands under ideal circumstances.

Emergency Any natural or manmade situation that results in severe injury, harm, or loss to humans or property.

Epidemic The occurrence of a disease or condition at higher than normal levels in a population.

Epidemiologists An investigator who studies the occurrence and control of disease or other health conditions or events in defined populations.

Epidemiology The study of the distribution of determinants and antecedents of health and disease in human populations, the ultimate goal of which is to identify the underlying causes of a disease, then apply findings to disease prevention and health promotion.

Epidemiologic transition A shift in the pattern of disease from largely communicable diseases to non-communicable diseases.

Eradication Termination of all transmission of infection by extermination of the infectious agent through surveillance or containment.

***Escherichia coli (E. coli)* O57:H7** A bacterial pathogen that can infect humans and cause severe bloody diarrhea (hemorrhagic colitis) and serious renal disease (hemolytic uremic syndrome).

Essential public health services A formulation of the processes used in public health to prevent epidemics and injuries, protect against environmental hazards, promote healthy behaviors, respond to disasters, and ensure quality and accessibility of health services. Ten essential services have been identified:

1. Monitoring health status to identify community health problems
2. Diagnosing and investigating health problems and health hazards in the community
3. Informing, educating, and empowering people about health issues
4. Mobilizing community partnerships to identify and solve health problems

5. Developing policies and plans that support individual and community health efforts
6. Enforcing laws and regulations that protect health and ensure safety
7. Linking people to needed personal health services and ensuring the provision of health care when otherwise unavailable
8. Ensuring a competent public health and personal health care work force
9. Evaluating effectiveness, accessibility, and quality of personal and population-based health services
10. Conducting research for new insights and innovative solutions to health problems

Family planning The conscious effort of couples to regulate the number and spacing of births through artificial and natural methods of contraception. Family planning connotes conception control to avoid pregnancy and abortion, but it also includes efforts of couples to induce pregnancy.

Female genital cutting(also called female circumcision and female genital mutilation) A collective term for various traditional practices which are all related to the cutting of the female genital organs. Four different forms and grades of female genital cutting are usually distinguished.

Foodborne illness Illness caused by the transfer of disease organisms or toxins from food to humans.

Global health Health problems, issues, and concerns that transcend national boundaries and may best be addressed by cooperative actions.

Goals For public health programs, general statements expressing a program's aspirations or intended effect on one or more health problems, often stated without time limits.

Gross domestic product The total market value of all the goods and services produced within a country during a specified period of time.

Gross national product A measure of the incomes of residents of a country, including income they receive from abroad but subtracting similar payments made to those abroad.

Group association Two factors such as a characteristic and a disease occur together more often than expected by chance alone in the same group or population. This does not require that the investigator have data on the characteristics of the individuals that make up the group or population (*Synonym*: ecological association).

Hazard A possible source of harm or injury.

Health The state of complete physical, mental, and social well-being and not merely the absence of disease or infirmity. It is recognized, however, that health has many dimensions (anatomic, physiologic, and mental) and is largely culturally defined. The relative importance of various disabilities will differ, depending on the cultural milieu and on the role of the affected individual in that culture. Most attempts at measurement have been assessed in terms of morbidity and mortality.

Health-adjusted life expectancy (HALE) A composite health indicator that measures the equivalent number of years in full health that a newborn can expect to live, based on current rates of ill health and mortality.

Health disparity Difference in health status between two groups, such as the health disparity in mortality between men and women, or the health disparity in infant mortality between African-American and white infants.

Healthcare safety net The provision of services for those who cannot afford to purchase the services.

Health education Any combination of learning opportunities designed to facilitate voluntary adaptations of behavior (in individuals, groups, or communities) conducive to good health. Health education encourages positive health behavior.

Health planning Planning concerned with improving health, whether undertaken comprehensively for an entire community or for a particular population, type of health services, institution, or health program. The components of health planning include data assembly and analysis, goal determination, action recommendation, and implementation strategy.

Health policy Social policy concerned with the process whereby public health agencies evaluate and determine health needs and the best ways to address them, including the identification of appropriate resources and funding mechanisms.

Health problem A situation or condition of people (expressed in health outcome measures such as mortality, morbidity, or disability) that is considered undesirable and is likely to exist in the future.

Health promotion An intervention strategy that seeks to eliminate or reduce exposures to harmful factors by modifying human behaviors. Any combination of health education and related organizational, political, and economic interventions designed to facilitate behavioral and environmental adaptations that will improve or protect health. This process enables individuals and communities to control and improve their own health. Health promotion approaches provide opportunities for people to identify problems, develop solutions, and work in partnerships that build on existing skills and strengths.

Health status indicators Measurements of the state of health of a specified individual, group, or population. Health status may be measured by proxies such as people's subjective assessments of their health; by one or more indicators of mortality and morbidity in the population, such as longevity or maternal and infant mortality; or by the incidence or prevalence of major diseases (communicable, chronic, or nutritional). Conceptually, health status is the proper outcome measure for the effectiveness of a specific population's health system, although attempts to relate effects of available medical care to variations in health status have proved difficult.

Health system (or healthcare system) The combination of resources, organization, and management that culminate in the delivery of health services to the population. The health system includes population-based preventive services, clinical preventive and other primary medical care services, and all levels of more sophisticated treatment and chronic care services.

Home rule Authority granted to local jurisdictions such as cities or countries by state constitutions or state legislative actions.

Hookworm A parasite that lives in the small intestine of its host, which may be a mammal such as a dog, cat, or human.

Hypertension High blood pressure.

Incidence A measure of the disease or injury in the population, generally the number of new cases occurring during a specified time period.

Indicator A measure of health status or a health outcome.

Infant mortality rate The number of live-born infants who die before their first birthday per 1,000 live births; often broken into two components, neonatal mortality (deaths before 28 days per 1,000 live births) and postneonatal mortality (deaths from 28 days through the rest of the first year of life per 1,000 live births).

Infectious disease A disease caused by the entrance into the body of organisms (such as bacteria, protozoans, fungi, or viruses) that then grow and multiply there (often used synonymously with communicable disease).

Infrastructure The systems, competencies, relationships, and resources that enable performance of public health's core functions and essential services in every community. Categories include human, organizational, informational, and fiscal resources.

Injury The result of an act that damages, harms, or hurts; unintentional or intentional damage to the body resulting from acute exposure to thermal, mechanical, electrical, or chemical energy or from the absence of such essentials as heat or oxygen.

Intervention A generic term used in public health to describe a program or policy designed to have an impact on a health problem. For example, a mandatory seat belt law is an intervention designed to reduce the incidence of automobile-related fatalities. Five categories of heath interventions are: (1) health promotion, (2) specific protection, (3) early case finding and prompt treatment, (4) disability limitation, and (5) rehabilitation.

Leading causes of death Those diagnostic classifications of disease that are most frequently responsible for deaths (often used in conjunction with the top 10 causes of death).

Life expectancy The number of additional years of life expected at a specified point in time, such as at birth or at age 45.

Life expectancy at birth The average number of years a newborn baby could expect to live if current mortality trends were to continue for the rest of the newborn's life.

Local public health agency (LPHA) Functionally, a local (county, multicounty, municipal, town, other) health agency, operated by local government, often with oversight and direction from a local board of health, that carries out public health's core functions throughout a defined geographic area. A more traditional definition is an agency serving less than an entire state that carries some responsibility for health and has at least one full-time employee and a specific budget.

Low birthweight A birthweight less than 2500 grams.

Malaria A disease of humans caused by blood parasites of the species *Plasmodium falciparum*, vivax, ovale, or malariae and transmitted by anopheline mosquitoes.

Maternal death The death of a woman while pregnant, during delivery, or within 42 days of delivery, irrespective of the duration and the site of pregnancy. The cause of death is always related to or aggravated by the pregnancy or its management; it does not include accidental or incidental causes.

Maternal mortality ratio The number of women who die as a result of pregnancy and childbirth complications per 100,000 live births in a given year.

Measles A highly communicable disease characterized by fever, general malaise, sneezing, nasal congestion, a brassy cough, conjunctivitis, and an eruption over the entire body, caused by the rubeola virus.

Measure An indicator of health status or a health outcome, used synonymously with *indicator* in this text.

Mission For public health, assuring conditions in which people can be healthy.

Mitigation Measures taken to reduce the harmful effects of a disaster or emergency by attempting to limit the impact on human health and economic infrastructure.

Morbidity A measure of disease incidence or prevalence in a given population, location, or other grouping of interest.

Mortality Expresses the number of deaths in a population within a prescribed time. Mortality rates may be expressed as crude death rates (total deaths in relation to total population during a year) or as death rates specific for diseases and sometimes for age, sex, or other attributes (e.g., the number of deaths from cancer in white males in relation to the white male population during a given year).

Natural experiment A change that occurs in one particular population but not another similar population without the intervention of an investigator.

Necessary cause If the "cause" is not present the disease or "effect" will not develop.

Neonatal mortality rate Number of deaths to infants under 28 days of age in a given year per 1000 live births in that year.

Neonatal tetanus A bacterial infection usually contracted by a puncture wound with a dirty object.

Non-communicable disease Illness that is not spread by any infectious agent.

Non-governmental organization (NGO) A non-profit group or association organized outside of institutionalized political structures to realize particular social objectives, such as environmental protection, or serve particular constituencies, such as indigenous peoples

Obesity Excessive body fat content.

Objectives Targets for achievement through interventions. Objectives are time-limited and measurable in all cases. Various levels of objectives for an intervention include outcome, impact, and process objectives.

Odds ratio A measure of the strength of the relationship that is often a good approximation of the relative risk. This ratio is calculated as the odds of having the risk factor if the disease is present divided by the odds of having the risk factor if the disease is absent.

Outcomes Indicators of health status, risk reduction, and quality-of-life enhancement (sometimes referred to as results of the health system). Outcomes are long-term objectives that define optimal, measurable future levels of health status; maximum acceptable levels of disease, injury, or dysfunction; or prevalence of risk factors.

Overweight Excess weight relative to height.

Parasite An animal or vegetable organism that lives on or in another and derives its nourishment therefrom.

P.E.R.I. process A mnemonic which summarizes the evidence-based public health process including problem description, etiology, recommendations based upon evidence, and implementation.

Pneumonia An inflammation, usually caused by infection, involving the alveoli of the lungs

Policy development One of public health's three core functions. Policy development involves serving the public interest by leading in developing comprehensive public health policy and promoting the use of the scientific knowledge base in decision making.

Poliomyelitis (polio) Infantile paralysis, a viral paralytic disease.

Population-based public health services Interventions aimed at disease prevention and health promotion that affect an entire population and extend beyond medical treatment by targeting underlying risks, such as tobacco, drug, and alcohol use; diet and sedentary lifestyles; and environmental factors.

Population comparisons A type of investigation in which groups are compared without having information on the individuals within the group (*Synonym*: ecological study).

Population health approach As used here, a term used to describe an evidence-based approach to problem solving that considers a range of possible interventions including health care, traditional public health and social interventions (*Synonyms*: ecological approach, socio-ecological approach).

Preparedness All measures and policies taken before an event occurs that allow for prevention, mitigation, and readiness.

Prevalence A measurement of the number of people suffering from a certain condition over a specific time period. The "prevalence rate" is the share of the population, which is being measured, who have the condition.

Prevention Anticipatory action taken to prevent the occurrence of an event or to minimize its effects after it has occurred. Prevention aims to minimize the occurrence of disease or its consequences. It includes actions that reduce susceptibility or exposure to health threats (primary prevention), detect and treat disease in early stages (secondary prevention), and alleviate the effects of disease and injury (tertiary prevention). Examples of prevention include immunizations, emergency response to epidemics, health education, modification of risk-prone behavior and physical hazards, safety training, workplace hazard elimination, and industrial process change.

Preventive strategies Frameworks for categorizing prevention programs, based on how the prevention technology is delivered—provider to patient (clinical preventive services), individual responsibility (behavioral prevention), or alteration in an individual's surroundings (environmental prevention)—or on the stage of the natural history of a disease or injury (primary, secondary, tertiary).

Primary intervention An intervention that occurs before the onset of the disease.

Primary medical care Clinical preventive services, first-contact treatment services, and ongoing care for commonly encountered medical conditions. Basic or general health care focuses on the point at which a patient ideally seeks assistance from the medical care system. Primary care is considered comprehensive when the primary provider takes responsibility for the overall coordination of the care of the patient's health problems, whether these are medical, behavioral, or social. The appropriate use of consultants and community resources is an important part of effective primary health care. Such care is generally provided by physicians but can also be provided by other personnel, such as nurse practitioners or physician assistants.

Primary prevention Prevention strategies that seek to prevent the occurrence of disease or injury, generally through reducing exposure or risk factor levels. These strategies can reduce or eliminate causative risk factors (risk reduction).

Proportion A fraction in which the numerator is made up of observations that are also included in the denominator.

Protective factor A factor which is associated with a reduced probability of disease.

Public health The science and art of preventing disease; prolonging life; and promoting physical health and mental health and efficiency through organized community efforts toward a sanitary environment, control of community infections, education in hygiene, and the development of social machinery to ensure capacity in the community to maintain health. These include organized community efforts to prevent, identify, and counter threats to the health of the public.

Public health agency A unit of government (federal, state, local, or regional) charged with preserving, protecting, and promoting the health of the population through assuring delivery of essential public health services.

Public health in America A document developed by the Core Functions Project that characterizes the vision, mission, outcome aspirations, and essential services of public health. Also see *essential public health services.*

Public health organization A nongovernmental entity (e.g., not-for-profit agency, association, corporation) participating in activities designed to improve the health status of a community or population.

Public health practice The development and application of preventive strategies and interventions to promote and protect the health of populations.

Public health system That part of the larger health system that seeks to assure conditions in which people can be healthy by carrying out public health's three core functions. The system can be further described by its inputs, practices, outputs, and outcomes.

Public health workforce The public health workforce includes individuals:

- Employed by an organization engaged in an organized effort to promote, protect, and preserve the health of a defined population group. The group may be public or private, and the effort may be secondary or subsidiary to the principal objectives of the organization
- Performing work made up of one or more specific public health services or activities
- Occupying positions that conventionally require at least 1 year of postsecondary specialized public health training and that are (or can be) assigned a professional occupational title

Randomized clinical trial An investigation in which individuals are assigned to study or control groups using a process of randomization. (*Synonym*: experimental study).

Rate A mathematical expression for the relation between the numerator (e.g., number of deaths, diseases, disabilities, services) and denominator (population at risk), together with specification of time. Rates make possible a comparison of the number of events between populations and at different times. Rates may be crude, specific, or adjusted.

Randomization As part of a randomized clinical trial, assignment of participants to study and control groups using a chance process in which the participants are assigned to a particular group with a known probability (*Synonym*: Random assignment).

Recommendations Statements based upon evidence indicating that actions such as cigarette cessation will improve outcomes such a reducing lung cancer.

Recovery Actions of responders, government, and victims that help return an affected community to normal by stimulating community cohesiveness and governmental involvement. The recovery period falls between the onset of an emergency and the reconstruction period.

Rehabilitation An intervention strategy that seeks to return individuals to the maximum level of functioning possible.

Relative risk A ratio of the probability of the outcome if a factor known as a risk factor is present compared to the probability of the outcome if the factor is not present.

Response The phase in a disaster or public health emergency when relief, recovery, and rehabilitation occur.

Reverse causality The situation in which the apparent "cause" is actually the "effect."

Risk The probability that exposure to a hazard will lead to a negative consequence.

Risk assessment A determination of the likelihood of adverse health effects to a population after exposure to a hazard.

Risk factor An aspect or personal behavior or lifestyle, an environmental exposure, or an inborn or inherited characteristic that, on the basis of epidemiologic evidence, is known to be associated with health-related conditions.

Risk indicator A characteristic such as gender or age that is associated with an outcome but is not considered a contributory cause (*Synonym*: risk marker).

Screening The use of technology and procedures to differentiate those individuals with signs or symptoms of disease from those less likely to have the disease. Then, if necessary, further diagnosis and, if indicated, early intervention and treatment can be provided.

Score In the context of evidence-based recommendations, a measurement of the quality of the evidence and a measurement of the magnitude of the impact.

Secondary intervention Early detection of disease or risk factors and intervention during an asymptomatic phase.

Secondary prevention Prevention strategies that seek to identify and control disease processes in their early stages before signs and symptoms develop (screening and treatment).

Sex selective abortion The practice of aborting a fetus after a determination, usually by ultrasound but also rarely by amniocentesis or another procedure, that the fetus is an undesired sex, typically female.

Sexually transmitted infections (STIs) Diseases, also known as sexually-transmitted diseases (STDs), that are commonly transmitted between partners through some form of sexual activity, most commonly vaginal intercourse, oral sex, or anal sex.

Social justice A philosophy that aims to provide fair treatment and a fair share of the reward of society to individuals and groups.

Society A group of people who occupy a specific locality and share the same cultural traditions

Strength of the relationship A supportive or ancillary criteria implying that a measurement of the strength of an association such as a relative risk or odds ratio is large or substantial.

Stroke Temporary or permanent loss of the blood supply to the brain.

Sufficient cause If the "cause" is present the disease or "effect" will occur.

Supportive criteria Criteria that may be used to argue for a cause and effect relationship when the definitive requirements have not been fulfilled (*Synonym*: ancillary criteria).

Surrogate outcome A measurement of outcome that looks at short term results such as changes in laboratory tests that may not reflect longer term or clinical important outcomes.

Surveillance Systematic monitoring of the health status of a population through collection, analysis, and interpretation of health data in order to plan, implement, and evaluate public health programs, including determining the need for public health action.

Tertiary intervention An intervention that occurs after the initial occurrence of symptoms but before irreversible disability occurs.

True rate A measurement that has a numerator which is a subset of the denominator and a unit of time, such as a day or a year, over which the number of events in the numerator is measured.

Under-five child mortality rate The annual number of deaths in children under five years, expressed as a rate per thousand live births, averaged over the previous 5 years.

Undernutrition Low weight-for-age; two z-scores below the international reference for weight-for-age.

Victim blaming Placing the responsibility or blame for a bad outcome on the individual who experiences the bad outcome due to their behavior.

Vulnerability The susceptibility of a population to a specific type of event, generally associated with the degree of possible or potential loss from a risk that results from a hazard at a given intensity. Vulnerability can be influenced by demographics, the age and resilience of the environment, technology, social differentiation and diversity, as well as regional and global economics and politics.

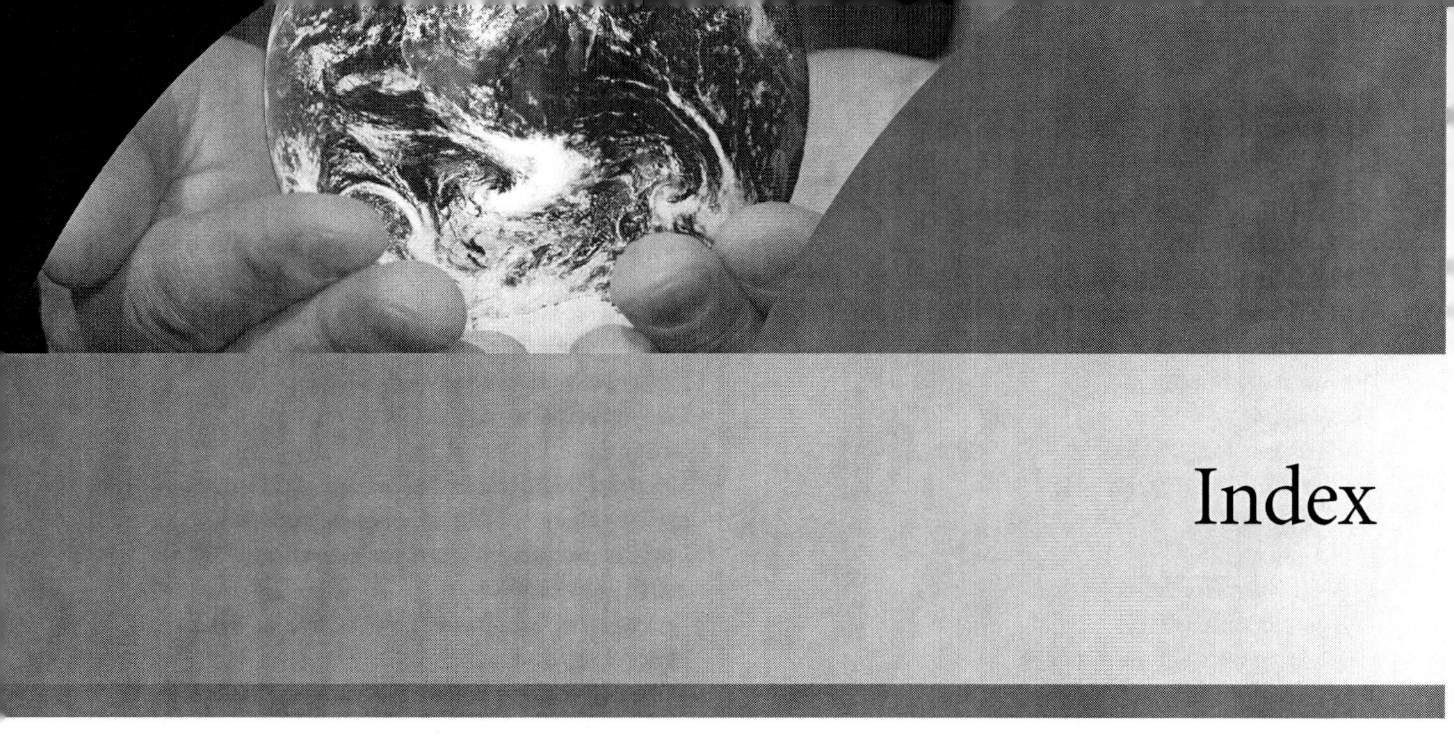

Index

Page numbers in italic denote figures; those followed by *n* denote footnotes, and those followed by *t* denote tables

A

Absolute risk, 46*nj*
Abuja Declaration of 2000, 151
Access, to healthcare, 17
Acquired Immune Deficiency Syndrome. *See* AIDS
Administrative occupations, 98–99
African American men, in Tuskegee study, 81–82
African Development Bank, 198
African Programme for Onchocerciasis Control, 208
Age, causes of death by, 27
Age adjustment, 43
Age distribution, 43
Agency for Healthcare Research and Quality (AHRQ), 66*t*
AIDS, 5, 24, 29, 43, 84, 206
  addressing burden of, 148–150
  basic facts about, 142*t*
  burden of, 140–143
  costs and consequences of, 146–148
  future challenges to control of, 156, 157
  human rights and, 78–79
  tuberculosis and, 158
Air pollution
  indoor, 163, 165, 166, 170, 174, 218
  outdoor, 166, 169, 174
  reducing levels of, 5
  urban, 167
Alcohol abuse
  addressing burden of, 125
  burden of, 123
  costs and consequences of, 124
American Cancer Society, 45
American public health agencies, brief history of, 64 (box 4–1)
American Public Health Association
  ethical principles, 94–96
  formation of, 4
American public health movement, history behind, 3–4
American Red Cross, 70
Ancillary criteria, 45
  cigarettes, lung cancer and, 45–47, 47*t*
Angiosarcoma, 42 (box 3–1)
Antibiotics, 4
APHA. *See* American Public Health Association
APOC. *See* African Programme for Onchocerciasis Control
Artemisinin, 151
Artifactual, 40
Asbestosis, 42 (box 3–1)
Asian Development Bank, 198
ASPH. *See* Association of Schools of Public Health
Assessment, 60
Association of Schools of Public Health, 109
Assurance, 60
Asthma, determinants of disease and, 11–12 (box 1–1)
At-risk population, 41
Attributable risk percentage, 50*n*
Avian influenza, 155–156, 206

B

Bacterial infections, 146
Behaviors
  disease and, 10
  understanding, 221

Belmont Report, 81, 82*t*
Bilateral development assistance agencies, 198–199, 198*t*
Bill & Melinda Gates Foundation, 70, 199–200, 201, 205, 208
Biological plausibility, 46
Bioterrorism, 5
Bioterrorism preparedness, 106
Bipolar disorder, 122*t*, 127
Birth records, 4
Blood glucose, 118*t*
BLS. *See* Bureau of Labor Statistics
Branch office model, 63
Built environment, disease and, 10
Burden of disease
  by group of cause, percent of deaths, 2001, *32*
  in terms of morbidity and mortality, 41–42
Bureau of Labor Statistics, 99, 101

C

Cancer, 25, 118*t*, 132
  burden of, 120–121
  leading causes of death, by region, 2001, 121*t*
  prevention of, tobacco control and, 127
Carbon monoxide, 166*t*
Cardiovascular disease, 118*t*, 132
  burden of, 118–119
  costs and consequences of, 123
  as leading cause of death worldwide, 35
CARE, 70
Careers in public health, 97, 100*t*, 104–105
Case, 139*t*
Case-control studies, 44
Case-fatality, 41
Case fatality rate, 139*t*, 180
Cataract blindness control, in India, 129–130
Cataract Blindness Control Project, 129, 130
Causation, 44, 49 (box 3–3)
Centers for Disease Control and Prevention (CDC), 65, 66*t*, 67 (box 4–2), 107
Certified Health Education Specialists, 113
CEUs. *See* Continuing education units
Chadwick, Edwin, 4
Chagas disease, controlling in Southern Cone of South America, 153–154
CHES. *See* Certified Health Education Specialists
CHEs. *See* Complex humanitarian emergencies
Chest X-rays, 4
Childhood healthcare, as health determinant, 17
Child mortality, environmental health and reduction in, 164*t*
Child oral health, community oriented public health and, 73 (box 4–6)
Children, second-hand smoke and, 48
China, tuberculosis in, 153
Cholera, 4
Cholesterol, high, addressing burden of, 125–126
Chronic pulmonary disease, smoking and, 48
Cigarettes, women and mass consumption of, 39
Cigarette smoking
  examples of "who" and "how" related to, 54*t*
  lung cancer and
    ancillary or supportive criteria and, 45–47, 47*t*
    establishing cause and effect, 47–49, 48*t*
    as risk factor for, 45
  recommendations related to reducing health impact of, 49–52
  steps after implementation relative to, 54–56
  victim blaming and, 54
Civil conflict, complex humanitarian emergencies and, 178
Civil War, 4
Close calls, 51
Cohort studies, 44, 45
Communicable diseases, 22, 137–159
  addressing burden of, 148–152
  avian influenza, 155–156
  burden of, 139–140
  case studies, 152–155
  costs and consequences of, 146–148
  deaths from selected infectious and parasitic diseases, 140*t*
  defined, 118
  diarrheal disease, 145
  future challenges to control of, 156–158
  HIV/AIDs, 141–143
  importance of, 137–138
  key terms, definitions, and concepts, 138–139, 139*t*
  leading causes of death from, 2001, 140*t*
  malaria, 145
  MDGs and, 139*t*
  neglected diseases, 145–146
  tuberculosis, 143–145
  vignettes, 137
Community mobilization, health behavior changes and, 221, 224
Community-oriented primary care, 70, 72 (box 4–5)
Community-oriented public health, 71
  child oral health and, 73 (box 4–6)

Community partnerships, mobilizing, public health and, 71–72
Competencies
preparedness management system for public health workforce and, *113*
for public health practitioners, 108–109, 110–111*t*, 111–112
Complex humanitarian emergencies, 178, 189
addressing health effects of, 185–187
assessment and surveillance, 185–186
disease control, 186–187
food, 186
safe and healthy environment, 186
case studies, 187–188
characteristics of, 181
health effects of, 182–184
causes of death, 182–183
mental health, 183–184
violence against women, 183
importance of, to global health, 177–178
key terms related to, 178–180
selected, 179*t*
Confounding variable, 44
Consistency, 46
Contagion control, 6*t*
Continuing education, for public health workers, 97
Continuing education units, 97, 114
Contributory cause(s), 9
establishing, 44–45
fulfilling requirements for, *46*
implication of, 47–49
inability to definitely establish, 45–47
lightning, thunder, and, 44 (box 3–2)
Control (disease control), 139*t*
Convention on the Elimination of all Forms of Discrimination Against Women, 77
Convention on the Rights of the Child, 77
COPC. *See* Community-oriented primary care
COPH. *See* Community-oriented public health
Core functions
IOM-defined, 60
public health workforce and, 90
Coronary artery disease, smoking and, 48
Cost-effectiveness analysis, 83
Council on Linkages between Academia and Public Health Practice, 109, 112
CRC. *See* Convention on the Rights of the Child
Credentials, for public health workers, 113
Crude mortality rate, 179
Culture
health and, 223–224
health beliefs and practices and, 215–217
diagnosis and treatment of illness, 216–217
folk illness, 216
health providers, 217
perceptions of disease, 215–216, 217*t*
perceptions of illness, 215
prevention of illness, 216
importance of, to health, 213–214
social impact assessment and, 222–223, 223*t*
in various domains, 214
vignettes, 213
CVD. *See* Cardiovascular disease

D

DANIDA, 129
Death
causes of
in adults, 15-59 years, by broad income group, 2001, 27*t*
by age, 27
in children, ages 0-14, by broad income group, 2001, 27*t*
by gender, 28
by region, 26–27
ten leading, 25*t*
determinants of, 9–11
Death records, 4
Declaration of Helsinki, 80–81, 81*t*
Demographic characteristics, 40
Demographic transition, 30–31
fertility/mortality percentages, *31*
implications of, 32–33
Department of Energy, 69
Department of Health and Human Services, 65, 66*t*, 107
Department of Homeland Security, 69
Department of Housing and Urban Development, 69
Depression, 6, 122*t*, 127
Determinants, of disease, disability, and death, 9–11
Determinants of health, 16–18, 17*t*
Development assistance, positive outcomes in, 207*t*
Diabetes, 118*t*, 120*t*, 126–127, 132
burden of, 119–120
costs and consequences of, 123–124
Diarrhea, 24, 140
addressing burden of, 151
burden of, 145
oral rehydration therapy for, 151, 158

reducing burden of water-related disease and, 174
Diet, healthy, 126
Diffusions of Innovations model, 220, 224
Disability, 9–11, 20, 22, 24
Disability Adjusted Life Year (DALY), 22
burden of deaths and disease within countries, 29
calculating, 23–24
ten leading causes of, 25*t*
Disaster, defined, 178. *See also* Natural disasters
Disease(s), 22. *See also* Communicable diseases; Non-communicable diseases
culture and perceptions of, 215–216, 217*t*
determinants of, 9–11
distribution of, 40
differences in, 42–43
global burden of, 24–29
measuring burden of, 22–24
Distribution of disease, 40
Distributions of person and place, generating hypotheses from, 42 (box 3–1)
Doctors Without Borders, 188, 200–201, 205, 208
Dose-response relationship, 46
DOTS, TB treatment strategy, 150, 153, 158
Drug resistance
description of, 138–139
HIV/AIDS and, 157
tuberculosis and, 144–145

E

Earthquake in Pakistan, 187–188
Earthquake Rehabilitation and Reconstruction Authority, 188
Ebola virus, 155, 206
Ecological perspective, 219, 219*t*
Ecological studies, 43
Economic recession of 2009, worker displacement and, 114
Education
as health determinant, 16–17
for public health workers, 102, 109, 111–112
Effectiveness, 50
Efficacy, 45, *46*
Emergency management specialists, 106
Eminence-based recommendation, 50
Environment, as health determinant, 16
Environmental factors, disease and, 10
Environmental health
future challenges to, 173
global burden of disease and, 173–174
importance of, 163–165
key concepts in, 165
poor women and children and, 173–174
typical issues, determinants and health consequences, 65*t*
UN Millennium Goals and, 164*t*
vignettes, 163
Environmental health problems, costs and consequences of, 168–169
Environmentally-related diseases, burden of, 167–168
Environmental Protection Agency (EPA), 69
Epidemiological transition, 30, 31–32
Epidemiologists, 40, 108
Epidemiology, history behind, 4
Eradication (of disease), 139*t*
ERRA. *See* Earthquake Rehabilitation and Reconstruction Authority
Essential public health services, public health workforce and, 90
Ethical rights, global health and importance of, 75–76
Ethics
investment choices in health and, 83–84
key challenges for the future and, 84–85
public health workers and, 94–97
Etiology, establishing contributory cause, 44–45
European Convention on the Protection of Human Rights, 76
Evidence-based health, 5
complete P.E.R.I. approach to, *55*
questions to ask, 55*t*
Evidence-based medicine, 5
Evidence-based public health, 39–57
Evidence-based recommendations, 50–51, 51 (box 3–4)
Exercise, 17, 126
Experimental studies, 44

F

Farmer, Paul, 205
Farr, William, 4
Federal public health agencies, roles of, 65
Federal Relief Commission, 188
Fertility, demographic and epidemiologic transitions and, 30–33
Fluoride, cavities and, 42 (box 3–1)
Folk illness, 216
Food and Drug Administration, 1, 5, 64 (box 4–1), 66*t*
Food-borne disease, 138
Foundations, global health and, 199–200
Framework Convention on Tobacco Control (WHO), 55
FRC. *See* Federal Relief Commission
Full time equivalent (FTE) workers

of federal, state, and local government health agencies, 91*t*
of state and local health agencies by state, 2003 and 2008, 93–94*t*
of state and local health agencies per 10,000 population, 1998-2008, U.S., *92*

G

Gates Foundation. *See* Bill & Melinda Gates Foundation
GAVI. *See* Global Alliance for Vaccines and Immunization
Gebbie, Kristine, 89
Gender
causes of death by, 28
determinants of health and, 16
ten leading causes of death ordered by, in low- and middle-income countries, 2001, 28*t*
Gender equality, environmental health and, 164t
Genetics, disease and, 10
Geography, disease and, 10
Germ theory of disease, 4
Global Alliance for Vaccines and Immunization, 193, 201–202, 209
Global burden of disease, 24–29
burdens of deaths and disease within countries, 29
causes of death by age, 27
causes of death by gender, 28
causes of death by region, 26–27
overview, 24–26
ten leading causes of, in low- and middle-income by region, 2001, 26*t*
trends in, 28–29
Global Fund, The, 201, 202, 206, 209
Global health
agenda setting for, 205–206
bilateral development assistance agencies and, 198–199, 198*t*
cooperating for improvement in, 194
future challenges to, 206–207
intellectual property rights and, 79–80
key actors in, 194–200
organizational actors in, 195*t*
trends in, 204–205
Global health organizations and agencies, roles of, 65, 68
Global public health organizations, 68t
Government agencies, health issues and, 69
Government public health agencies
goals and roles of, 59–60
viewing, framework for, *63*
Gross domestic product per capita, female life expectancy at birth, selected countries, 2004, *33*
Group associations, 40
differences/changes used in suggesting, artifactual or real, 43
implication of, 43–44
Guide to Community Prevention Services, The (CDC), 51

H

HALE. *See* Health-Adjusted Life Expectancy
Hand washing, 4
Health
culture and, 213–214, 223–224
as human right, 78
Health-Adjusted Life Expectancy, 22
selected countries, 2004, 23*t*
Health behaviors
changing, 221–222
community mobilization, 221
health education, 222
mass media, 221–222
social marketing, 222
success in health promotion, 222
culture, behavior change and, 218–219
improving
Diffusions of Innovations model, 220, 220*t*
ecological approach, 219, 219*t*
Health Belief model, 219, 224
Stages of Change model, 220, 220*t*
Health Belief model, 219, 224
Health care, 8–9, 9*t*
Healthcare safety net, 64
Health disparities, global, 15
Health education, 222, 224
Health educators, 101
Health impact, reducing, what works, 49–52
Health insurance, universal, 17–18
Health issues, 5
Health problems
addressing and describing, 40
rates and, 40–41
Health promotion
achieving success in, 222, 222*t*, 224
approaches to, 8–9
disease prevention and, 5, 6*t*
Health protection, 6*t*
Health providers
cultural beliefs about, 217
examples of, 218*t*

Health reform legislation (2010), public health workforce and, 114–115
Health Resources and Services Administration, 65, 66*t*, 89, 92, 96
Health services, culture and use of, 216–217
Health services administrators, 101
Health status, measuring, importance of, 16
Health status indicators, key, 18, 18*t*, 20, 22
Heart disease, 25
Helicobacter pylori, 121, 127
Helminthic infections, 146
  burden of, in Africa, by % of global burden of condition, 147*t*
Hepatitis B, 11
HHS. *See* Department of Health and Human Services
High blood pressure, addressing burden of, 125–126
High-risk approach, 8, *8*
HIV/AIDS, 5, 7, 11, 24, 29, 43, 84
  addressing burden of, 148–150
  basic facts about, 142*t*
  burden of, 140–143
  costs and consequences of, 146–148
  culture, behavior change and, 218
  environmental health and control of, 164*t*
  future challenges to control of, 156, 157
  human rights and, 78–79
  prevalence by country, 2005, *143*
  risk factors for, 142
  in Thailand, 152–153
  tuberculosis and, 158
Home rule model, 63
HRSA. *See* Health Resources and Services Administration
Human Immunodeficiency Virus. *See* HIV/AIDS
Human research cases, key, 81–83
  Jewish Chronic Disease Hospital, 82–83
  Milgram obedience study, 83
  Tuskegee study, 81–82
  Willowbrook School study, 82
Human rights
  foundations for health and, 76–77
  global health and importance of, 75–76
  health as, 78
  health interventions and, 77–78
  HIV/AIDS and, 78–79
  key challenges for the future, 84–85
  temporary suspension of, 79
Human subjects
  foundations for research on, 80–81
    Declaration of Helsinki, 80–81
    Nuremberg Code, 80
  institutional review boards and, 83, 84
Hygiene
  culture, health behaviors and, 218
  environmental health and, 167, 168, 172, 174
  integrating investment choices about, 172–173
Hygiene movement, 4, 6*t*
Hypertension, 118*t*, 125–126
Hypotheses, generating, distributions of person and place and, 42 (box 3–1)

I

IAVI. *See* International AIDS Vaccine Initiative
ICCPR. *See* International Covenant on Civil and Political Rights
ICD. *See* International Classification of Diseases
ICESR. *See* International Covenant on Economic, Social, and Cultural Rights
IDP. *See* Internally displaced people
IHD. *See* Ischemic heart disease
IHS. *See* Indian Health Service
Illness
  culture and diagnosis/treatment of, 216–217
  culture and perceptions of, 224
  culture and prevention of, 216
Immunization, 28, 193
Implementation
  framework of options for, 53*t*
  interventions and, 52–54
  steps after, 54–56
Improving-the-average approach, 8, *8*
Incidence, 22
Incidence rates, 22, 41
India, cataract blindness control in, 129–130
Indian Health Service, 65, 66*t*
Infant mortality rate, 18, 18*t*
  by region, 2004, *19*
Infection, disease and, 10
Influenza, 28
  avian, 155–156
  1918 pandemic, 156
Inhalation-related communicable disease, 138
Institute for One World Health, 203
Institute of Medicine, 89
  core public health functions defined by, 60, *63*
Institutional review boards, human subjects research and, 83, 84
Insulin, 119
Insulin-dependent diabetes mellitus, 120

Intellectual property rights, global health and, 79–80
Inter-American Development Bank, 198
Internally displaced people, 179, 179*t*, 189
International AIDS Vaccine Initiative, 198, 203, 208
International Classification of Diseases, 41
International Commission on Epidemics, 204
International Committee of the Red Cross, 181
International Covenant on Civil and Political Rights, 76–77
International Covenant on Economic, Social, and Cultural Rights, 76, 77
International Partnership on Microbicides, 208
Interventions, 5
  implementation and, 52–54
  motivational, 53–54
  primary, 52
  secondary, 52
  tertiary, 52
IRBs. *See* Institutional review boards
Ischemic heart disease, 118*t*, 119

J

Jenner, Edward, 3
Jewish Chronic Disease Hospital, 82–83
Journal of the American Medical Association, 114
Juvenile diabetes, 120

K

Kellogg Foundation, 70
Kerala, case study, 33–34
Kim, Jim, 205

L

Lead, 5, 166*t*
Legionnaire's disease, 155
Life expectancy
  at birth, 18, 18*t*
    by region, 2004, *19*
    selected countries, 2004, 23*t*
    for world, 28
  increase in, during 20th century, 2
  1960-2002, 28*t*
Lightning and thunder, contributory cause and, 44 (box 3–2)
Lind, James, 3
Local autonomy model, 63
Local health departments
  with employees in selected occupations, by size of population serviced, U.S., 2008, 96*t*
  estimated size and composition of workforce, U.S., 2008, 97*t*
  general patterns of staffing in, 94
  percentage of, employing selected professional occupations, 1990 and 2005, 198*t*
Local public health agencies, 91
  roles of, 60, 63–65
Lung cancer
  cigarette smoking and, 39
    ancillary or supportive criteria and, 45–47, 47*t*
    establishing cause and effect, 47–49, 48*t*
    as risk factor for, 45
Lymphatic filariasis, 146, 152

M

"Mad cow" disease, 3*n*b
MADD. *See* Mothers Against Drunk Driving
Magnitude of impact, 50
Malaria, 11, 24, 28, 140, 215
  addressing burden of, 151
  burden of, 145
  costs and consequences of, 148
  environmental health and control of, 164*t*
Mass media, health behavior changes and, 221–222, 224
Master's of Public Health, 90, 113
Maternal and child health, 7, 164*t*
Maternal mortality, by region, 2000, *21*
Maternal mortality ratio, 20
MDGs. *See* Millennium Development Goals
Medicaid, 65
Medical anthropologists, disease defined by, 215
Medical care, disease and, 10
Men, determinants of health and, 16
Mental disorders, 127, 132
  burden of, 121–122
  costs and consequences of, 124
Mental health, 6
  integrating into primary care in Uganda, 130–131
  key terms and definitions, 122*t*
Milgram, Stanley, 83
Milgram obedience study, 83
Millennium Development Goals
  communicable diseases and, 139*t*
  environmental health and, 164*t*
Morbidity, 9, 20, 41–42
Morbidity and Mortality Weekly Report, 65
Morocco, trochoma control in, 154–155
Mortality, 9, 20
  burden of disease in terms of, 41–42

demographic and epidemiologic transitions and, 30–33
Mortality rates, 41
Mothers Against Drunk Driving, 70
Motivational interventions, 53–54
MPH. *See* Master's of Public Health
MSF. *See* Doctors Without Borders
Multilateral development banks, 197–198
Mycobacterium tuberculosis, 143

N

NAACP. *See* National Association for the Advancement of Colored People
NACCHO. *See* National Association of County and City Health Officials
National Association for the Advancement of Colored People, 82
National Association of County and City Health Officials, 93, 94, 96, 114
National Institutes of Health, 66*t*
National Public Health Performance Standards Program, 113–114
National Vaccine Plan, 71 (box 4–4)
Natural disasters, 189
addressing health effects of, 184–185
case studies, 187–188
characteristics of, 180–181
future challenges in meeting health needs after, 188–189
health burden of, 181–182
importance of, to global health, 177–178
key terms related to, 178–180
selected, 2004 and 2005, 178*t*
Natural experiment, 45*ni*
Necessary cause, 47
Neglected diseases, 145–146
addressing burden of, 152
burden of, 145–146
costs and consequences of, 148
Neonatal mortality, by WHO region, 2000, *20*
Neonatal mortality rate, 18, 18*t*
Newborn screening, 5
NGOs. *See* Nongovernmental organizations
NIH. *See* National Institutes of Health
Nitrogen dioxide, 166*t*
Non-communicable diseases, 22, 24, 25, 117–133
addressing burden of, 124–127
burden of, 118–123
alcohol abuse, 123
cancer, 120–121
cardiovascular disease, 118–119
diabetes, 119–120
mental disorders, 121–122
tobacco use, 122–123
case studies, 127–131
costs and consequences of, 123–124
death and DALYs from leading cause, by region, 2001, 119*t*
defined, 118
future challenges, 131–133
importance of, 117–118
key definitions, 118, 118*t*
vignettes, 117
Nongovernmental organizations, 208
global health and, 200–201, 200*t*
public health and, 70
Nuremburg Code
research on human subjects and, 80
standards of, 80*t*
Nutritionists, 101

O

Obesity, 125–126, 219
Obligation, 53, 54
Occupational classifications, for public health workers, 98–99, 101
Occupational Safety and Health Administration, 69
OCP. *See* Onchocerciasis Control Program
Odds ratio, 46*nj*
Onchocerciasis Control Program, 207, 208
Onchocerciasis (river blindness), case study, 207–288
Oral rehydration therapy (ORT), for diarrhea, 151, 158
OSHA. *See* Occupational Safety and Health Administration
OXFAM, 70
Ozone, 166*t*

P

Pakistan, earthquake in, 187–188
Palliative care, 139*t*
Pandemic flu, 7
Panic disorder, 122*t*, 127
Parasite, 139*t*
Particulate matter, 166*t*
Partners in Health, 205
Pasteur, Louis, 4
"Patterns of resort," 217
Pellagra, 4
Penicillin, 4, 139
Percent efficacy, 50*nm*
P.E.R.I. process

circular nature of, 56
evidence-based public health and, 40, *40, 55*
Pharmaceutical firms, global health and, 203
Physical inactivity, diseases associated with, 126
Physicians, 101
Pneumonia, 24
Point prevalence, 22
Poland, curbing tobacco use in, 128–129
Policy development, 60
Polio, 4–5, 28, 193, 215
Polyvinyl chloride, angiosarcoma and exposure to, 42 (box 3–1)
Population comparisons, 43
Population health, 6*t*
approaches to, 3, 9*t*
components of, 7*t*
implications, 6–7
full spectrum of, *6*
what is meant by, 5
Population pyramids, demographic transition, *31*
Population(s), 5, 7
Post-traumatic stress disorder, 183–184
Poverty, environmental health and eradication of, 164*t*
PPPs. *See* Public-private partnerships
Premature death, 24
Present value, Disability Adjusted Life Year as, 23
Prevalence, 22, 41
Primary education, universal, environmental health and, 164*t*
Primary interventions, 52, 53*t*
Professional occupations, 98
Proportion, 41*n*b
Prospective studies, 44
Protective factor, 46*n*k
Protozoan infections, 146
PTSD. *See* Post-traumatic stress disorder
Public health. *See also* Evidence-based public health
approach of, changes over time, 3–5
eras of, 6*t*
importance of work in, 89
often ignored history of, 1–2
traditional, population health and, 9*t*
Turnock's meanings of, 3*n*a
what is meant by, 2–3
Public health agencies
American, brief history of, 64 (box 4–1)
collaboration among, 68
health care partnerships with, 70
"Public Health in America Statement," 60
Public health occupations
characteristics of, 97–105
career prospects, 104–105
composite public health practice profiles, 103–104*t*
important and essential duties, 102
minimum qualifications, 102
occupational classifications, 98–99, 101
public health practice profile, 101–102, 102*t*
salary estimates, 103–104
workplace considerations, 103
Public health practice, 90
Public health practitioners, competencies for, 108–109, 110–111*t*, 111–112
Public Health Ready, 114
Public health services, ten essential, 60, 61–62*t*, *63*
Public Health Training Centers, funding for, 112
Public health work, public health workers and, 90
Public health workers
ethics and, 94–97
number of, in selected occupational categories and titles, U.S., 2000, 95*t*
Public health workforce, 89–115
components of preparedness management system, *113*
composition of, 93–94
development of, 112–114
future, distribution and composition of, 107–108
growth prospects for, 105–108
health reform legislation (2010) and, 114–115
size and distribution of, 90–93
Public Health Workforce Enumeration 2000, 90, 101, 105
Public-private partnerships, global health and, 202–203, 203*t*
Puerperal fever, 4

Q

Qualifications, for public health occupations, 102
Quarantine, 3

R

Radon, 5
Randomization, 45
Randomized clinical trials, 44
Rape, as weapon of war, 183
Rates, 40
describing health problems and, 40–41
true, 41*n*b
Recommendations
classification of, 51*t*
eminence-based, 50

evidence-based, 50–51
what works to reduce health impact, 49–52
Refugees, 189
complex humanitarian emergencies and, 178–179
selected populations and source of, 2006, 180*t*
Region, causes of death by, 26–27
Registered nurses, 99, 101
Relative risk, for cigarette smoking, 46
Retrospective studies, 44
Reverse causality, 45*n*h
Risk factors, 8, 29–30, 45
defined, 29
leading, for burden of disease, low-, middle- and high-income countries, 2001, 30*t*
Risk indicators, 40
Risk markers, 40
RNs. *See* Registered nurses
Robert Wood Johnson Foundation, 70
Rockefeller Foundation, 70, 109, 199, 204, 206
Roll Back Malaria, 201
Rwanda, case study, 187

S

Sachs, Jeff, 205
SAEFA. *See* South Asia Earthquake Flash Appeal
Salary estimates
mean salary for full-time equivalent workers of state and local health agencies, 1998-2008, U.S., *105*
public health occupations and, 103–104
SAMHSA. *See* Substance Abuse and Mental Health Services Administration
Sanitation
environmental health and, 167, 168, 170–171
integrating investment choices about, 172–173
Sanitation technologies, selected, 171*t*
SARS. *See* Sudden Acute Respiratory Syndrome
Save the Children, 200
Schistosomiasis, 146, 152, 215
Schizophrenia, 122*t*, 127
Score, 50
Scurvy, 3, 11
Secondary interventions, 52, 53*t*
Second-hand smoke, 48
Semmelweis, Ignaz, 4
September 11, 2001 terrorist attacks, public health occupations in aftermath of, 108
Sexual or blood-borne disease, 138
Sexual violence, against women in complex humanitarian emergencies, 183
Shattuck Commission, 64 (box 4–1)
Silicosis, 42 (box 3–1)
Smoking
culture, health behaviors and, 218–219
reducing health impact of, 49–52
Snow, John, 4
Social-ecological model, 3
Social-economic-cultural factors, disease and, 10–11
Social impact assessment, culture and, 222–223, 223*t*
Social interventions, population health and, 9*t*
Social justice, 4
Social marketing, health behavior changes and, 222, 224
Social Security Act of 1935, 64 (box 4–1)
Social status, as health determinant, 16
Social support, as health determinant, 16
Society's shared health concerns, 5
Society's vulnerable groups, 5
South America, Southern Cone of, Chagas disease in, 153–154
South Asia Earthquake Flash Appeal, 188
Stages of Change model, 220, 224
State public health agencies, roles of, 60, 63–65
Stop TB, 201
Strength of the relationship, 45
Stroke, 25, 118*t*
Substance abuse, 6
Substance Abuse and Mental Health Services Administration, 65, 66*t*
Sudden Acute Respiratory Syndrome, 69 (box 4–3), 155, 194, 206
Sufficient cause, 47
Sulfur dioxide, 166*t*
Supportive criteria, 45
cigarette smoking and, ancillary or supportive criteria and, 45–47, 47*t*
Surgeon General's *Report on Smoking and Health*, 48
Surrogate outcomes, 50*n*l
Syphilis, Tuskegee study and, 81–82

T

TB. *See* Tuberculosis
Technical occupations, 99
Tertiary interventions, 52, 53*t*
Thailand, HIV/AIDS in, 152–153
Tobacco control, cancer prevention and, 127
Tobacco use
addressing burden of, 125
burden of, 122–123
costs and consequences of, 124

culture, health behaviors and, 218–219
curbing in Poland, 128–129
history behind, 39
Trachoma, controlling in Morocco, 154–155
Training, for public health workers, 97, 109, 111–112
TRIPS Agreement, 79
True rate, 41*n*b
Tuberculosis, 4, 24, 140, 193, 194, 206
addressing burden of, 150
basic facts about, 144*t*
burden of, 143–145
in China, 153
costs and consequences of, 148
death rates, reducing, 11
DOTS and, 150, 153, 158
HIV/AIDS and, 158
addressing burden of, 150
Tuskegee study, 81–82
Type I diabetes, 119, 120, 126
Type II diabetes, 119, 120, 126

U

U. S. Office of Personnel Management, 98
UDHR. *See* Universal Declaration of Human Rights
Uganda, integrating mental health into primary care in, 130–131
UNAIDS, 65, 68*t*, 197, 197*t*, 205, 208
Under-five child mortality
rate of, 18*t*, 20
by region, 2006, *20*
Underweight infants, culture, health behaviors and, 218
UNHCR. *See* United Nations High Commissioner for Refugees
UNICEF, 65, 68*t*, 182, 196–197, 201, 204, 205, 208
Uninsured population, 18
United Nations, 77
agencies of, 195–197, 195*t*
United Nations High Commissioner for Refugees, 179
United States Agency for International Development, 65
United States Public Health Service, 4
"Public Health in America Statement," 60
Universal Declaration of Human Rights, 76, 77
Universal health insurance, 17–18
Urban air pollutants, selected, 166*t*
Urban air pollution, 167, 168
U.S. Department of Labor, 99
USAID. *See* United States Agency for International Development

V

Vaccinations, 3, 138, 193
Vector-borne disease, 138
Victim blaming, cigarette smoking and, 54
Violence against women, in complex humanitarian emergencies, 183
Vital statistics, 4
Volatile organic chemicals, 166*t*
Vulnerable groups, focusing on needs of, 7–8

W

War, complex humanitarian emergencies and, 178
War on Poverty, 64 (box 4–1)
Waterborne diseases, 4, 138, 167, 167*t*, 174
Waterborne pathogens, selected, 169*t*
Water-related infections, classification of, 167*t*
Water supply
environmental health and, 167, 168, 171–172
excellent, potential morbidity reductions from, 172*t*
integrating investment choices about, 172–173
"When-Who-How" approach, 52, 53
WHO. *See* World Health Organization
Willowbrook School study, 82
Women
cigarette smoking and, 39
determinants of health and, 16
empowerment of, environmental health and, 164*t*
violence against, in complex humanitarian emergencies, 183
Workplace considerations public health occupations and, 103
World Bank, 65, 68*t*, 198, 201, 204, 205, 206, 208
World Health Organization, 20, 65, 68*t*, 80, 127, 194, 201, 204, 208
description and role of, 195–196
on environmental health, 165
Framework Convention on Tobacco Control (WHO FCTC), 55
partnerships related to, 201
regional offices, 196*t*
World Medical Association, 80
World Trade Organization, 79
World War II, 4
WR. *See Morbidity and Mortality Weekly Report*

CPSIA information can be obtained at www.ICGtesting.com
Printed in the USA
LVOW021407141011

250535LV00001B/4/P

9 781449 621957